Current Topics in Pathology

Continuation of Ergebnisse der Pathologie

65

Editors

E. Grundmann W. H. Kirsten

Correlations Between Morphologic and Clinical Features in Idiopathic Perimembranous Glomerulonephritis

Human Parathyroid Gland: A Freeze-Fracture and Thin Section Study

Malignant Nephrosclerosis in Patients with Hemolytic Uremic Syndrome (Primary Malignant Nephrosclerosis)

Liver Carcinogenesis in Rats After Aflatoxin B_1 Administration

Blastomycosis

Contributors

A. Adam, K. D. Bock, A. Bohle, P. Bünger, M. Bulla, H. Christ, L. Diekmann, H. H. Edel, U. Frotscher, H. -V. Gärtner, K. E. Grund, K. Hayduk, U. Helmchen, R. Kluthe, W. Kösters, D. Meyer, A. M. Novi, V. Ott, E. Renner, K. Salfelder, F. Scheler, R. M. Schmülling, J. Schwarz, H. G. Siebert, M. Strauch, J. Thiele, T. Watanabe

With 119 Figures

Springer-Verlag Berlin Heidelberg New York 1977

E. Grundmann, Professor Dr., Pathologisches Institut der Universität, Westring 17, D-4400 Münster/Westf., Germany

W.H. Kirsten, Professor Dr., Department of Pathology, The University of Chicago, 950 East 59th Street, Chicago, IL 60637, USA

ISBN-13: 978-3-642-66705-3 **eISBN-13: 978-3-642-66703-9**
DOI: 10.1007/978-3-642-66703-9

Softcover reprint of the hardcover 1st edition 1977
Library of Congress Catalog Card Number 56-49162.

Offsetprinting and bookbinding: Universitätsdruckerei H. Stürtz AG., Würzburg

2122/3130 — 543210

Contents

List of Contributors

Adam, Annemarie	Niethammerstr. 6, D-7400 Tübingen
Bock, Prof. Dr. K.D.	Medizinische Klinik des Universitätsklinikums, Hufelandstr. 55, D-4300 Essen 1
Bohle, Prof. Dr. A.	Pathologisches Institut, Universität Tübingen, Liebermeisterstr. 8, D-7400 Tübingen
Bünger, Dr. P.	Allg. Krankenhaus Heidberg, Tangstedter Landstr. 400, D-2000 Hamburg 62
Bulla, Dr. M.	Universitäts Kinderklinik, Josef-Stelzmann-Str. 9, D-5000 Köln 41
Christ, Dr. Dr. H.	Bahnhofstr. 58, D-7457 Bisingen
Diekmann, Dr. L.	Universitäts Kinderklinik, D-4400 Münster
Edel, Prof. Dr. H.H.	Städtisches Krankenhaus–Medizinische Klinik München-Harlaching, Sanatoriumsplatz 2, D-8000 München 90
Frotscher, Doz. Dr. U.	Medizinische Unviersitäts Klinik, D-5300 Bonn-Venusberg
Gärtner, Dr. Hermine V.	Pathologisches Institut, Universität Tübingen, Liebermeisterstr. 8, D-7400 Tübingen
Grund, Dr. K.E.	Chirurgische Universitäts Klinik, D-6500 Mainz
Hayduk, Doz. Dr. K.	Medizinische Universitäts Klinik, Otfried-Müller-Straße, D-7400 Tübingen
Helmchen, Doz. Dr. U.	Pathologisches Institut der Universität Tübingen, Liebermeisterstr. 8, D-7400 Tübingen
Kluthe, Prof. Dr. R.	Medizinische Klinik und Poliklinik der Universität, Sonnhalde 1-5, D-7800 Freiburg

Kösters, Doz. Dr. W.	Städtische Krankenanstalten, Medizinische Klinik, D-6800 Mannheim
Meyer, Prof. Dr. D.	Pathologisches Institut, Kreiskrankenhaus, D-7140 Ludwigsburg
Novi, Dr. Anna M.	Pathologisches Institut der Universität Düsseldorf, Moorenstr. 5, D-4000 Düsseldorf
Ott, Dr. V.	Filderklinik, Haberschlaihalde, D-7000 Stuttgart-Bolanden
Renner, Prof. Dr. E.	Städtisches Krankenhaus, Medizinische Klinik, D-5000 Köln-Merheim
Salfelder, Dr. K.	Pathology Department, Universidad de los Andes, Merida, Venezuela
Scheler, Prof. Dr. F.	Medizinische Klinik und Poliklinik der Universität Göttingen, Humboldtallee 1, D-3400 Göttingen
Schmülling, Dr. R.M.	Medizinische Universitäts Klinik, Otfried-Müller-Straße, D-7400 Tübingen
Schwarz, Dr. J.	Clinical Laboratories, Jewish Hospital Association, Cincinnati, OH 45229, USA
Siebert, Prof. Dr. H.G.	Medizinische Universitäts Klinik, Josef-Stelzmann-Str. 9, D-5000 Köln 41
Strauch, Prof. Dr. M.	Städtische Krankenanstalten, Medizinische Klinik, D-6800 Mannheim
Thiele, Dr. J.	Pathologisches Institut der Medizinischen Hochschule, Karl-Wiechert-Allee 9, D-3000 Hannover 61
Watanabe, Dr. T.	Department of Pathology, Faculty of Medicine, Kyushu University, Maidashi 3-1-1, Higashi ku, Fukuoka 812, Japan

Correlations Between Morphologic and Clinical Features in Idiopathic Perimembranous Glomerulonephritis

A Study on 403 Renal Biopsies of 367 Patients

H.V. GÄRTNER, T. WATANABE*, V. OTT, A. ADAM, A. BOHLE*, H.H. EDEL,
R. KLUTHE, E. RENNER, F. SCHELER, R.M. SCHMÜLLING, H.-G. SIEBERTH

I. Introduction

Perimembranous glomerulonephritis (PGN), also called extramembranous glomerulonephritis (*Berger* et al., 1961; *Royer* et al., 1962; *Ducrot* et al., 1963), or epimembranous (*White*, 1969; *Seymour* et al., 1971), or membranous nephropathy (*Ehrenreich* and *Churg*, 1968; *Cameron*, 1970), is a morphologically well-defined disease occurring in both idiopathic and nonidiopathic forms. Together, they constitute about 9% of all inflammatory glomerular diseases in the patients examined by us over the past years (*Bohle* et al., 1974).

Little has been reported to date concerning the relationship between the morphologic and clinical findings of this disease entity (*Ehrenreich* and *Churg*, 1968; *Ducrot* et al., 1969; *Churg* and *Ehrenreich*, 1973; *Franklin* et al., 1973; *Gluck* et al., 1973; *Habib* et al., 1973; *Row* et al., 1975).

Our previous investigations of 100 patients with PGN (*Gärtner* et al., 1974) demonstrated along with *Ehrenreich* and *Churg* (1968), *Ducrot* et al. (1969), *Rosen* (1971), *Gluck* et al., (1973), that PGN may occur at any age, more often, however, between 31 and 60, and nearly twice as frequently in males as in females (*Pollak* et al., 1968; *Ducrot* et al., 1969; *Habib* et al., 1971; *Rosen*, 1971). The disease begins insidiously with no characteristic history of illnesses. Anamnestically dominant initial symptoms are edema or edema and proteinuria (*Ehrenreich* and *Churg*, 1968; *Pollak* et al., 1968; *Ducrot* et al., 1969; *Foreland* et al., 1969; *Gluck* et al., 1973). The disease climaxes in a fully developed nephrotic syndrome (*Ehrenreich* and *Churg*, 1968; *Pollak* et al., 1968; *Habib*, 1970) combined in about half of the patients with minor hypertension and hematuria. In accordance with *Ehrenreich*

* Supported by the Deutsche Forschungsgemeinschaft.

and *Churg*, we subdivided the developing progressive changes in the glomerular basement membrane into four stages to demonstrate, in agreement with these authors, as well as with *Hatta* (1972), that the degree of transformation of the basement membrane was dependent on the duration of the disease. The results of the morphometric examinations confirm, in contrast to the opinion of other authors (*Cameron*, 1970; *Churg* et al., 1970; *Habib*, 1970; *Murphy* et al., 1973) that PGN belongs to the proliferative glomerular disorders. The prognosis of PGN is unfavorable, regardless of the therapy administered. Till now, it remains to be answered whether the specific morphologic changes, classified by *Ehrenreich* and *Churg*, into four stages, are paralleled by specific clinical symptoms and whether an alteration in these symptoms correlates with changes in morphologic structures, thus allowing a prognosis on the basis of the morphologic picture. Furthermore, it is unknown whether nonspecific morphologic changes, in addition to the typical progressive basement membrane lesions, have an influence on the course and prognosis of the disease, and whether a patient's sex affects the features and course of the disease. To examine the correlations between morphologic findings and clinical features at the time of biopsy, and to determine the further morphologic and clinical course of PGN by serial renal biopsies, we have evaluated our experience of the past ten years with 367 patients with idiopathic PGN.

II. Material and Methods

Renal biopsies of 439 patients with PGN, diagnosed between 1964 and 1974, served as the starting point for our study. Because only patients with idiopathic PGN should be considered, 72 patients with nonidiopathic PGN were eliminated, thus providing a total of 367 patients for our examination. Nonidiopathic PGN occurred either in connection with drug therapy (D-penicillamine, gold, tridione), or SLE, diabetes mellitus, or a malignant tumor. D-penicillamine-induced PGN has been reported on elsewhere (*Gärtner* et al., 1975).

Of the 367 patients 38 were serial biopsied, 31 of them twice, 5 three times, and, in two cases, four biopsies were performed, so that a total of 414 biopsies were available for the following study. Because, for technical reasons, the silver staining did not succeed in 11 cases, the morphologic and clinical analysis could be performed on only 403 renal biopsies, taking into account 13 autopsies—55 cases were additionally examined immunohistologically in 15 cases electron-microscopically.

Microscopic examinations were performed on PAS-stained sections, embedded in paraffin, and on Movat silver-stained semithin sections (1 μ thick) to characterize the typically occurring morphologic changes in the glomerular basement membrane in PGN, according to the classification of *Ehrenreich* and *Churg*. FITC-labeled antisera were supplied by Behring for the immunohistologic studies (antihuman-IgG, IgM, IgA, IgD, IgE, -HAA, albumin, and complement). Electron-microscopic examinations were performed in paraffin-embedded tissues, inlaid in plexiglass.

In evaluating the clinical data, the following parameters were considered:

1. Age and sex
2. History of illnesses
3. First subjective and objective symptoms of the disease
4. Period of observation, i.e., the time between the appearance of the first renal symptoms and the renal biopsy, subsequently referred to as duration of the disease

5. Clinical symptoms and laboratory findings at the time of the biopsy

The morphologic changes in each renal biopsy were simultaneously classified into stages without knowledge of the clinical data, thus allowing the following correlations between the morphology and clinical features to be examined:

1. Stage, age, and sex
2. Stage and duration of the disease
3. Stage and proteinuria
4. Stage and nephrotic syndrome
5. Stage, blood pressure, serum creatinine, and creatinine clearance
6. Stage and clinical course of the disease
7. Stage and therapy.

In addition, the morphologic and clinical results from 38 cases with serial renal biopsies were analyzed.

The nephrotic syndrome was defined as follows–proteinuria more than 3 g/24 h, total serum protein less than 6 g/100 ml, albuminemia less than 3 g/100 ml. Edema and hyper-cholesterinemia were not obligatory. A blood pressure with a systolic value greater than 140 mm Hg and a diastolic value more than 90 mm Hg was considered to be elevated. Creatinine clearance values less than 80 ml/min/1.73 m^2 were regarded as being mildly limited and less than 40 ml/min/1.73 m^2 as markedly limited. Serum creatinine values up to 1.2 mg% were normal. The erythrocyturia was classified in three degrees of severity:

1. 3-10 erythrocytes/field of vision = mild (+)
2. 11-20 erythrocytes/field of vision = medium (++)
3. more than 20 erythrocytes/field of vision = severe (+++)

This classification of the erythrocyturia refers to the sediment obtained from freshly collected urine samples centrifuged under standard conditions and examined under 40-fold magnification.

The evaluation of clinical criteria of the clinical course of the disease was based on the proposals of *Renner* et al. (1969)–an improvement or deterioration occurred by an alteration in the creatinine clearance values of more than 15 ml/min, in the proteinuria by more than 50% of the starting value, in the total serum protein by more than 1 g/100 ml, in arterial systolic blood pressure by more than 20 mmHg, in diastolic blood pressure by more than 10 mm Hg, and in increase or decrease in eryhtrocyturia. Differences in the mean values were considered significant if the level of significance in the F-test according to R.A. Fischer was $2P \leqq 0.05$.

III. Results

1. Clinical Findings

a) Age, Sex (Fig. 1): Idiopathic PGN occurs in every age group, ranging between 1 and 75, with a peak between 31 and 50 years. The average age is 39. Males are afflicted twice as frequently as females (67% males : 33% females).

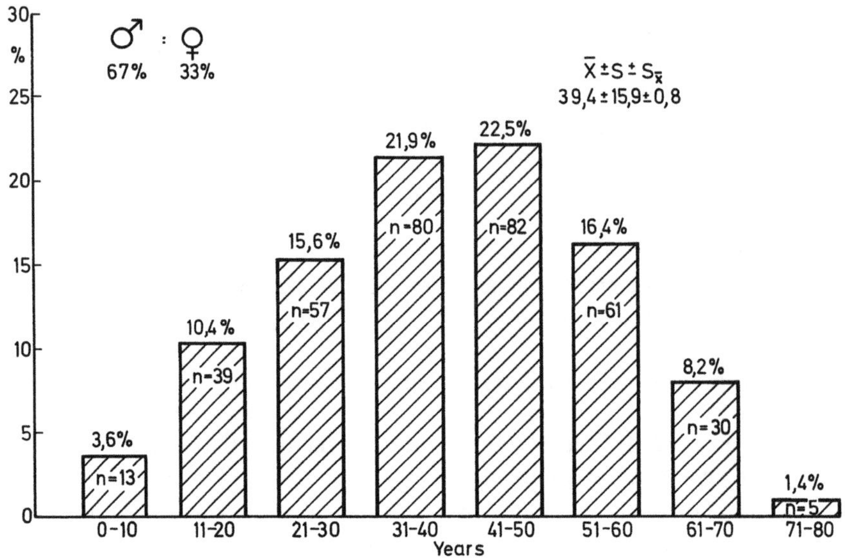

Fig. 1. Distribution of sex and age of 367 patients with idiopathic PGN at time of first renal biopsy

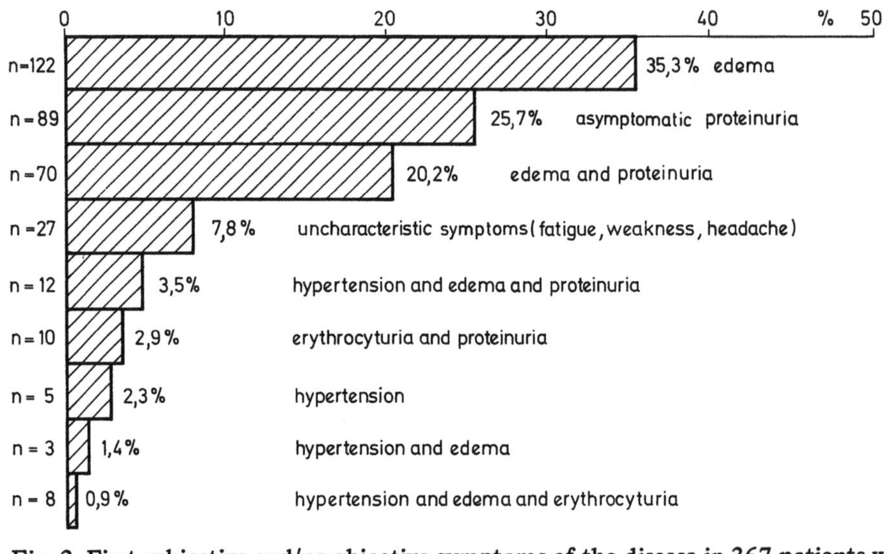

Fig. 2. First subjective and/or objective symptoms of the disease in 367 patients with idiopathic PGN

b) Previous Diseases: Tonsillitis (37%), bacterial and viral infections (22%), as well as scarlet fever and rheumatic fever (4%), are most often revealed in the past history. Approximately a third of the recorded previous diseases are heterogeneous disorders which sometimes occurred so long ago that no connection with the PGN can be established. In 15% of the cases, there is no history of illnesses.

c) Initial Subjective and/or Objective Clinical Symptoms of the Disease (Fig. 2). The first clinical symptoms, associated with an acute nephrotic syndrome, are most often anamnestically reported as edema, either alone or combined with proteinuria, if a medical examination took place at that time. In a quarter of the patients, an asymptomatic proteinuria characterized the insidious beginning of the disease.

Hypertension or hypertension with proteinuria and erythrocyturia, as well as uncharacteristic symptoms as fatigue and weakness, are rarely reported as initial symptoms.

d) Duration of the Disease, or the period of observation from the first appearance of subjective and/or objective symptoms to the renal biopsy is an average of 21 months. Nearly two-thirds of the patients are biopsied in the first year.

e) Clinical Findings at the Time of the Biopsy (Table 1). This table shows that a nephrotic syndrome exists in 70% of the patients at the time of biopsy (average proteinuria 6.9 g/24 h).

Table 1. Clinical findings of 367 patients with idiopathic PGN at time of first renal biopsy

Proteinuria (g/day)	Nephrotic syndrome	Erythrocyturia	
1- 3 : 33%	70%	No	31%
4- 6 : 32%	No nephrotic syndrome at any time (18%)	Mild (+)	53%
7-12 : 25%		Medium (++)	12%
13-50 : 10%	Initial nephrotic syndrome, later disappearing (12%)	Severe (+++)	4%
$\bar{x} \pm s \pm s_{\bar{x}}$:		Macrohematuria	–
6.9 ± 5.8 ± 0.3			

Blood pressure (mm Hg)	Creatinine clearance ($ml/min/1.73\ m^2$)		Serum creatinine (mg %)
Systolic blood pressure $\bar{x} \pm s \pm s_{\bar{x}}$	< 120	59%	to 1,2 : 70%
	80 - 120		1.3 - 1.4 : 13%
154 ± 22 ± 1	40 - 79	23%	1.5 - 5 : 14%
Diastolic blood pressure $\bar{x} \pm s \pm s_{\bar{x}}$	< 40	6%	5.1 - 30 : 3%
	Not determined	12%	$\bar{x} \pm s \pm s_{\bar{x}}$
95 ± 12 ± 1			1.6 ± 2.5 ± 0.13

$\bar{x}$ = means; s = SD (standard deviation); $s_{\bar{x}}$ = SEM (standard error of the mean)

Of the 30% who had no nephrotic syndrome at the time of the biopsy, 12% showed a nephrotic syndrome at the beginning of the disease which then disappeared with or without therapy as the disease progressed, and 18% showed no nephrotic syndrome at any time. Most of the patients (53%) had only a mild erythrocyturia, if any at all. Severe erythrocyturia was observed in only a few patients and a macrohematuria was not observed.

The average systolic, as well as diastolic, blood pressure at the time of the biopsy was slightly elevated. Most patients had normal serum creatinine (70%) and creatinine clearance values (59%).

2. Morphologic Findings

The progressive morphologic changes, developing during the course of PGN, were classified on silver-stained semithin sections, according to *Ehrenreich* and *Churg*, into four stages. We introduced a fifth stage, designated as a reparation stage, in contrast to the fifth stage of *Ehrenreich* and *Churg*, which is defined as an end stage. The following findings could therefore be reported:

1. The semithin sections of 85 biopsies (21% of the total number) exhibit alterations representing stage I, as described by *Ehrenreich* and *Churg*, with scattered, distinctly vis-

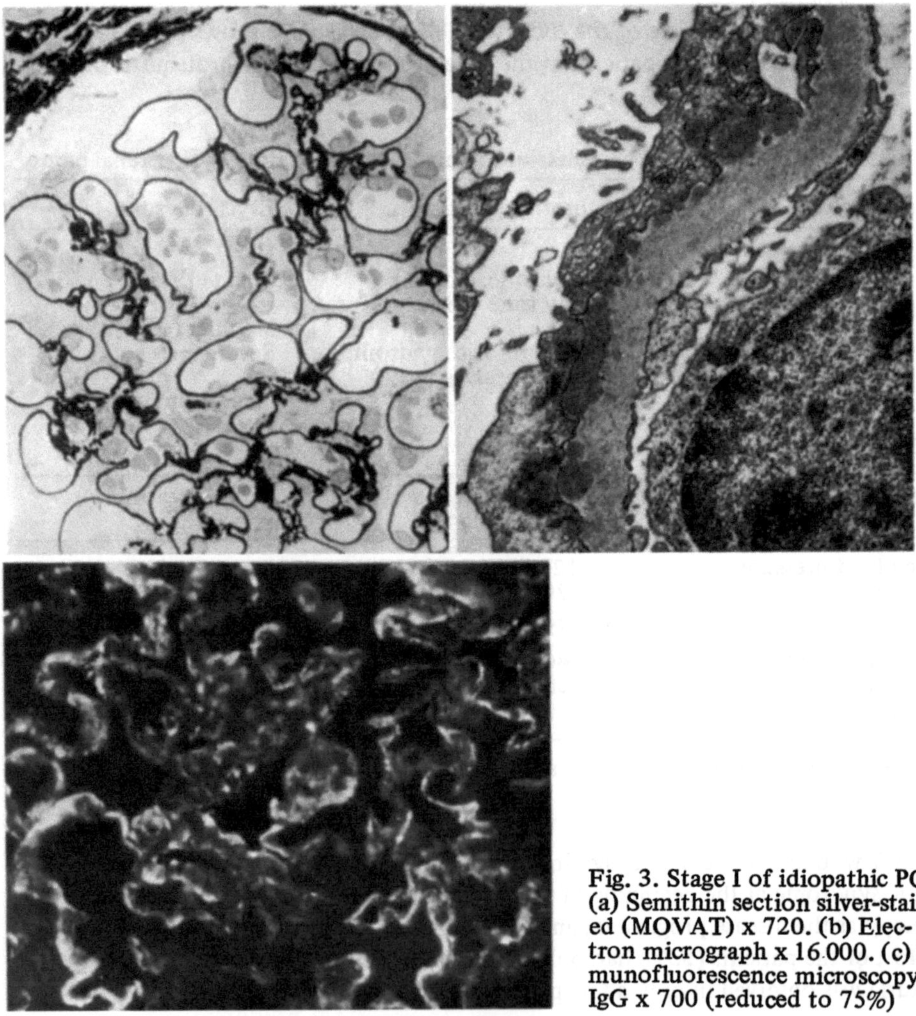

a b c

Fig. 3. Stage I of idiopathic PGN. (a) Semithin section silver-stained (MOVAT) x 720. (b) Electron micrograph x 16.000. (c) Immunofluorescence microscopy IgG x 700 (reduced to 75%)

ible projections (spikes) on the epithelial side of the glomerular basement membrane (Fig. 3a). Electron-microscopic examinations of five biopsies in this stage showed several subepithelial electron-dense deposits (Fig. 3b). The foot processes over the deposits were always fused and swollen or distorted. In 19 cases, the alterations observed microscopically were so minor that a final diagnosis could be established only by immunohistologic methods, showing a fine granular fluorescence along the glomerular capillary wall (Fig. 3c). As Table 2 indicates, IgG was deposited in combination with β_{1C} in all cases, with two exceptions. Six cases showed an additional deposition of IgM, four cases of IgA.

Table 2. Immunohistologic findings in 55 cases of PGN

Stage Detection of	Stage I n = 19	Stage II n = 22	Stage III n = 8	Stage IV n = 4	Stage V n = 2
IgG	19/19	21/22	7/8	4/4	1/2
IgM	6/19	8/22	5/8	1/4	∅
IgA	4/19	6/22	3/8	3/4	∅
β_{1C}	17/19	22/22	8/8	3/4	∅
Fibrinogen	∅	1/22	1/8	∅	∅
Negative	∅	∅			1/2
Special findings			3 cases: IgG, IgM, β_{1C} 2 cases: 1 IgG, IgM, IgA, β_{1C} 1 case: IgA, β_{1C}	1 case: 1 IgG, IgA	

2. In 170 biopsies (42% of the total), the typical morphologic alterations of stage II were fully developed and, often, the entire glomerular capillary walls were covered with numerous brown deposits, dispersed with argyrophilic spikes on the epithelial side of the tooth-like basement membrane (Fig. 4a). In three cases examined electron-microscopically (Fig. 4b), newly formed basement membrane material was found between the subepithelial electron-dense deposits, some of which were already incorporated into the basement membrane. The immunohistologic picture of 22 stage II cases (Fig. 4c) showed an intensive, granular, pearl necklace fluorescence along the capillary wall with evidence of IgG + β_{1C} or IgM, respectively, IgA and β_{1C}, or several immunoglobulins + β_{1C} (Table 2). The most frequent deposition in this stage was also IgG and β_{1C}. IgG was found either as sole immunoglobulin or in combination with others.

3. In 82 biopsies (20% of the total), stage III was observed, characterized by an extensive incorporation of brown deposits by adjacent spikes (Fig. 5a). Three cases examined electron-microscopically showed numerous electron-dense deposits incorporated into the basement membrane (Fig. 5b). In addition, isolated electron-lucent areas within the basement membrane were found. Immunohistologic investigations of eight cases (Fig. 5c) indicated an intense, coarse, pearl necklace fluorescence along the capillary wall. A deposition of IgG

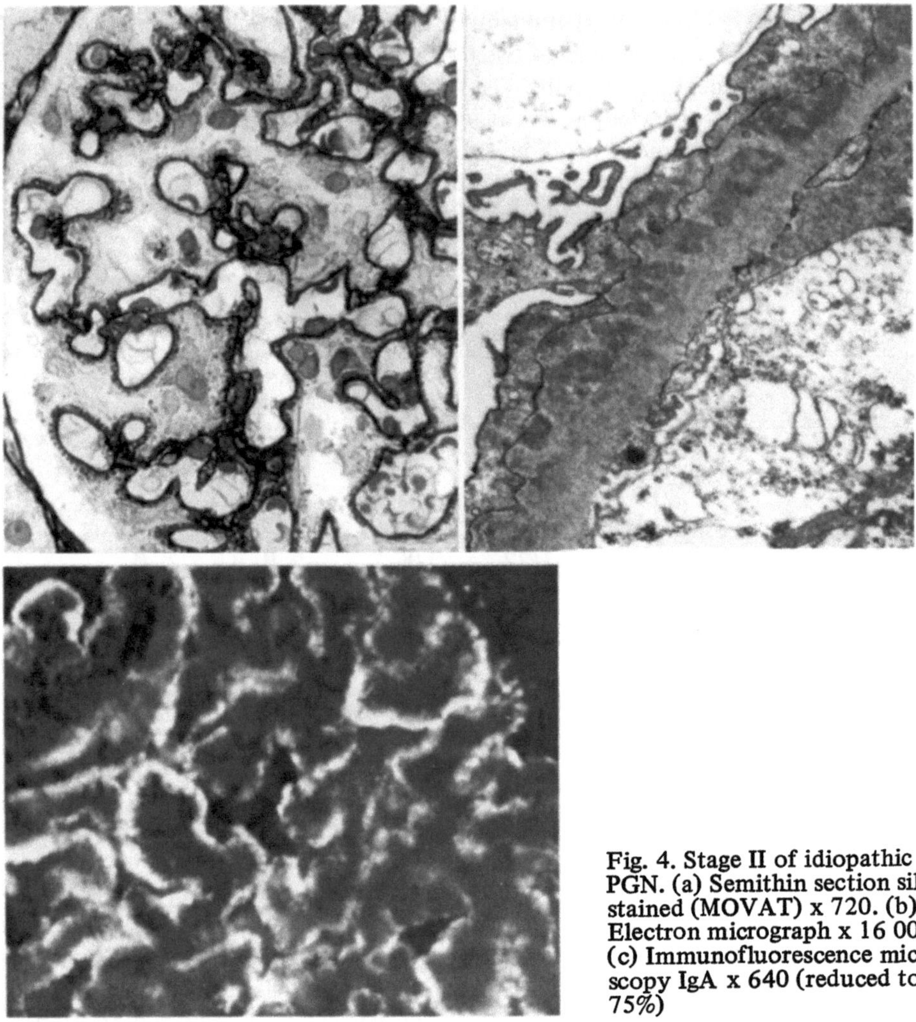

a b c

Fig. 4. Stage II of idiopathic PGN. (a) Semithin section silver-stained (MOVAT) x 720. (b) Electron micrograph x 16 000. (c) Immunofluorescence microscopy IgA x 640 (reduced to 75%)

and β_{1C} was found in most cases, however, an additional deposition of IgM was detected more often than in stages I and II.

4. In 45 biopsies (12% of the total), alterations representing stage IV were observed, characterized by a chain-like transformation of the basement membrane which appeared split and contained oval holes (Fig. 6a). Only a few isolated brown deposits, considerably smaller than those in stage III could still be found within the chain-like structure. In addition, six cases showed along with the alterations of stage IV, a segmental accumulation of deposits and some spikes, characteristic of stage II. In the two cases examined electron-microscopically, the chain-like parts of the basement membrane corresponded to numerous electron-lucent vacuolated areas, often located near the endothelial part of the basement membrane (Fig. 6b). The four cases examined immunohistologically demonstrated a coarse granular fluorescence along the capillary wall, subjectively less intensive and irregular than in the stage described above (Fig. 6c).

a b c
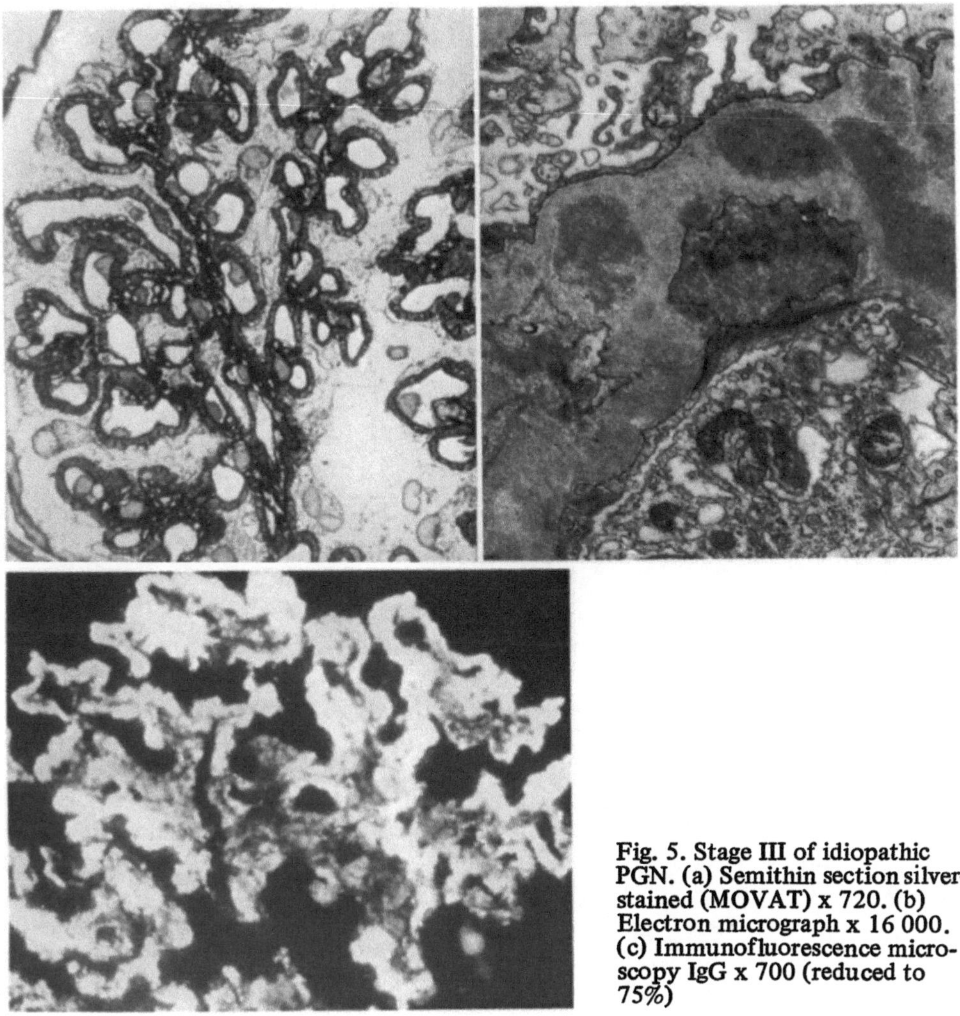

Fig. 5. Stage III of idiopathic PGN. (a) Semithin section silver-stained (MOVAT) x 720. (b) Electron micrograph x 16 000. (c) Immunofluorescence microscopy IgG x 700 (reduced to 75%)

In one case, complement was no longer detected (Table 2). In all other cases, it was present along with IgG.

5. In 21 cases (4% of the total biopsies), the alterations, designated by us for stage V, were found. In contrast to the end stage V of *Ehrenreich* and *Churg*, we considered it a reparation stage when an extensive normalization of the basement membrane occurs. In the semithin section, the basement membrane appeared to be very delicate and still only partially thickened or chain-like transformed (Fig. 7a).

The electronmicroscopic pictures of the four cases examined again showed electron-lucent areas of various sizes along with entirely normal basement membrane parts (Fig. 7b). Electron-dense deposits were no longer visible. Of the two cases examined immunohistologically, one showed negative results, whereas the presence of IgG in the area of the capillary wall could be demonstrated in the other but without complement (Table 2).

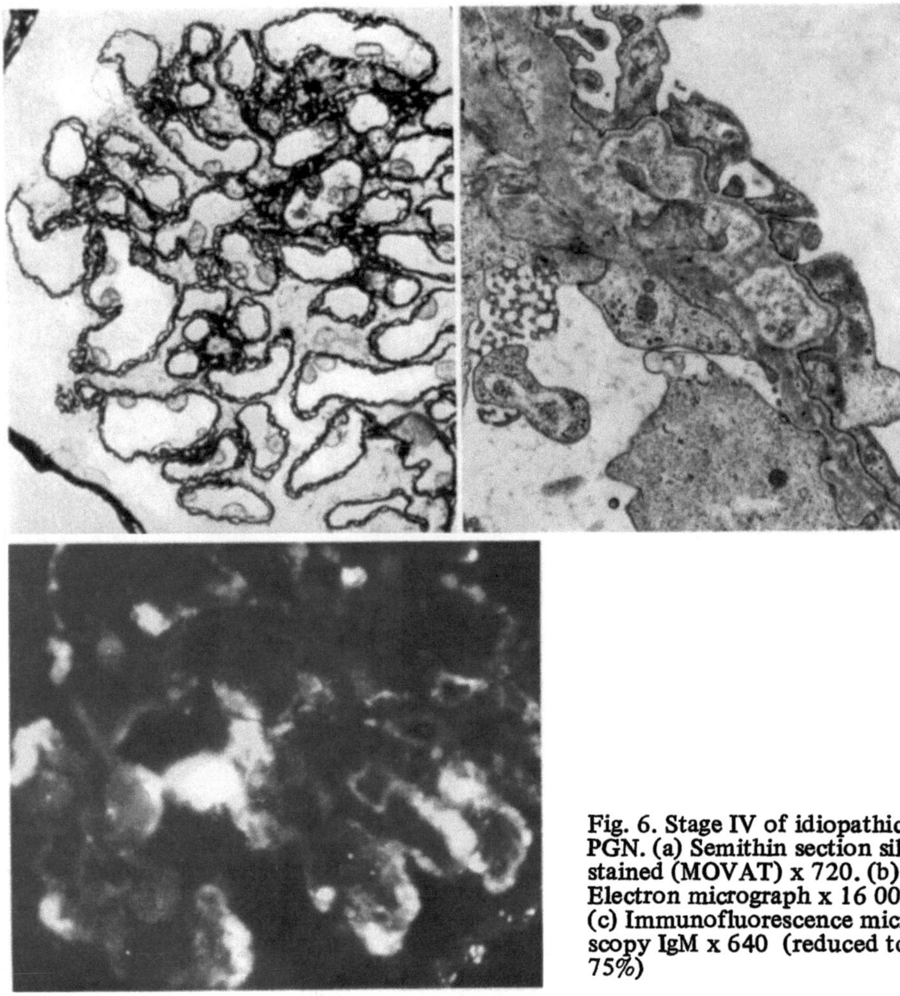

a b c

Fig. 6. Stage IV of idiopathic PGN. (a) Semithin section silver-stained (MOVAT) x 720. (b) Electron micrograph x 16 000. (c) Immunofluorescence microscopy IgM x 640 (reduced to 75%)

3. Correlations Between the Morphologic Stage and Clinical Parameters (Fig. 8)

1. Figure 8 illustrates the correlation between the morphologic stages of PGN and the duration of the disease. The duration of the disease (period between the first appearance of clinical symptoms and the renal biopsy) was shortest in stages I and II and longest in stages IV and V. It can, therefore, be concluded that the morphologic changes in the basement membrane were dependent upon the duration of the disease and that the degree of basement membrane transformation increased the longer the disease persisted.

2. Between the morphologic stages of PGN and the degree of proteinuria, as well as the appearance of the nephrotic syndrome, exists an inverse relationship (Fig. 9). Whereas, in stages I and II, the highest proteinuria values were observed, in stage V, only a minor proteinuria existed. The frequency of the nephrotic syndrome declined correspondingly with the decrease in proteinuria in relation to the duration of the disease, and to the degree of

a 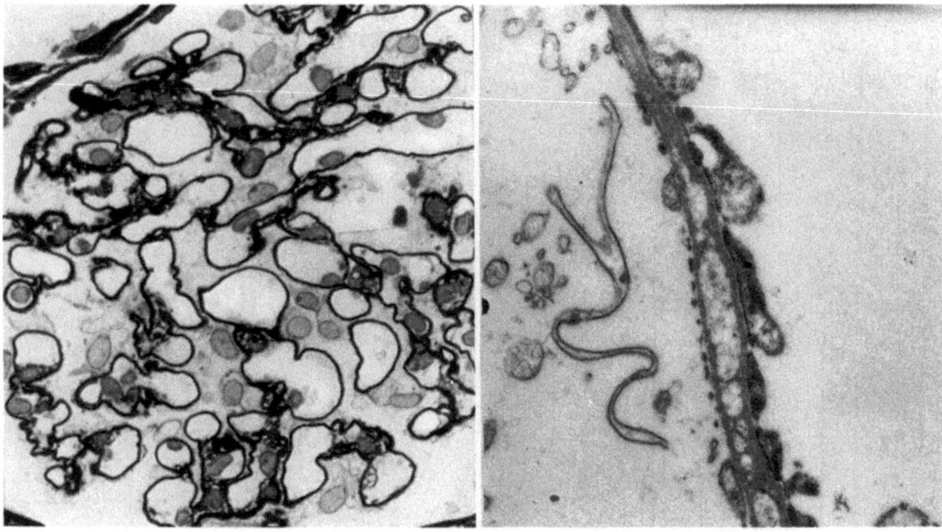 b

Fig. 7. Stage V of idiopathic PGN. (a) Semithin section silver-stained (MOVAT) x 720. (b) Electronmicrograph x 16 000 (reduced to 75%)

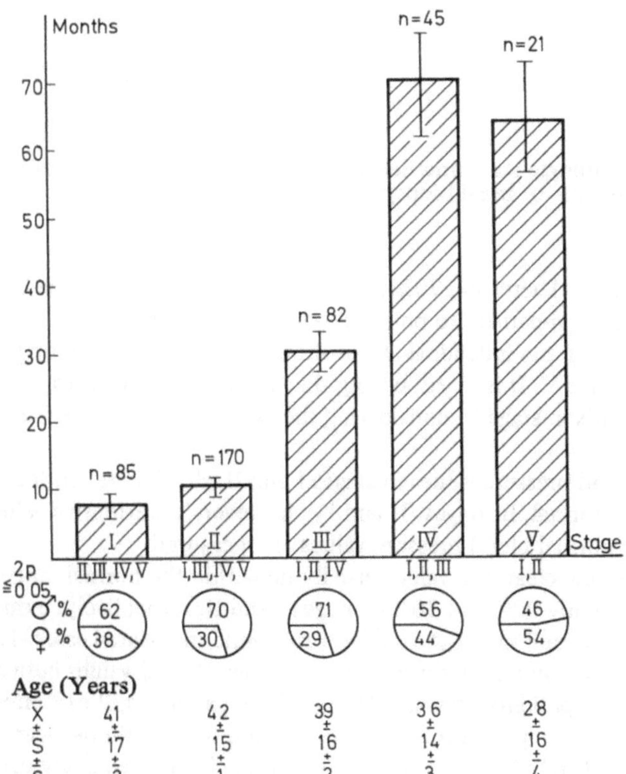

Fig. 8. Correlation between morphologic stage and duration of disease, at time of renal biopsy and relationships of sex ratio and age to different stages in idiopathic PGN ($\overline{x}$ = mean, s = SD = standard deviation, $s_{\overline{x}}$ = SER = standard error of the mean)

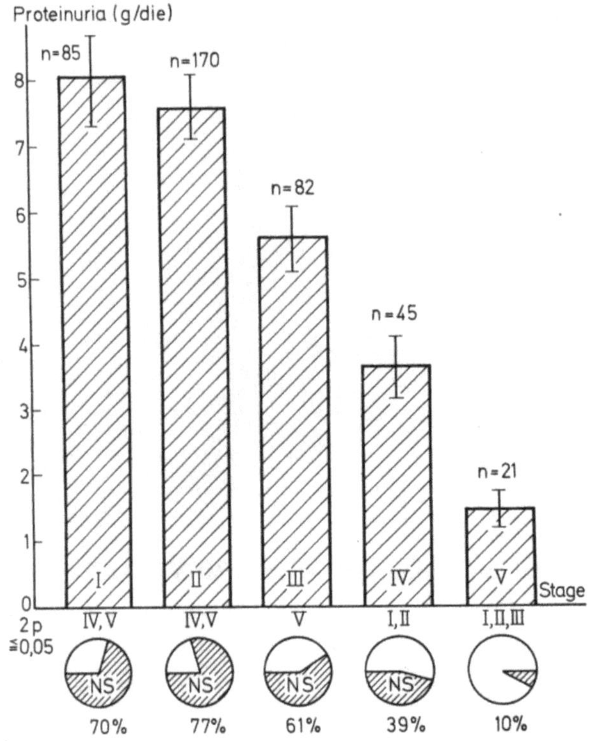

Fig. 9. Correlation between morphologic stage and degree of proteinuria as well as frequency of nephrotic syndrome at time of renal biopsy

basement membrane transformation. Therefore, 70% of stage I cases and 77% of stage II cases had a nephrotic syndrome in comparison to only 10% of stage V cases.

3. The distribution of sexes within the individual stages showed males predominating in stages I and II and females in stage V. It is worth noting that the patients in stages I and II were generally older than patients in stage V, considering the average age of the 367 patients to be 39 (Fig. 8).

4. As Figure 10 shows, the blood pressure values in stages I and II of PGN are, on the average, only slightly elevated or normal. In stages III and IV, however, hypertensive values are present, whereas, in stage V, normal blood pressure values are measured.

5. Serum creatinine and creatinine clearance values usually lie within the normal range in the individual stages (Table 3). Only 22% and 30% of stages I and II, respectively, exhibited elevated serum creatinine values and values $\geqq$3 mg/% were found in isolated cases. The most frequently elevated serum creatinine values were found in stage III and values between 5-30 mg/% were found in 8% of the patients. In stage IV, 2% of the patients still exhibited serum creatinine values between 5-5.5 mg/% (Table 3). Accordingly, the creatinine clearance was most frequently reduced (40%) in stages III and IV, although, also relatively often in stage II. As expected, nearly all cases in stage V exhibited normal values.

Table 3. Correlation between morphologic stage and serum creatinine and creatinine clearance

Serum creatinine (mg%)	Stage I n = 76 (9)[a]	Stage II n = 160 (10)	Stage III n = 74 (8)	Stage IV n = 40 (5)	Stage V n = 21
0 – 1.2	78%	70%	62%	68%	95%
1.3 – 2.9	20%	29%	27%	27%	5%
3.0 – 4.9	1%	–	3%	3%	–
$\geq$ – 5.0	1%	1%	8% (5-30 mg/%)	2% (5-5.5 mg/%)	–
$\bar{x} \pm s \pm s_{\bar{x}}$	1.3 ± 1.3 ± 0.1	1.3 ± 0.9 ± 0.1	2.5 ± 4.8 ± 0.1	1.3 ± 1 ± 0.2	0.9 ± 0.2 ± 0.1
Creatinine clearance (ml/min/1.73 m^2)	**Stage I n = 56 (29)**	**Stage II n = 127 (43)**	**Stage III n = 63 (19)**	**Stage IV n = 32 (13)**	**Stage V n = 15 (6)**
> – 120					
80 – 120	73%	62%	60%	63%	80%
40 – 79	23%	29%	35%	18%	20%
0 – 39	4%	9%	5%	9%	–

[a] Figures in parentheses represent number of cases without informations.

6. Table 4 shows the clinical course of PGN in 223 patients after renal biopsy, correlating to the stage of the disease (mean observation period of 27 months). From this table, it can be concluded that the further clinical course was most unfavorable for those patients with alterations in stage III at the time of the renal biopsy. The clinical manifestations of 30% of the patients had deteriorated after an average of 29 months and 15% of the patients had died. Remarkably, most deaths during a later course were observed in patients whose glomerular alterations in stages I and II were seen at the time of the biopsy. On the contrary, none of the patients in stages IV and V died during a later course after an average of 29 and 24 months respectively. As would be expected, the further clinical course of patients in stage V at the time of the biopsy, with one exception, could be considered especially favorable. This would be shown by the data of most clinical remissions in this stage. Remissions during a later course will also be relatively often observed in patients demonstrating stage I alterations at the time of the biopsy. Taking into consideration the 223 patients with known clinical data, collectively, one finds after an average observation period of 27 months, improvement or no change in 39% or 24% of the patients, respectively, whereas 22% had deteriorated, 11% died, and only 4% could be considered clinically cured.

7. The clinical course, in the different stages after the biopsy, did not seem to be significantly influenced by the type of therapy—72-79% of the patients in the different stages had already been treated before the first biopsy (Table 5). Most frequently, steroids alone (15-27%), or in combination with immunosuppressive or cytotoxic drugs (3-23%) were given.

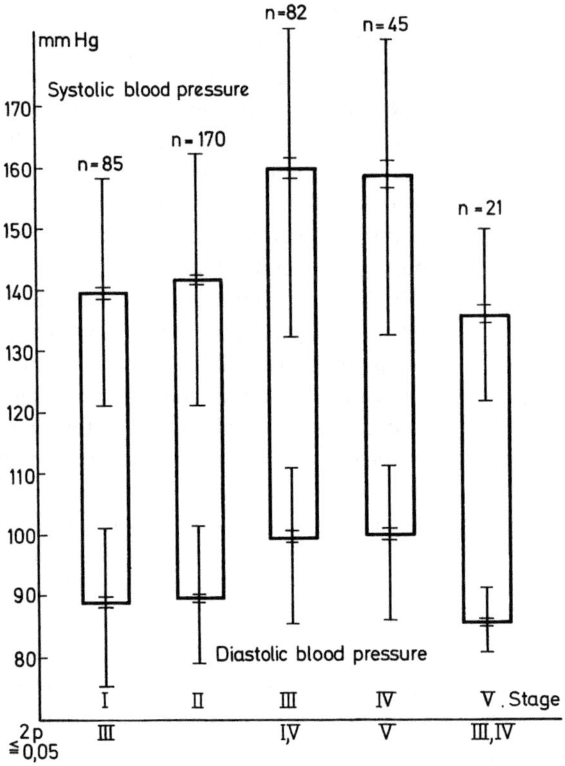

Fig. 10. Correlation between morphologic stage and systolic and diastolic blood pressure at time of renal biopsy

Table 4. Clinical course in relation to stage of disease (n = 223)

Clinical course	Stage I n	(%)	Stage II n	(%)	Stage III n	(%)	Stage IV n	(%)	Stage V n	(%)	Stages I-V n	(%)
Remission	4	(10)	2	(2)	1	(2)	–	–	3	(22)	10	(4)
Improvement	16	(39)	35	(40)	17	(36)	12	(37)	7	(49)	87	(39)
No change	7	(17)	26	(30)	8	(17)	10	(30)	3	(24)	54	(24)
Deterioration	5	(12)	17	(19)	14	(30	11	(33)	1	(7)	48	(22)
Deaths	9	(22)	8	(9)	7	(15)	–	–	–	–	24	(11)
n : ♂ : ♀	9 : 0		7 : 1		5 : 2						21 : 3	
Total	41	(18)	88	(39)	47	(21)	33	(16)	14	(6)	223	(100)
Mean observation period	22		29		29		29		24		27	

Table 5. Correlation between morphologic stage and therapy in 280 patients before and 115 patients after first renal biopsy

Therapy	Stage I (%)		Stage II (%)		Stage III (%)		Stage IV (%)		Stage V (%)		Total number of patients Stages I-V	
	Before	After	Before	After	Before	After	Before	After	Before	After	Before % (n)	After % (n)
No therapy	21	7	28	4	27	4	27	27	23	75	24 (68)	12 (14)
Steroids	24	22	16	36	21	13	27	27	15	25	21 (57)	26 (30)
Steroids and saluretics/ antihypertensive drugs	7	19	13	15	15	13	9	9	8	–	12 (33)	14 (16)
Steroids and immuno-suppressive/cytotoxic drugs	3	30	5	15	2	27	14	9	23	–	5 (15)	19 (22)
Immunosuppressive or cytotoxic drugs	–	–	–	9	6	22	–	9	–	–	1 (3)	9 (10)
Antihypertensive drugs or saluretics	27	11	18	12	19	17	14	–	15	–	20 (56)	11 (13)
Antibiotics/unspecific therapy	18	11	20	9	10	4	9	19	15	–	17 (48)	9 (10)
Percentage (%) and number of patients	100	100	100	100	100	100	100	100	100	100	100 (280)	100 (115)
(n)	(69)	(27)	(123)	(46)	(53)	(23)	(22)	(11)	(13)	(8)		

Patients in stages I and II usually received a nonspecific or antibiotic therapy before the first biopsy or a therapy with saluretics or antihypertensive drugs. In contrast to the therapy before the first biopsy, the therapy after it, in all stages, consisted mainly of steroids and immunosuppressive drugs or steroids and cytotoxic drugs, or immunosuppressive or cytotoxic drugs alone.

In stage V, reflecting the most favorable clinical course, only one quarter of the patients remained under therapy after the first biopsy.

Table 6. Autopsy cases: Morphologic findings

Age of patient[a]	Stage	Glomeruli nonspecific additional lesions	Tubuli	Interstitial tissue fibrosis[b]	Other findings	Cause of death
59	I	–	Swollen	–		Acute renal failure pulmonary embolism
72	II	–	Atrophic	++	–	Uremia
51	II	Focal sclerosis	Swollen	–	–	Uremia pulmonary embolism
57	III	–	Atrophic	++		Myocardial infarction
57	III	50% hyalinized glomeruli	Atrophic	+++	Shrunken kidney	Uremia
60	III	Hypertensive lesions	Atrophic	++	–	Uremia
32	III	50% hyalinized glomeruli	Atrophic	+++	Shrunken kidney	Uremia
37	III	–	Atrophic	++	–	Uremia pulmonary embolism
28	III	Hypertensive lesions	Atrophic	++	Shrunken kidney	Uremia
59	III	–	Atrophic	+		Uremia
64	IV	50% hyalinized glomeruli	Atrophic	+++	Shrunken kidney	Uremia
20	IV	–	Swollen	+		Uremia
44	IV + II	–	Atrophic	++		Uremia

[a] Of the 13 patients, 9 were male, 4 female, classified as follows: Stage I = 1, stage II = 2, stage III = 7, stage IV = 2, stage IV + II = 1.

[b] + = mild; ++ = medium; +++ = severe.

8. Of the 13 autopsy cases available for examination (Table 6), most (seven cases) had lesions of stage III and, in three cases, renal shrinkage with pronounced (more than 50%) glomerular hyalinization was detected. These alterations are described by *Ehrenreich* and *Churg* as the end stage V, whereas we prefer to refer to them as stage III with focal glomerular scars. One case showed hypertensive glomerular lesions.

All seven cases showed a focal or diffuse interstitial fibrosis and varying degrees of tubular atrophy. Six of the seven patients in stage III died of uremia following progressive renal insufficiency. One patient, with hypertension, died after a myocardial infarction. Stage IV was found in three autopsy cases, in one, combined with stage II alterations corresponding to a recurrence. One of these cases showed renal shrinkage with numerous hyalinized glomerula. Two of the autopsies were also marked by a diffuse interstitial fibrosis and tubular atrophy. These patients died of uremia from chronic renal insufficiency. In one case, evidence of acute renal failure was observed, corresponding to the clinical picture. Symptoms of acute renal failure, predominating clinically as well, were found in two more cases with stages I and II modifications. One additional case, with stage II alterations, died of chronic renal insufficiency and showed tubular atrophy, as well as interstitial fibrosis.

4. Clinical and Morphologic Findings in Relation to the Sex (Table 7a and 7b)

More women than men were found in the younger age group (< 30 years) although the average ages were similar (Table 7a). As can be further concluded from Table 7a, the clinical picture of the female was less serious than that of the male (lower proteinuria, less often nephrotic syndrome, lower blood pressure, less frequently elevated retention values). The clinical course of 153 males and 74 females and the morphologic and clinical courses of serial renal biopsies also indicated that the prognosis was better for females than for males (Table 7b). The clinical picture, showing a milder course of the disease in the female, was also reflected by the relationship of the sex to deaths in the various stages. More men died in stages I, II, and III than women even when one considers the more frequent occurrence of idiopathic PGN in males.

Table 7a. Clinical features of idiopathic PGN at time of renal biopsy in relation to sex

	Males (n = 247)	Females (n = 120)
Mean age ($\overline{x} \pm s \pm s_{\overline{x}}$)	40 ± 16 ± 1	38 ± 16 ± 2
< 30 years (%)	26%	37%
Proteinuria ($\overline{x} \pm s \pm s_{\overline{x}}$) (g/day)	7.6 ± 6.4 ± 0.4	5.1 ± 3.8 ± 0.3
Nephrotic syndrome	71%	54%
Mean blood pressure (mm Hg)	156/96	140/91
Serum creatinine ($\overline{x} \pm s \pm s_{\overline{x}}$) (mg%)	1.6 ± 2.4 ± 0.2	1.3 ± 2.3 ± 0.2
Creatinine clearance (ml/min/1.73 m^2) < 120 80-120	53%	64%
< 80- 40	25%	19%
< 40	22%	17%

See footnote, Table 1.

Table 7b. Clinical course of idiopathic PGN after renal biopsy [mean observation period period $\overline{x} = 26$ months (1-109)] and morphologic and clinical course of serial renal biopsies [mean observation period $\overline{x} = 49$ months] in relation to sex

Clinical course	Males n = 153 (94 cases without information) %	n	Females n = 74 (46 cases without information) %	n
Remission	3	5	27	20
Improvement	35	53	47	35
No change	23	35	14	10
Deterioration	25	38	4	3
Deaths	14	22	8	6
Serial renal biopsies	**Males n = 34**		**Females n = 12 (2 cases without information)**	
1. Morphologic course:				
Improvement	8	3	58	7
No change	11	4	8	1
Deterioration	81	27	34	4
2. Clinical course:				
Improvement	35	12	58	7
No change	24	8	34	4
Deterioration	41	14	8	1

5. Observations on Serial Renal Biopsies

As examinations of the serial biopsy cases showed (Table 8), the morphologic transformations of the glomerular basement membrane progressed regularly as the PGN continued, whereas the duration in a particular stage probably varied.

The reparation stage V can be reached from all other stages, most rapidly (30 months) from stage I, and, most slowly, (76 months) from stage III (mean observation period of the 38 cases with serial renal biopsies of 49 months).

Table 8. Serial renal biopsies in idiopathic PGN: Relationship between morphologic stage at time of the first renal biopsy and later morphologic course ($\overline{x} = 49$, n = 38)

Stage	I	II	III	IV	V
First biopsy	n = 9				
At second biopsy		n = 5	n = 2	–	n = 2
Mean observation period		10	16.5		30
First biopsy		n = 19			
At second biopsy		n = 5	n = 7	n = 4	n = 3
Mean observation period		10	27	31	40
First biopsy			n = 6		
At second biopsy				n = 5	n = 1
Mean observation period				32	76
Fist biopsy				n = 4	
At second biopsy				n = 3	n = 1
Mean observation period				14	31

As can be seen in Table 9, more than 50% of the 21 cases, improving clinically between the first and second biopsy (mean observation period of 25 months), were found to be in stages IV and V at the time of the second biopsy. In contrast, more than half of the group, whose clinical course deteriorated between the first and second biopsy, remained in stage II (after a considerably longer mean observation period between the first and second biopsy of 65 months). In the group without clinical changes, a decrease in the early stages or an increase in stages IV and V, respectively, was observed at the time of the second biopsy in relation to the first after a short observation period (mean observation period of 20 months).

Table 9. Clinical course between first and second biopsy in relation to morphologic stages at time of first and second renal biopsy in serial renal biopsies (n = 38)

	First biopsy		Second biopsy				
	Stage	No. of patients	Stage I	II	III	IV	V
Improvement	I	5	–	1	2	–	2
n = 21	II	11	–	2	4	3	2
55%	III	4	–	–	–	4	–
	IV	1	–	–	–	1	–
	V	0					
Mean observation period between 1st and 2nd biopsy ($\overline{x}$) = 25 months (5-57)							
No change	I	1	–	1	–	–	–
n = 9	II	5	–	1	2	1	1
24%	III	0					
	IV	3	–	–	–	3	–
	V	0					
Mean observation period between 1st and 2nd biopsy ($\overline{x}$) = 20 months (8-37)							
Deterioration	I	3	–	3	–	–	–
n = 8	II	3	–	2	1	–	–
21%	III	2	–	–	–	2	–
	IV	0					
	V	0					
Mean observation period between 1st and 2nd biopsy ($\overline{x}$) = 65 months (1-83)							
Deaths n = 0							
Remission n = 0							

A final statement as to the prognosis of PGN can nevertheless not be made on the basis of the observation periods between the two biopsies (presented here). This is shown in Table 10, in which the clinical course between the first and second biopsy, as well as that after the second biopsy is shown. From this table, it is clear that the clinical course between the two biopsies improves, but that the clinical picture worsens at a later course. Therefore, even in the cases which improved during the period between the first and second biopsy, a deterioration in the clinical picture was noted at a later course in nearly 30% of the cases.

Table 11 shows the therapy administered to 38 patients with serial renal biopsies before and after the first biopsy. Most cases had already been treated before the biopsy with

Table 10. Change in clinical course in serial renal biopsies of idiopathic PGN after observation period between first and second biopsy

Clinical course between 1st and 2nd biopsy	Clinical course after 2nd and last biopsy				
	Remission	Improvement	No change	Deterioration	Deaths
Improvement n = 21	4	6	5	6	–
No change n = 9	–	3	1	3	–[a]
Deterioration n = 8			2	2	1[b]
Mean observation period between the 1st and 2nd biopsy in 38 cases with serial renal biopsies $\bar{x}$ = 21.4 months (1-83)	Mean observation period after the 2nd and last biopsy to date in 33 cases with serial renal biopsies $\bar{x}$ = 29.8 months (2-76)[c]				

[a] Two cases without information

[b] Three cases without information

[c] Five cases without information

steroids, either alone or in combination with immunosuppressive or cytotoxic drugs. After the biopsy, therapy with immunosuppressive or cytotoxic drugs (alone or in combination with steroids) predominates. The therapy is thus independent of the stage present at the time of the biopsy. No positive correlation can be made between the clinical course and the employed therapy (Table 12). In all three clinical course groups, that is, those with improved, deteriorated or stationary clinical pictures, nearly half of the cases were treated before and after the biopsy with steroids, immunosuppressive, or cytotoxic drugs or a combination thereof.

The four cases which went into clinical remission at a later course, after the second and third biopsy, were all treated with corticosteroids, immunosuppressive or cytotoxic drugs and steroids. In two of these cases, the treatment was discontinued after the second biopsy.

IV. Discussion

The preceding data and clinical findings, collected from 367 patients with PGN and 403 biopsies (average age, age range, sex range, clinical history, first symptoms, clinical symptoms at the time of the biopsy, course of the disease, and prognosis), agree essentially with the results of other authors (*Ehrenreich* and *Churg*, 1968; *Pollak* et al., 1968; *Ducrot* et al., 1969; *Foreland* et al., 1969; *Habib*, 1970; *Gluck* et al., 1973) as well as with our own preliminary studies (*Gärtner* et al., 1974).

1. Our present study supplementarily shows that the dynamics of the clinical course of PGN can be best comprehended by modifying the morphologic stage classification of *Ehrenreich* and *Churg* (1968). In our opinion, the processes of transformation of the basement membrane, leading to the characteristic late alterations of stage IV, cannot be assessed

Table 11. Therapy in serial renal biopsies before and after first renal biopsy (n = 38) (%)

	No therapy	Steroids	Steroids and saluretics or antihypertensive drugs	Immunosuppressive or cytotoxic drugs	Antihypertensive drugs or saluretics	Steroids and immunosuppressive or cytotoxic drugs	Antibiotics or unspecific therapy
Before 1st biopsy	26	32	8	5	8	5	16
After 1st biopsy	3	18	13	29	8	21	8

Table 12. Clinical course in serial renal biopsies (n = 38) in relation to therapy before and after biopsy [mean observation period between first and second biopsy $\bar{x}$ = 21,4 months (1-83)]

Clinical course	No therapy Before/After	Steroids Before/After	Steroids and saluretics or antihypertensive drugs Before/After	Immunosuppressive or cytotoxic drugs Before/After	Antihypertensive drugs or saluretics Before/After	Steroids and immunosuppressive or cytotoxic drugs Before/After	Antibiotics or unspecific therapy Before/After
Improvement n = 21	5/–	7/5	2/2	1/8	2/–	1/6	3/–
No change n = 9	3/1	3/1	–/2	–/1	1/1	1/2	1/1
Deterioration n = 8	2/–	2/1	1/1	1/2	–/2	–/–	2/2
Deaths n = 0							
Remission n = 0							

in every case as a deterioration in the disease, but can be interpreted also as the beginning of a reparation phase. As the reparation continues, stage IV gives rise to stage V, described by us as a reparation stage, characterized by an extensive normalization of the basement membrane structure. Probably by misinterpreting stage IV as one of exclusive morphologic deterioration, the frequently mentioned discrepancy in clinical improvement, in this stage, results (*Pollak* et al., 1968; *Foreland* et al., 1969; *Seymour* et al., 1971; *Row* et al., 1975). To enable an uniform evaluation of stage IV and an integration of the morphologic findings of the reparation stage V into the current classification of *Ehrenreich* and *Churg*, one should refer to a progression of the basement membrane transformation processes rather than to a progression of the disease with morphologic deterioration. To disregard the glomerular hyalinization processes by this classification is not considered by us to be a disadvantage because these processes which can occur, according to our findings, especially in stage III and IV of PGN, as well as in other glomerulonephrites, e.g., mesangioproliferative GN, should have been distinctly mentioned in the diagnosis.

2. As the results under consideration indicate, each stage is associated with different clinical symptoms, so that a morphologic classification of the glomerular basement membrane alterations, into five stages, is justified. An analysis of the clinical and morphologic findings in PGN, in relation to the various stages, indicates a strong correlation between the morphologic picture and the clinical symptoms. In agreement with *Ehrenreich* and *Churg* (1968), *Pollak* et al. (1968), *Ducrot* et al. (1969), *Hatta* (1972), the relationship between the duration of the disease and the stage shows that the degree of basement membrane transformation is dependent on the duration of the disease. The observation that the shortest duration of the disease is associated with stage I and the longest with stages IV and V supports the morphologic findings that the stages succeed one another and that the subepithelial-located electron-dense deposits occur earlier than the intramembranous electron-lucent deposits. This is in accordance with the findings of *Ehrenreich* and *Churg* (1968), *Bariéty* et al. (1970), *Hatta* (1972), *Gluck* et al. (1973), *Törnroth* et al. (1975). In addition, the correlation between the degree of proteinuria and the morphologic stage indicates that, in idiopathic PGN, the most severe proteinuria is present in stages I and II, and the nephrotic syndrome is thus most often found in these stages.

In agreement with earlier studies (*Gärtner* et al., 1974), the present findings show a decrease in proteinuria in relation to the duration of the disease or the degree of basement membrane transformation, respectively (*Hatta*, 1972), so that, in stage V, the proteinuria has essentially disappeared.

Correspondingly, the nephrotic syndrome occurs less frequently as the basement membrane transformation increases in relation to the disease duration, an observation made also by *Ducrot* et al. (1969). PGN usually proceeds monosymptomatically in stages I and II with clinical manifestations characterized by the nephrotic syndrome with high proteinuria but without significant increase in blood pressure or restruction of the filtration capacity. But the clinical features of stage III are defined by elevated retention values and blood pressure values combined with a retrogressive proteinuria in regard to stage II. Thus, most patients with a restricted creatinine clearance, elevated serum creatinine and blood pressure values, or compensated and decompensated renal insufficiency, are observed in this stage. As the autopsy findings show, glomerular alterations in stage III, were most often present in patients who died of chronic renal insufficiency, frequently in combination with glomerular hyalinization processes and interstitial fibrosis with tubular atrophy. Nevertheless, this renal insufficiency, may not be attributed primarily to the glomerular lesions as long as glomerular hyalinization processes do not predominate. A more essential role in the development of the renal insufficiency is played rather by interstitial fibrosis (*Pollak* et al., 1973) along with tubular atrophy which is often observed in PGN in the kidney whose glomeruli are not hyalinized. We suspect, that, in these cases, the interstitial fibroses are remnants of acute renal failure, sometimes observed in PGN (Table 6). In our opinion, acute renal failure, frequently follows an existing nephrotic syndrome, was not always observed clinically.

A comparison of the clinical and morphologic findings in stage IV with those in stage III supports the fact that, in stage III, the symptoms climax and, in some cases, the turning point of the disease is reached. Although the clinical manifestations in stage IV still consist relatively often of hypertension, a slightly restricted creatinine clearance and an elevation in retention values, renal insufficiency occurs more seldom. The generally less severe picture of the disease in stage IV in comparison to stage III, as well as the morphologic findings of an extensive disappearance of immune deposits from the basement membrane, can be interpreted as the beginning of a reparation phase.

In cases which continue to deteriorate clinically in this stage, interstitial fibrosis, tubular atrophy, and glomerular hyalinization processes predominate which we could not relate to the basement membrane transformation processes. On the other hand, we also observed cases which, in addition to the predominating basement membrane modifications of stage IV, showed stage II alterations, namely, formation of deposits and development of spikes. Clinically, a fully developed nephrotic syndrome exists, corresponding to a recurrence.

The reparative character of the transformation process is finally clear in stage V through the extensive normalization of the basement membrane. This is confirmed by the near absence of clinical symptoms. Morphologic, as well as clinical findings, justify defining this stage as a reparation stage.

3. It could further be shown that PGN, not only occurs more often in males than females, in accordance with the literature (*Pollak* et al., 1968; *Ducrot* et al., 1969; *Habib* et al., 1971; *Rosen*, 1971), but also more severely. In contrast to *Franklin* et al. (1973), who observed a course of the disease leading to death mainly in females, our study (Table 4) indicates a higher mortality in males which by far exceeds the frequency of PGN in this sex. This fact, combined with the less severe clinical features in the female (lower proteinuria, less occurrence of nephrotic syndrome, less severe clinical features in the female (lower proteinuria, less occurrence of nephrotic syndrome, less often elevated retention and blood pressure values), is one of the main reasons to consider more females than males as reaching the reparation stage.

This is, in a way, a contradiction of the results in Table 6, according to which males die more often of PGN only to the extent that they are afflicted more often than females. Substantially fewer patients are presented in Table 6, however, thus making it less representative than Table 4. Moreover, the data summarized in Table 4 refer to different patients than those in Table 6. No patients in Table 6, dying of PGN, were biopsied before their deaths.

4. As the present study indicates, the different morphologic stages proceed progressively and the rate of the basement membrane transformation processes, as well as the duration of a particular stage, can vary. Thus, after arriving at a diffuse stage III, several years could elapse before the typical stages IV and V basement membrane alterations develop. The variable durations of the individual stages are reflected also by the differential clinical course.

Improved clinical manifestations would thus be observed when stages IV and V are reached within a short period of time. This suggests that a quick completion of the morphologic transformation, i.e., a rapid succession of the various stages, expresses a more favorable prognosis for the disease. Conversely, most patients with progressively deteriorating clinical features continue to show the stage II histologic alterations even after a long observation period (Table 9), i.e., the unfavorable clinical course, over a long period of time, is associated with a very slow morphologic progression and persistence of early lesions.

5. The observation that stages I-V succeed one another and that the shortest duration of the disease is associated with stage I and the longest with stages IV and V, seems to contradict the fact that the average age does not increase but decreases with an increase in the duration of the disease, according to the findings of *Ducrot* et al. (1969). The evidence that the patients in our study in stage V are, on the average, 12 years younger, suggests that an early manifestation of the disease would be more favorable prognostically. Other explanations are that older patients could die from other causes before even reaching stage V, that females, represented in a larger number in stage V with known milder clinical manifestations than males, could be found more often in younger ages and, finally, among the cases in stage V, one finds those with a rapid course of the disease which progresses to stage V in a relatively short time by a favorable clinical picture.

6. An attempt to explain the variable rapid course of the disease, in connection with the somewhat shorter disease duration in stage V cases, yields the observation that initial segmental alterations in stage I of PGN need not develop into typical diffuse alterations of stages II and III, but can remain as segmental lesions. It can be expected that PGN, in a considerable number of patients, remains in a stage during which only a segmental deposition of immune precipitates occurs and the basement membrane transformations retain their segmental character. The segmental deposition of immune precipitates provokes in principle, a similar transformation of the basement membrane as in the diffuse deposition of immune precipitates. The segmental character of the basement membrane alterations enables the transformation processes to proceed more quickly toward the reparation stage, because large parts of the basement membrane show no microscopically visible transformation and do not seem to be affected by the disease, a fact which would indicate a favorable prognosis for the segmental forms (*Ducrot* et al., 1969; *Erwin* et al., 1973; *Habib* et al., 1973; *Murphy* et al., 1973).

7. At which stage of PGN can a reparation stage, combined with a clinical remission, develop? Our investigations show, in contrast to the view of *Gluck* et al. (1973) and in agreement with *Churg* (1973), that morphologic recovery is possible at any stage. Whether diffuse or segmental processes are involved, the stage of reparation will develop first through a stage of incorporation of deposits and then through one of vacuolation of the intramembranous deposits (*Bariéty* et al., 1970). Therefore, it is also possible for PGN, with the typical diffuse stage III transformations, to proceed into a reparation stage V, even if the period of time is much longer.

8. Idiopathic PGN is a disease often extending over a period of years with only a slight morphologic and clinical tendency toward a cure. The unfavorable prognosis is evidenced by the fact that, within an average observation period of 2 1/2 years, 11% of the patients died and only 4% of the 367 examined exhibited a reparation stage. The prognosis is probably even more unfavorable if one considers that the presented study consists of select material in so far as those patients sho were not biopsied in the stage of terminal renal insuffi-

ciency were not included in this study. As our observations of the course of the disease show, the cases with persisting early alterations in which the basement membrane transformation process did not progress, had an especially bad prognosis, as did those considered as recurrences which showed stage II alterations with basement membrane modifications in stages III and IV and whose clinical features consisted of high proteinuria, nephrotic syndrome and hematuria (*Hatta*, 1972). An unfavorable course is also to be expected when additional glomerular hyalinization processes, interstitial fibrosis and tubular atrophy are observed. In relation to other renal diseases, the prognosis for PGN is generally better than for membrane-proliferative GN (MPGN) and the rapidly progressive GN, however, clearly worse than for the minimal proliferative GN (MPs) + nephrotic syndrome.

9. The minor tendency toward a remission of PGN is probably not influenced by the usual current therapy. As the present study shows, the clinical course and administered therapy exhibit no positive correlation. In all clinical course groups of patients with serial renal biopsies, approximately half were treated with steroids, immunosuppressive drugs or a combination therapy. Four of the 38 cases observed which obtained a remission during a later course also received this therapy either after the first or before the second biopsy and clinical remission occurred in one case after the drug therapy had been discontinued for a longer period of time. Also, these findings justify the therapeutical scepticism of many authors (*Erwin* et al., 1973; *Gluck* et al., 1973; *Habib* et al., 1973; *Olbing* et al., 1973; *Pollak* et al., 1973; *Donadio* et al., 1974; *Row* et al., 1975).

10. An indirect proof that idiopathic PGN is an immune complex nephritis is provided by: (1) animal experiments (*Heyman*, 1959; *Grupe* et al., 1967; *Dixon*, 1968; *Dixon* et al., 1968; *Edgington* et al., 1968; *Glassock* et al., 1968), (2) immune complex nephritis with similar alterations by known antigens as DNA (*Koffler* et al., 1973), (3) identical transformations by tumors (*Lee* et al., 1966; *Lewis* et al., 1971), (4) immunohistologic findings (*Bariéty* et al., 1970, 1972; *Murphey* et al., 1973), (5) administration of certain drugs as D-penicillamine, (*Jaffe* et al., 1968; *Gärtner* et al., 1975) tridione, and gold. Considering the pathogenesis that PGN is a special form of an immune complex nephritis, the course of PGN is dependent on the quality and quantity of either antigens or the antigen-antibody complexes. The difference in the course of idiopathic PGN can be understood by assuming that one is dealing with a polyetiological disease, caused by several unknown antigens. Considering that PGN can be induced in animals by antigens obtained from the brush border of convoluted tubule I antigen and, furthermore, that the same disease is also inducible by exogenous antigens, it is understandable that the disease, as autoimmune disease, would have an unfavorable prognosis. The prognosis seems to be favorable if PGN develops after the confrontation of the organism with temporarily occurring exogenous antigens, e.g., drugs (*Gärtner* et al., 1975). In favor of this view, are the investigations of *Naruse* et al. (1974) who observed no remission in cases of PGN exhibiting the presence of a tubular antigen. In contrast, those cases in which a tubular antigen was not detected immunohistologically, went into remission.

V. Summary

The morphologic and clinical features of idiopathic perimembranous glomerulonephritis (PGN), as well as the correlations between them are reported. The study included 403 renal biopsies of 367 patients, 38 of whom were serial biopsied.

1. Idiopathic PGN is observed twice as often in males as in females. The disease occurs in every age group, reaches a peak between 31 and 50, the average age being 39.

2. The morphologic picture of idiopathic PGN is characterized by subepithelial immune deposits provoking glomerular basement membrane transformation.

3. The progressive changes in the basement membrane, occurring in the course of the disease, can be subdivided into 5 stages. The shortest duration of the disease is observed in patients whose renal biopsies showed morphologic alterations of stage I, the longest by those in stages IV and V. This indicates that the morphologic changes in the glomerular basement membrane are dependent on the duration of the disease, and the degree of the basement membrane transformation increases the longer the disease persists. The rate of the entire transformation, as well as the duration of a particular stage, can vary.

4. The transformation processes, leading to the late alterations of stage IV, represent the beginning of a reparation phase. In some cases, this could give rise to stage V. This stage, observed in 4% of the 367 patients, is considered a reparation stage and is characterized by an extensive normalization of the basement membrane where electron-dense deposits are no longer detected.

5. Along with these specific basement membrane alterations, other nonspecific morphologic findings are important for the course and prognosis of idiopathic PGN. These include glomerular hyalinization processes, and—as remnants of an acute renal failure—interstitial fibroses and tubular atrophy. These nonspecific alterations are most often observed in stages III and IV.

6. The clinical picture, considered collectively at the time of the first renal biopsy, consists of a nephrotic syndrome with a high proteinuria in 70% of the patients, slightly elevated blood pressure values, a mild erythrocyturia in 53% of the patients, and, in one-third of the patients, a restricted renal function.

7. An analysis of the clinical and morphologic findings in idiopathic PGN in relation to the different stages, shows strong correlations between the morphologic features and the clinical symptoms. In stages I and II, the monosymptomatic clinical picture is characterized by a NS with high proteinuria in 70% and 77% of the patients respectively, generally normal blood pressure values, and normal serum creatinine and endogenous creatinine clearance values in two-thirds of the cases. The clinical and morphologic climax and, in some cases, the turning point of the disease is reached in stage III where the clinical manifestations consist of only a slight retrogressive proteinuria and markedly elevated blood pressure values, as well as severe renal insufficiency with serum creatinine values > 5 mg % in 8% of the cases. Although the clinical prognosis for patients in stage III is often unfavorable and 15% died in a later course of the disease, the clinical course is much more favorable after stage IV has been reached. The reparative character of the transformation process in stage V is confirmed by the near absence of clinical symptoms in this stage. Morphologic and clinical findings justify defining this stage as a reparation stage. This stage can be reached from all other stages, most rapidly from stage I and most slowly from stage III.

8. The correlation between the degree of proteinuria, frequency of NS and the morphologic stage, indicates a decrease in proteinuria and NS in relation to the duration of the disease, or the degree of basement membrane transformation.

9. The disease entity of idiopathic PGN in the female is milder than in the male as indicated by the less serious clinical picture at the time of the first renal biopsy, as well as the

more favorable clinical and morphologic course and the lower mortality rate in the female. More females than males reach the reparation stage V.

10. As serial renal biopsy findings of idiopathic PGN show, the variable durations of the individual stages are reflected by the differential clinical course. A quick completion of the morphologic transformation, i.e., a rapid succession of the various stages, expresses a more favorable prognosis for the disease, whereas an unfavorable clinical course is associated with a very slow morphologic progression and persistence of early lesions. In addition, segmental forms seem to indicate a more favorable prognosis than diffuse forms.

11. Though reparation processes occur in some cases, idiopathic PGN is a disease often extending over a period of years with only a slight morphologic and clinical tendency toward a cure, which may not be influenced by the usual current therapy.

References

Bariéty, J., Antoine, B.: Les glomérulopathies humaines à "dépôts". (Maladies générales exclues). Ann. Biol. clin. 30, 481-498 (1972).

Bariéty, J., Druet, Ph., Lagrue, G., Samarcq, P., Milliez, P.: Les glomérulopathies "extramembraneuses" (GEM). Étude morphologique en microscopie optique, électronique et en immunofluorescence. Path. Biol. (Paris) 18, 5-32 (1970).

Berger, J., Michielsen, P., Galle, P.: Les syndromes néphrotiques avec dépôts intermembrano-épithéliaux. J. Urol. Nephrol. 67, 52-57 (1961).

Bohle, A., Eichenseher, N., Fischbach, H., Kronenberg, K.H., Wehner, H.: Glomerulonephritis in children and adults. In: Proc. Vth Internat. Congr. Nephrol. Mexico, 1972, Basel: Karger, 1974, Vol. I, pp. 44-49.

Cameron, J.S.: Nephrotic syndrome. Brit. med. J. **1970 IV**, 350-353.

Churg, J.: Discussion about membranous nephropathy (Extramembranous Glomerulonephritis). In: Glomerulonephritis, Morphology, Natural History and Treatment. Kincaid-Smith, P., Mathew, T.H., Becker, E.L. (eds.). New York: John Wiley and Sons, 1973, p.481.

Churg, J., Ehrenreich, T.: Membranous nephropathy. In: Glomerulonephritis, Morphology, Natural History and Treatment. Kincaid-Smith, P., Mathew, T.H., Becker, E.L. (eds.). New York: John Wiley and Sons, 1973, pp. 443-448.

Churg, J., Habib, R., White, R.H.: Pathology of the nephrotic syndrome in children. Lancet **1970 II**, 1299-1302.

Dixon, F.J.: The pathogenesis of glomerulonephritis. Amer. J. Med. 44, 493-498 (1968).

Dixon, F.J., Edgington, T.S., Lambert, P.H.: Non-glomerular antigen-antibody complex nephritis. Immunopathology. In: Mechanisms of Inflammations Induced by Immune Reactions. Proc. Vth Internat. Symp. Miescher, P., Graber, P. (eds.). Basel: Schwabe, 1968, pp. 17-28.

Donadio, J.V., Holley, K.E., Anderson, C.F., Taylor, W.F.: Controlled trial of cyclophosphamide in idiopathic membranous nephropathy. Kidney Int. 6, 431-439 (1974).

Ducrot, H., Jungers, P., Hinglais, N., Demontera, H., Galle, P., Hamburger, J.: Les syndromes néphrotiques primitifs de l'adulte. In: Les Syndromes Néphrotiques. 34e Congr. Franç. Méd. Lyon, 1963. Paris: Masson, 1963, p. 289.

Ducrot, H., Tsomi, C., Jungers, P., Demontera, H., Hinglais, N., Giromini, M.: Étude anatomo-clinique des glomérulonéphrites extramembraneuses. Act. Néphrol. Hôp. Necker 1, 115-140 (1969).

Edgington, T.S., Glassock, R.J., Dixon, F.J.: Autologous immune complex nephritis induced with renal tubular antigen. I. Identification and isolation of the pathogenetic antigen, J. exp. Med. 127, 555-572 (1968).

Ehrenreich, T., Churg, J.: Pathology of membranous nephropathy. In: Sommer's Pathology Annual. New York: Appleton-Century-Crofts, 1968, Vol. II, pp. 145-186.

Erwin, D.T., Donadio, J.V., Holley, K.E.: The clinical course of idiopathic membranous nephropathy. Mayo Clin. Proc. **48**, 697-712 (1973).
Forland, M., Spargo, B.H.: Clinicopathological correlations in idiopathic nephrotic syndrome with membranous nephropathy. Nephron **6**, 498-525 (1969).
Franklin, W.A., Jennings, R.B., Earle, D.P.: Membranous glomerulonephritis: Long-term serial observations on clinical course and morphology. Kidney Int. **4**, 36-56 (1973).
Gärtner, H.V., Fischbach, H., Wehner, H., Bohle, A., Edel, H.H., Kluthe, R., Scheler, F., Schmülling, R.M.: Comparison of clinical and morphological features of peri- (epi-extra) membranous glomerulonephritis. Nephron **13**, 288-301 (1974).
Gärtner, H.V., Neild, G.H., Bohle, A.: Eine vergleichende Untersuchung klinisch-morphologischer Korrelationen bei idiopathischer und postmedikamentöser perimembranöser Glomerulonephritis (PGN). Verh. dtsch. Ges. Path. **59**, 537 (1975).
Gärtner, H.V., Neild, G.H., Bohle, A., Hallauer, W., Hoppe-Seyler, G., Lüttgen, F.M., Schollmeyer, P.: Perimembranöse Glomerulonephritis nach Penicillamintherapie. Klin. Wschr. **53**, 835-837 (1975).
Glassock, R.J., Edgington, T.S., Watson, J.J., Dixon, F.J.: Autologous immune complex nephritis induced with renal tubular antigen. II. The pathogenetic mechanism. J. exp. Med. **127**, 573-588 (1968).
Gluck, M.C., Gallo, G., Lowenstein, J., Baldwin, D.S.: Membranous glomerulonephritis. Evolution of clinical and pathologic features. Ann. int. Med. **78**, 1-12 (1973).
Grupe, W.E., Kaplan, M.H.: A proximal tubular antigen in the pathogenesis of autoimmune nephritis (Abstr.) Fed. Proc. **26**, 573 (1967).
Habib, R.: Classification anatomique des néphropathies glomérulaires. In: Päd. Fortbildungskurse. Basel-München-New York: Karger, 1970, Vol. XXVIII, pp. 3-47.
Habib, R., Kleinknecht, C.: The primary nephrotic syndrome of childhood. Classification and clinicopathology study of 406 cases. Path. Ann. **6**, 417-474 (1971).
Habib, R., Kleinknecht, C.: Idiopathic Extramembranous Glomerulonephritis in Children. In: Glomerulonephritis, Morphology, Natural History, and Treatment. Kincaid-Smith, P., Mathew, T.H., Becker, E.L. (eds.). New York: John Wiley and Sons, 1973, pp. 449-459.
Habib, R., Kleinknecht, C., Gubler, M.C.: Extramembranous glomerulonephritis in children: Report of 50 cases. J. Pediat. **82**, 754-766 (1973).
Hatta, J.: Electron microscopic analysis of glomerular basement membrane in membranous nephropathy. Jap. Circulat. J. **36**, 137-152 (1972).
Heyman, W., Hackel, D.B., Harwood, S., Wilson, S.G.F., Hunter, J.L.P.: Production of nephrotic syndrome in rats by Freund's adjuvants and rat kidney suspensions. Proc. soc. exp. Biol. (N.Y.) **100**, 660-664 (1959).
Jaffe, J.A., Treser, G., Suzuki, Y., Ehrenreich, T.: Nephropathy induced by D-penicillamine. Ann. intern. Med. **69**, 549 (1968).
Koffler, D., Agnello, V., Kunkel, H.G.: Polynucleotide immune complexes in serum and glomeruli of patients with systemic lupus erythematosus. Amer. J. Path. **74**, 109-124 (1973).
Lee, J.C., Yamauchi, H., Hopper, J., Jr.: The association of cancer and the nephrotic syndrome. Ann. intern. Med. **64**, 41 (1966).
Lewis, M.G., Loughridge, L.W., Phillips, T.M.: Immunological studies with extrarenal malignant disease. Lancet **1971 II**, 134.
Murphey, W.M., Deodhar, S.D., McCormack, L.J., Osborne, D.G.: Immunopathologic studies in glomerular disease with membranous lesions. Amer. J. clin. Path. **60**, 364-376 (1973).
Naruse, T., Miyakawa, Y., Kitamura, K., Shibata, S.: Membranous glomerulonephritis mediated by renal tubular epithelial antigen-antibody complex. J. Allergy clin. Immunol. **54**, 311-318 (1974).
Olbing, H., Greifer, J., Bennett, B.P., Bernstein, J., Spitzer, A.: Idiopathic membranous nephropathy in children. Kidney Int. 3, 381-390 (1973).
Pollak, V.E., Pirani, C.L., Clyne, D.H.: The natural history of membranous glomerulonephropathy. In: Glomerulonephritis, Morphology, Natural History, and Treatment. Kincaid-Smith, P., Mathew, T.H., Becker, E.L. (eds.). New York: John Wiley and Sons, 1973, pp. 429-442.
Pollak, V.E., Rosen, S., Pirani, C.L., Muehrcke, R.C., Kark, R.M.: Natural history of lipoid nephrosis and of membranous glomerulonephritis. Ann. intern. Med. **69**, 1171-1196 (1968).

Renner, E., Edel, H.H., Eigler, J., Buchborn, E.: Klinische und prognostische Bedeutung der histologischen Klassifizierung von Glomerulonephritiden. Klin. Wschr. **14**, 752-759 (1969).
Rosen, S.: Membranous glomerulonephritis. Current status. Human Path. **2**, 209-231 (1971).
Row, P.G., Cameron, J.S., Turner, D.R., Evans, D.J., White, R.H.R., Ogg, C.S., Chantler, C., Brown, C.B.: Membranous nephropathy. Quart. J.Med., N.S. XLIV, **174**, 207-239 (1975).
Royer, P., Habib, R., Vermeil, G., Mathieu, H., Alizon, M.: Les glomérulonéphrites prolongées de l'enfant. Ann. Pédiat. (Paris) 38, 793-807 (1962).
Seymour, A.E., Spargo, B.H., Penksa, R.: Contributions of renal biopsy studies to the understanding of disease. Amer. J. Path. **65**, 550-588 (1971).
Törnroth, T., Skrifvars, B.: The development and resolution of glomerular basement membrane changes associated with subepithelial immune deposits. Amer. J. Path. **79**, 219-230 (1975).
White, R.H.: Epimembranous nephropathy. Lancet **1969 I**, 746.

Human Parathyroid Gland: A Freeze Fracture and Thin Section Study

J. THIELE

I. Introduction

In all vertebrates the subtle balance of the ionized fraction of the total serum calcium is equilibrated by a hormone produced and secreted by the parathyroid glands (review by *Aurbach* et al., 1969). Although vitamin D with its metabolites and calcitonin play a certain role in the control of the calcium level, parathormone still remains the most decisive one for the preservation of calcium homeostasis. An unique feature of parathyroid physiology is that there is direct inverse feedback control by the ionized calcium itself (also by magnesium), as demonstrated by numerous animal experiments (review by *Capen* and *Roth*, 1973). Parathormone maintains the calcium balance by increasing the rate of bone resorption, and additionally by elevating the level of calcium absorption through the intestine and by renal tubular reabsorption. The activities of this hormone are mediated by activation of the enzyme adenyl cyclase and formation of cyclic adenosine monophosphate in the target cells of bone, small intestine and kidney (review by *Liddle* and *Hardman*, 1971).

Human parathyroid hormone isolated from adenomatous and hyperplastic glands consists of a polypeptide (molecular weight about 7,000) with an almost known amino acid composition and sequence (*O'Riordan* et al., 1971; *Arnaud* et al., 1971). The molecular weight of the purified, gland-extracted hormone differs from that secreted into the culture medium of parathyroid tissue slices (*Arnaud* et al., 1971). This observation suggests a possible precursor of the parathormone in the gland. It is suggested that this pro-parathyroid hormone is cleaved into smaller fragments before it is secreted into the culture medium of tissue slices, and, in patients with hyperparathyroidism, before release into the circulation (*Arnaud* et al., 1971; *Habener* et al., 1971; *Kemper* et al., 1972; *Jacobs* et al., 1974). More recent investigations emphasize a considerable heterogeneity of the circulating human parathyroid hormone (*Arnaud*, 1973; *Silverman* and *Yalow*, 1973; *Hesch* et al., 1975) and an important role of microtubules in the intracellular transport and conversion of parathyroid hormone precursor compounds (*Kemper* et al., 1975).

The chief cells of the parathyroid gland have been shown to synthesize and excrete parathormone (*Munger* and *Roth*, 1963). Numerous papers deal with the morphology of the normal and pathologically altered human parathyroid gland (reviews by *Thiele* et al., 1975 and *Altenähr*, 1972), as well as with the fine-structural changes of this organ in experimental animals (reviews by *Capen* and *Roth*, 1973 and *Roth* and *Capen*, 1974). Analysis of the fine structure reveals that the chief cells contain all organelles generally thought to take part in proteohormone synthesis (review by *Palade*, 1966; *Fawcett* et al., 1969). Deductions from many different animal experiments and findings in human hyperplastic glands suggest a secretory cycle which involves every single cell (*Roth* and *Raisz*, 1966; *Thiele* et al., 1974). This functional cycle can be divided into several successive steps: the resting, synthesizing, transferral, packing, secretory and involuting phases (*Roth* and *Capen*, 1974). All these steps or phases are characterized by certain alterations of the cytoplasmic organelles concerned with parathormone production and excretion. In the human parathyroids only a few steps of this functional cycle are clearly distinguishable: these are the resting phase (inactive chief cell), and a period of packing the secretory granules and their exocytosis (active chief cell). In between there are at least two other steps consistent with parathormone synthesis and involution (gradual regression) of the protein-synthesizing apparatus. A separate storage phase, as sometimes postulated in animals (*Capen* and *Roth*, 1973), is unlikely in man due to the high turnover rate of parathormone (*Potts* et al., 1968). All the parameters of physiology and normal and pathological morphology, as well as clinical findings pertaining to the parathyroid glands, make the chief cell an excellent model in the study of the fine structure and functional relationships of a proteohormone-producing cell.

Moreover, pathological alterations in man offer the opportunity to examine the functional morphology under different conditions and aspects of endocrine activity, and to compare it with similar experimentally induced effects in animals. Comprehensive fine-structural morphology will only be achieved by combination of different methods that include extensive serial sectioning, special staining and tissue preparation, and freeze-fracture, besides conventional thin sections. Since freeze-fracture preparation avoids the artefacts of double fixation, dehydration, and embedding, the replicas obtained by this method probably reflect the structures of the cells more precisely than thin sections. In addition, freeze-fracture partially retrieves the three-dimensional image lost by sectioning and presents the best way to investigate the fine structure of cellular membranes, consequently offering an insight into aspects of endocrine activity not easily achieved by conventional methods.

II. Materials and Methods

This study is based on the examination of 29 parathyroid glands removed surgically from 20 patients for conditions listed in Table 1. In addition, 2 glands resected in a patient during an exploratory neck operation were normal. Gross findings at surgery, clinical data, light microscopy of the glands and (as the most important indicator of parathormone action) the histomorphology of iliac crest biopsies were investigated to evaluate endocrine function. Clinical and morphological findings in a case of parathyroid carcinoma and a primary water-clear hyperplasia associated with a hyperparathyroid crisis are recorded elsewhere (*Thiele* et al., 1973b; *Thiele* and *Pichlmayr*, 1974).

Table 1. Parathyroid gland pathology of surgical specimens investigated by electron microscopy (thin sections) and freeze-fracture (asteriks)

Diagnosis	Number	Patients (initials)	Sex	Age (years)
	1	Ch.S.	F	60
	2	M.K.	F	50
Chief cell adenomas	3	* E.R.	F	50
Primary hyper-parathyroidism	4	Ch.P.	F	70
	5	G.H.	F	52
	6	G.S.	F	62
	7	H.W.	F	35
	8	R.K.	M	46
Carcinoma		A.R.	F	76
Primary water-clear cell hyperplasia		H.T.	F	56
	1	G.K.	F	33
	2	R.K.	F	36
	3	* D.K.	M	21
	4	G.A.	M	37
Diffuse secondary hyperplasias	5	H.K.	M	29
Secondary hyper-parathyroidism	6	J.K.	M	32
	7	D.T.	M	32
	8	H.B.	F	43
	9	* A.K.	F	21
	10	H.H.	M	32

Immediately following surgical removal, samples of parathyroid glands were immersed and minced in fixation solution (2.5% glutaraldehyde and 2% formaldehyde in 0.1 M sodium cacodylate buffer at pH 7.3; *Cotran* and *Karnovsky*, 1968). For *thin sections* aldehyde fixation lasted about 90-120 min followed by osmium tetroxide for 60 min (*Millonig*, 1961), dehydration by ethanol and Epon embedding (*Luft*, 1961). Thin sections were stained with uranyl acetate (*Watson*, 1958) and lead citrate (*Reynolds*, 1963). For further details see *Thiele* et al. (1973a). The ribbons of serial sections were mounted on formvar-carbon membranes (*Dowell*, 1964). Both the silver proteinate method (*Thiery*, 1967, 1969) and the alkaline bismuth procedure (*Ainsworth* et al., 1972) were also applied, to achieve a specific (histochemical) and a nonspecific enhancement of staining of the glycogen particles. For *freeze-fracture* preparation small tissue blocks were transferred to 30% Ringer's solution after aldehyde fixation of about 60 min, placed on specimen holders, and quickly frozen in liquid monochlorodifluoromethane (Freon 22) at −150°C. Fracturing and shadowing with platinum-carbon were performed following the method of *Moor* and *Mühlethaler* (1963) in a Balzers BA 360 M apparatus (Balzers AG, Liechtenstein). The carbon-platinum replicas were cleaned with hypochlorite bleach and chromic acid, repeatedly rinsed in distilled water and collected on formvar-carbon membranes (*Dowell*, 1964).

Electron microscopes: Siemens Elmiskop I a and 101.

III. Interpretation of Thin Sections and Freeze-Fracture Replicas of Parathyroid Parenchyma and Stroma Cells

In the normal, hyperplastic, and adenomatous glands of the human parathyroids, thin section and freeze-fracture may reveal and clearly differentiate at least four types of cells by reasons of their size, organelles, contents of secretory granules, glycogen accumulation, and appearance of the plasma membranes. These cell types are consistent with functionally and morphologically different aspects of the chief cells, including oxyphil cells. In the following chapters a more detailed survey is given, dealing with the fine structure of these different cell types. The appearance of their cytoplasmic components is noted with a view towards their identification in freeze-fracture replicas. Thereafter alterations of each of the most important organelles and other cell constituents are described, together with the new results obtained by comparison of thin sections and freeze-fracture replicas. The last part of this report is devoted to the interpretation of freeze-fracture morphology of the interstitial space, with particular emphasis on the fine structure of the vessels and the possible functional role as deduced from their morphology.

Interpretation of the freeze-fracture replicas has to take into account that the cleavage plane may run across the cell, exposing intercellular structures and organelles in a similar way to thin sections. Frequently, however, the fracture runs within the bimolecular lipid layer of the plasma membrane, splitting it into two leaflets (*Branton*, 1966). These two new leaflets of each plasma membrane are termed "face A" and "face B" (*McNutt* and *Weinstein*, 1970). One leaflet of the cleaved membrane adheres to the cytoplasm and corresponds to "face A," the other leaflet borders the extracellular space and corresponds to "face B;" the two faces are complementary (*Chalcroft* and *Bullivant*, 1970; *McNutt* and *Weinstein*, 1973; *Staehelin*, 1974).

IV. Parenchyma

1. General Aspects of the Different Cell Types

a) Active Chief Cell

According to extensive thin section studies by many authors (review by *Roth* and *Capen*, 1974), active or stimulated chief cells of the normal, primary and secondary hyperplastic and adenomatous human parathyroid gland exhibit an identical fine structure. They measure about 15 μm in diameter and contain large ovoid nuclei (diameter about 8 μm) with a least one (Fig. 1a), but often two nucleoli. The cytoplasm is filled with organelles, secretory granules, dense bodies of various content and structure (possibly lysosomes), and glycogen accumulation. These are responsible for the clear and vacuolated appearance in light microscopy. Many of the cytoplasmic components are also identified in freeze-fracture replicas (Figs. 2a-c). The most conspicuous organelles are mitochondria, cisternae of the rough surfaced endoplasmic reticulum arranged in parallel stacks, and numerous secretory granules (Fig. 1a, 2b), besides small bundles of microfilaments (Figs. 4b, 17a, b). The Golgi apparatus is extensively developed and always associated with many vesicles, secretory granules and a few dense bodies, probably lysosomes. In some small areas accumulations of glycogen granules (β-particles) are sometimes recognized. The plasma membranes show infoldings with neighboring cells (Figs. 1b, 2c). Almost every chief cell has an area of close attachment to a capillary wall, separated by only a small extracellular space.

b) Inactive Chief Cell

The fine structure of the inactive (resting or suppressed) chief cell is best studied in atrophic glands removed on the same occasion as the parathyroid adenoma in patients presenting a highly active hyperparathyroidism (*Roth* and *Munger*, 1962; *Black*, 1969). In these glands freeze-fracture generally confirms the findings established by examination of thin sections (Fig. 3a). Thus, the average cell diameter is smaller than that in active chief cells and the plasma membranes are straight, with minimal interdigitations. The cytoplasm contains only a few small, dispersed cisternae of the rough-surfaced endoplasmic reticulum, and mitochondria in varying amounts. The Golgi apparatus is inconspicuous and it is very rare for

---

Fig. 1a and b. Thin section of active chief cells. (a) Section showing oval nucleus containing a large nucleolus with a sponge-like structure, adjacent to the marginal chromatin layer. Cytoplasm with many mitochondria, large Golgi apparatus (arrow), small glycogen accumulations *(G)* and several secretory granules *(S)*. (b) Extensive infoldings of the plasma membranes with a small desmosome (arrow). a x 13,000; b x 48,000

Fig. 2a-c. Freeze-fracture of active chief cells. (a) Replica showing spherical nucleus, displaying outer and inner membranes of nuclear envelope with crowded pores and some areas devoid of particles (arrow). Cytoplasm with a stack of cisternae of endoplasmic reticulum showing smooth area on the cleaved surface (arrow). Large area of glycogen *(G)*. (b) Spherical bodies corresponding to secretory granules. Cell processes of interdigitating plasma membranes (arrows). (c) Interdigitating plasma membranes of several transversally cleaved chief cells; glycogen *(G)*. a x 18,500; b x 16,500; c x 17,500

All micrographs of freeze-fracture replicas are mounted in such a way that shadowing is directed from below

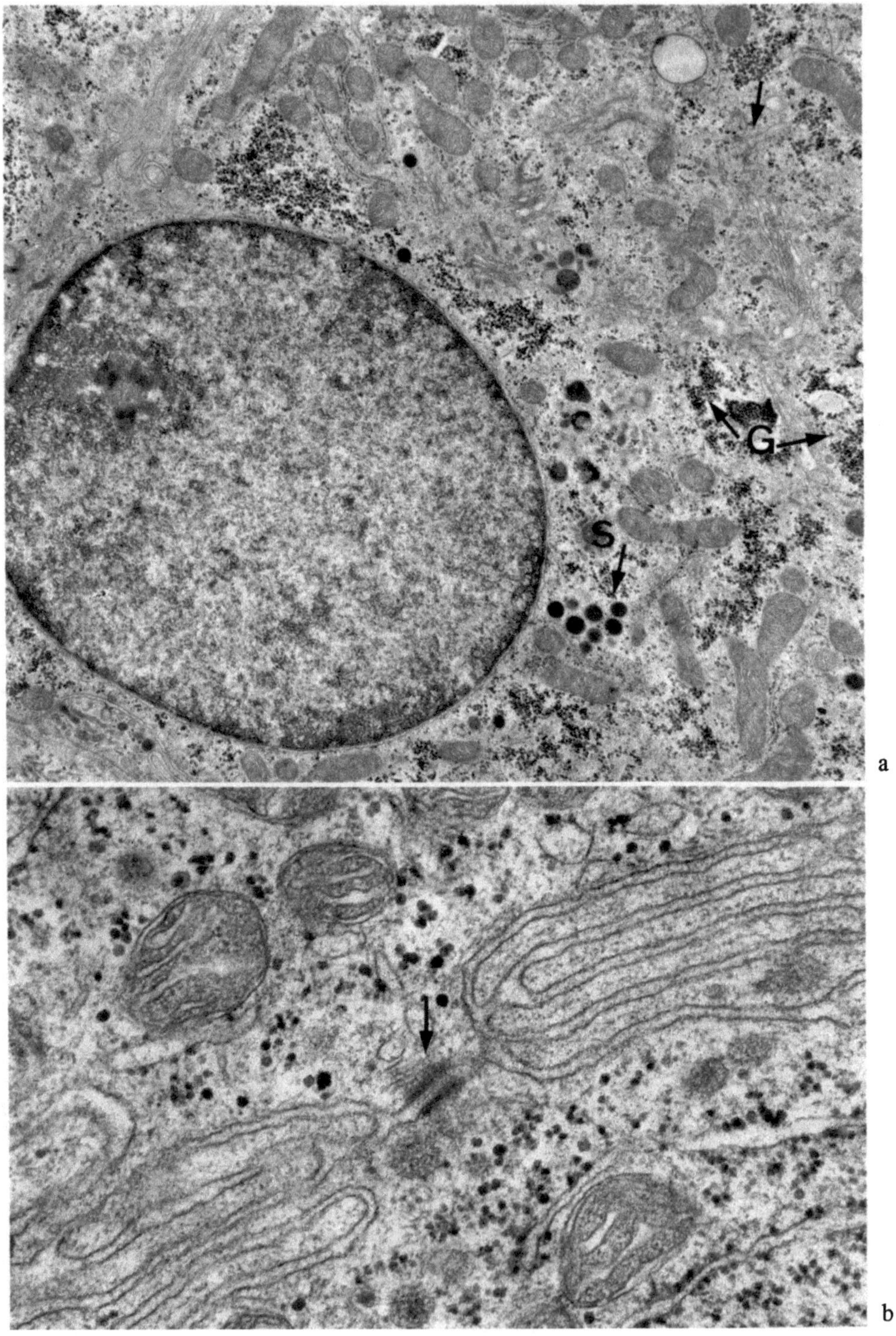

Fig. 1a-b. (Legend see p. 35)

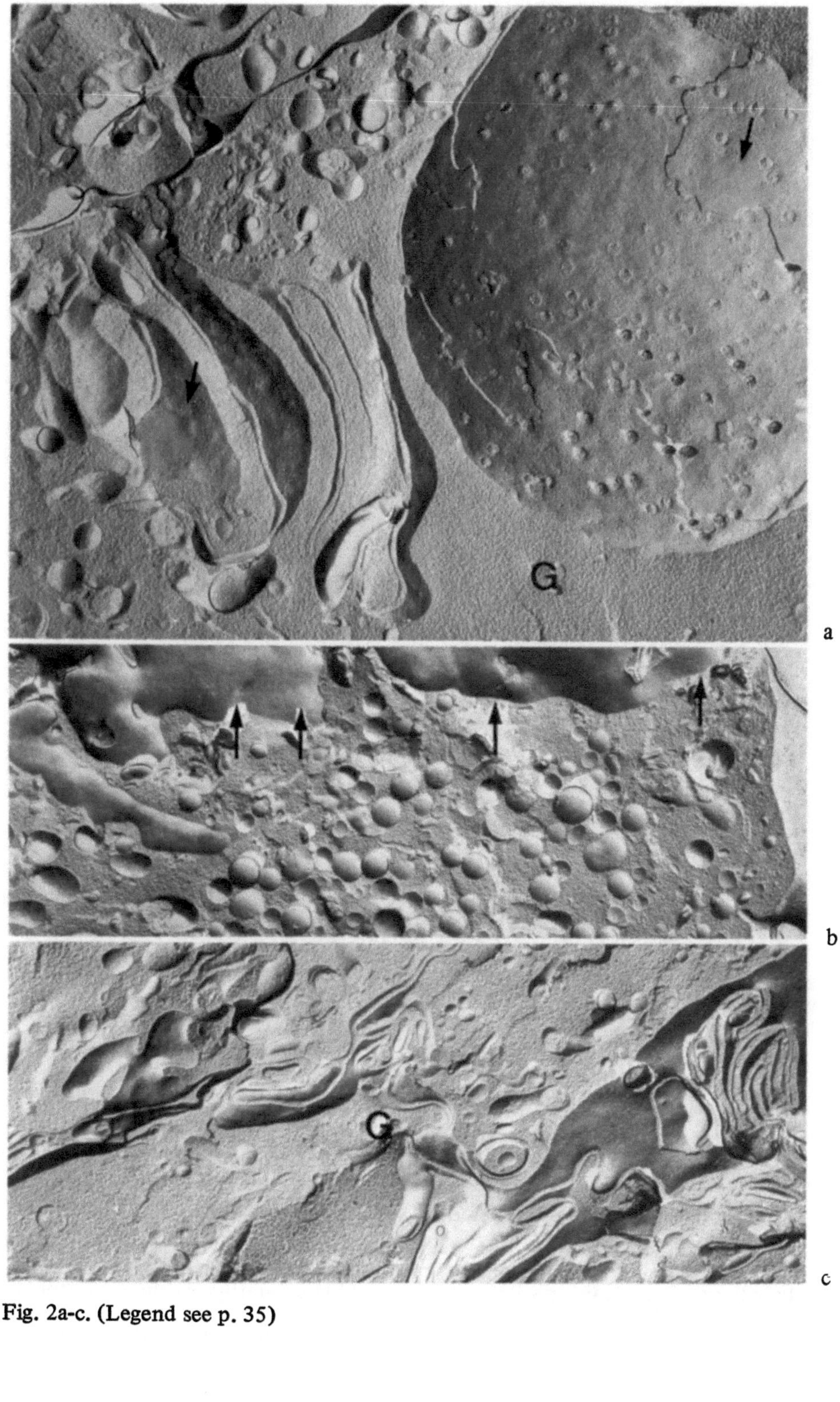

Fig. 2a-c. (Legend see p. 35)

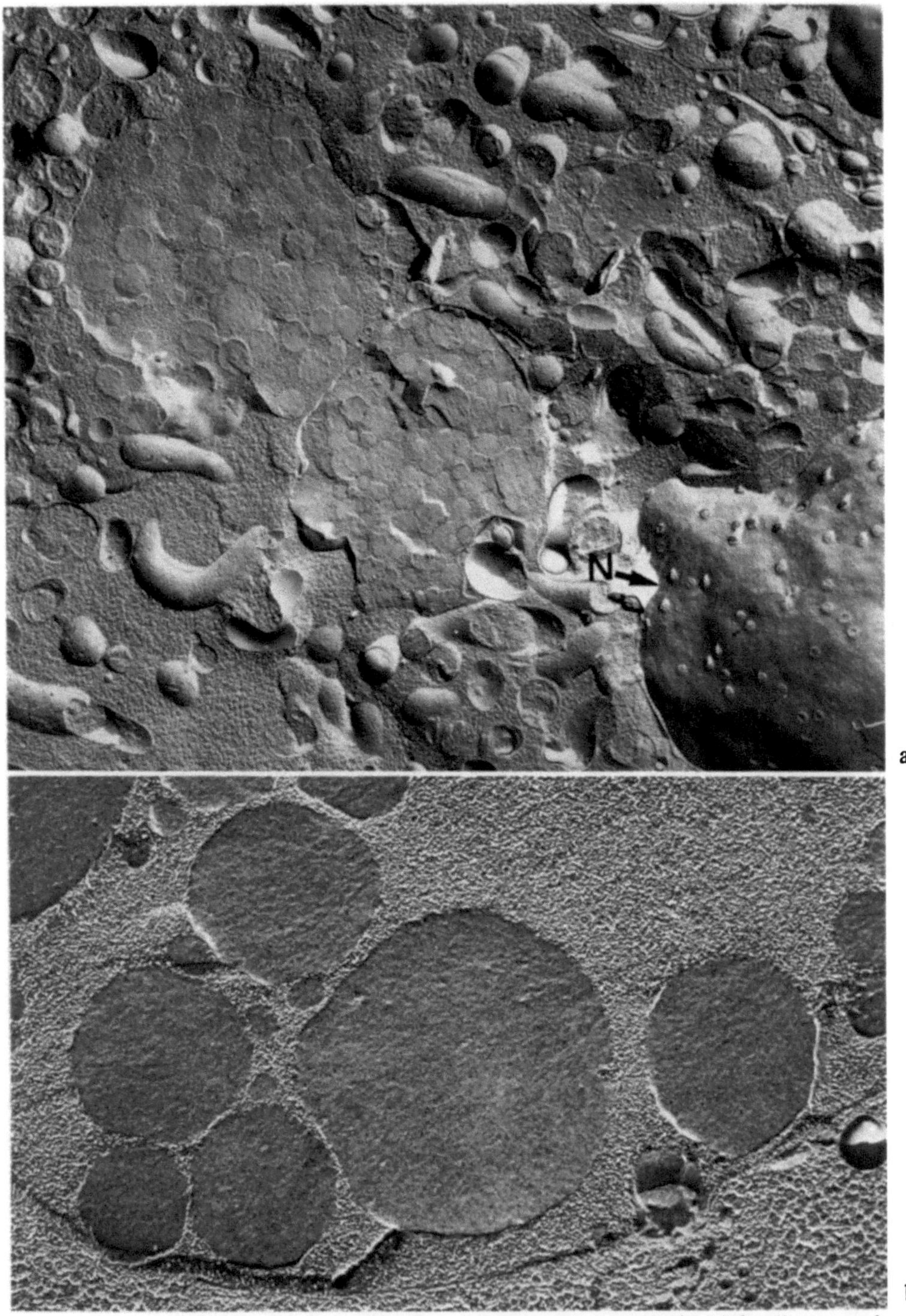

Fig. 3a and b. Freeze-fracture of an inactive (suppressed or resting) chief cell removed concomitantly with an adenoma in a patient with primary hyperparathyroidism. (a) Cytoplasm containing mitochondria and large complex bodies with lipid inclusions. Nucleus with several pores *(N)*. (b) High magnification of a lipid body, exhibiting a completely smooth cleavage plane. a x 16,000; b x 38,000

secretory granules to be seen. The most remarkable and characteristic features of inactive chief cells are large aggregates of complex lipid bodies (possibly residual bodies, see later section), and large areas of glycogen (Figs. 3b, 22b, c).

c) Small Water-Clear Cell

In chronically stimulated chief cells of secondary hyperplastic glands, and even in a very few adenomas, so-called small water-clear cells (*Eger* and *van Lessen*, 1954) have been identified in light microscopy. The very clear or highly vacuolated appearance is easily understood when it is taken into consideration that the large glycogen content in this cell type is dissolved by the conventional processing methods of paraffin wax histology. In thin sections and freeze-fracture replicas this cell type exhibits cytoplasm almost completely occupied by glycogen accumulations (Figs. 4a, 5a). Among the areas of glycogen there are always solitary lipid droplets to be seen (Fig. 5a). A few mitochondria and small cisternae of the rough-surfaced endoplasmic reticulum are located in the periphery of the cell; secretory granules are infrequent.

Most probably this distribution of cytoplasmic components denotes a cell whose endocrine function is more or less exhausted due to the long-lasting hyperstimulation of the glands in secondary hyperparathyroidism. These water-clear cells take no part in the normal secretory cycle of the other chief cells, although reversibility and transformation into cyclically excreting chief cells seems to be possible by mobilization of the glycogen and lipids, provided the abnormal parathyroid stimulation ceases.

Fig. 4a and b. Thin section of a small water-clear cell. (a) Extensive accumulation of β-glycogen granules in the cytoplasm. Between the crowded glycogen granules several membrane-bound translucent vacuoles, probably containing lipids and a very few secretory granules. (b) A grazing section of the nuclear surface with several pores at different levels of secretion, exhibiting electron-dense annuli of the pore complex, a few with a central granule (arrows). The nucleus is surrounded by many polysomes with formation of rosettes and a felt-like arrangement of microfilaments. a x 16,000; b x 40,000

Fig. 5a and b. Freeze-fracture of a small water-clear cell. (a) View showing extensive glycogen accumulation almost completely occupying the cytoplasm. The cleavage plane runs across some lipid droplets (arrow) or along their surface *(L)*. (b) Nuclear envelope *(N)* with several pores and perinuclearly arranged cisternae of the endoplasmic reticulum ("A- and B-faces") with a pore (arrow). a x 16,000; b x 40,000

Fig. 6a-c. Thin sections of oxyphil cells of a secondary hyperplastic parathyroid gland. (a) View showing cytoplasm filled by crowded mitochondria. In between, part of the Golgi complex (arrow) and small accumulations of glycogen. (b) Desmosome connecting an oxyphil cell (on the right) with a large mitochondrium and an active chief cell (on the left) with glycogen granules and cisternae of the rough-surfaced endoplasmic reticulum. (c) High magnification of large crowded mitochondria with numerous densely packed cristae, in between β-glycogen granules and a secretory granule. a x 12,500; b and c x 38,000

Fig. 7a-c. Freeze-fracture of oxyphil cells of the normal parathyroid gland. (a) View with nucleus *(N)* and cleaved membranes of the nuclear envelope, exposing several pores. Cytoplasm with crowded mitochondria and cleavage plane running across the mitochondria or within their membranes. (b) Numerous tiny particles are exposed on "A-" and "B-faces" of the inner mitochondrial membranes. Additionally there are small depressions on the "A-faces" and elevations on the "B-faces" of this membrane, probably corresponding to cross fractured pediculi cristae. One transversely cleaved mitochondrium exposes a crista arising from the inner membrane (arrow). (c) Cross-fractured mitochondrium ("A-face") with elongated cristae. Glycogen *(G)* with polygonal fracture plane of the β-particle. a x 16,000; b x 52,000; c x 42,000

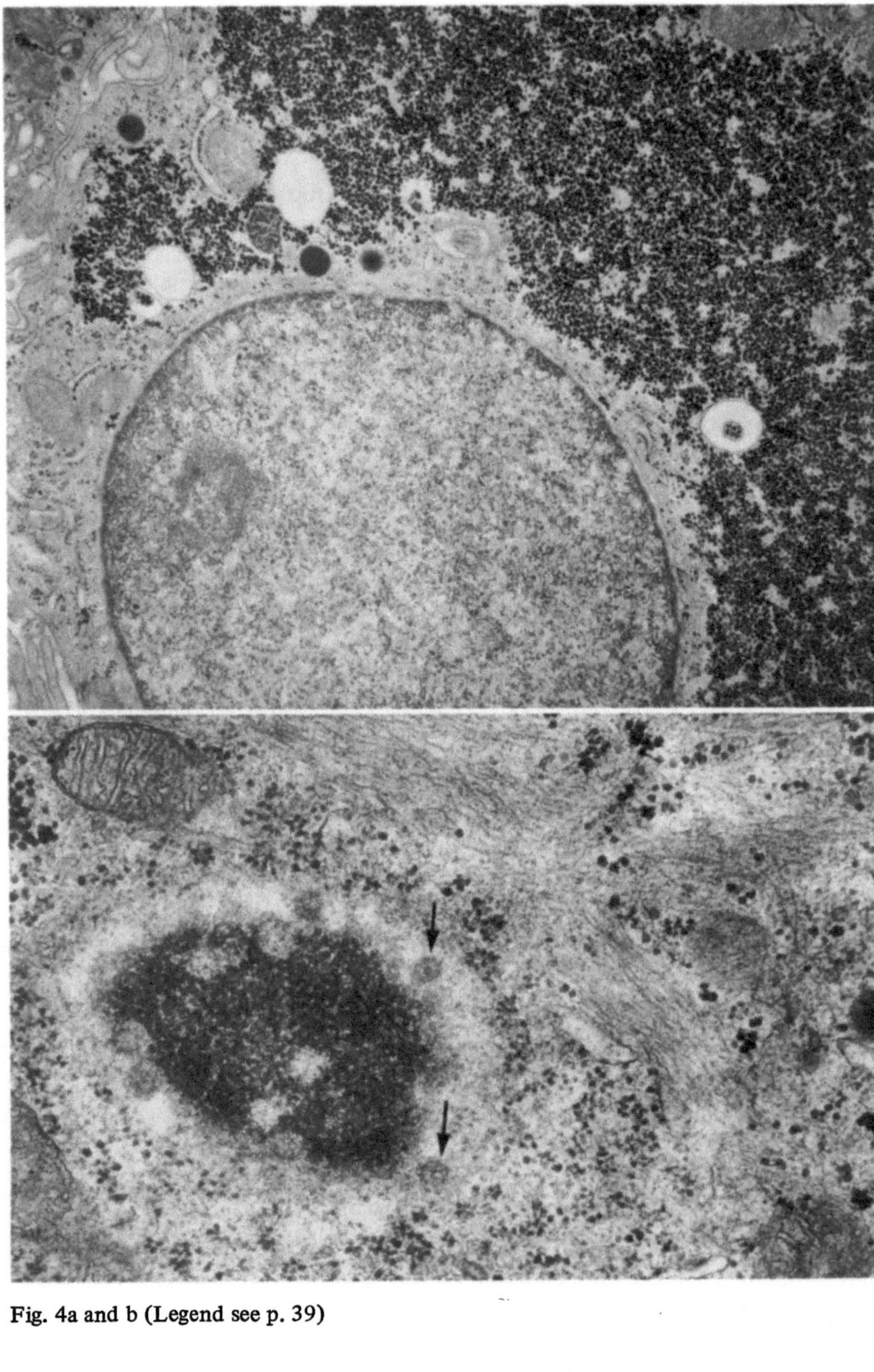

Fig. 4a and b (Legend see p. 39)

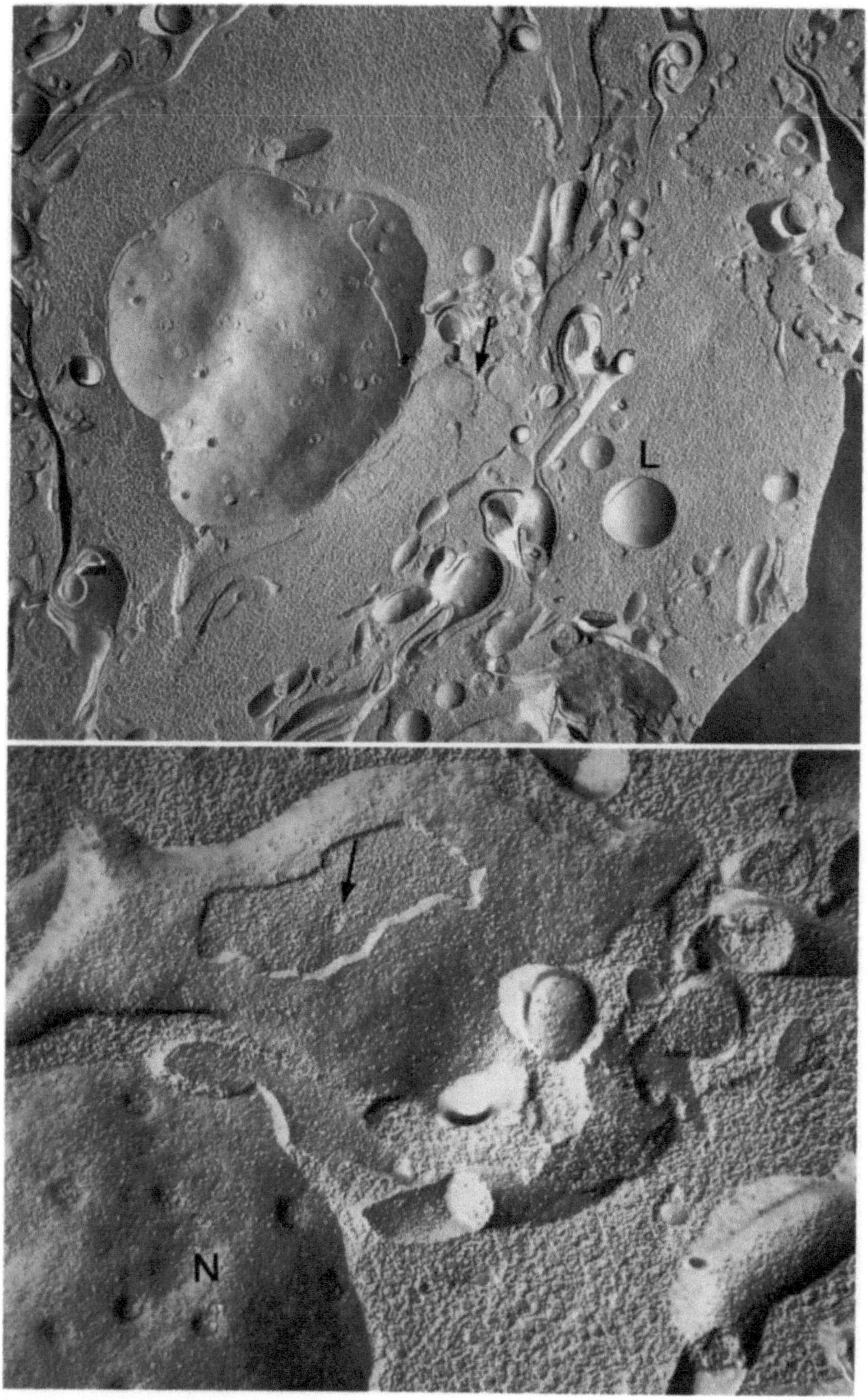

a

b

Fig. 5a and b (Legend see p. 39)

a

b

c

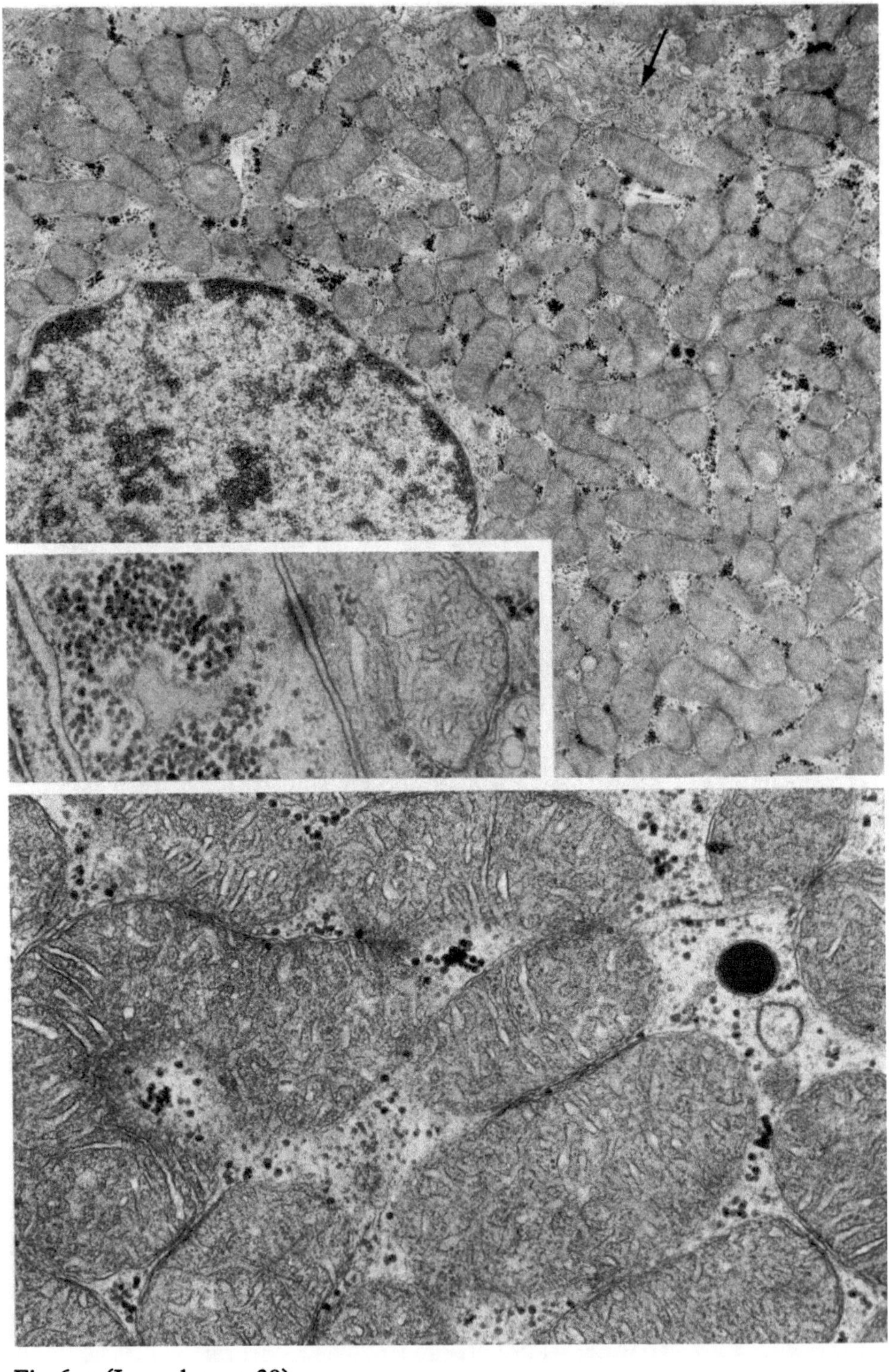

Fig. 6a-c (Legend see p. 39)

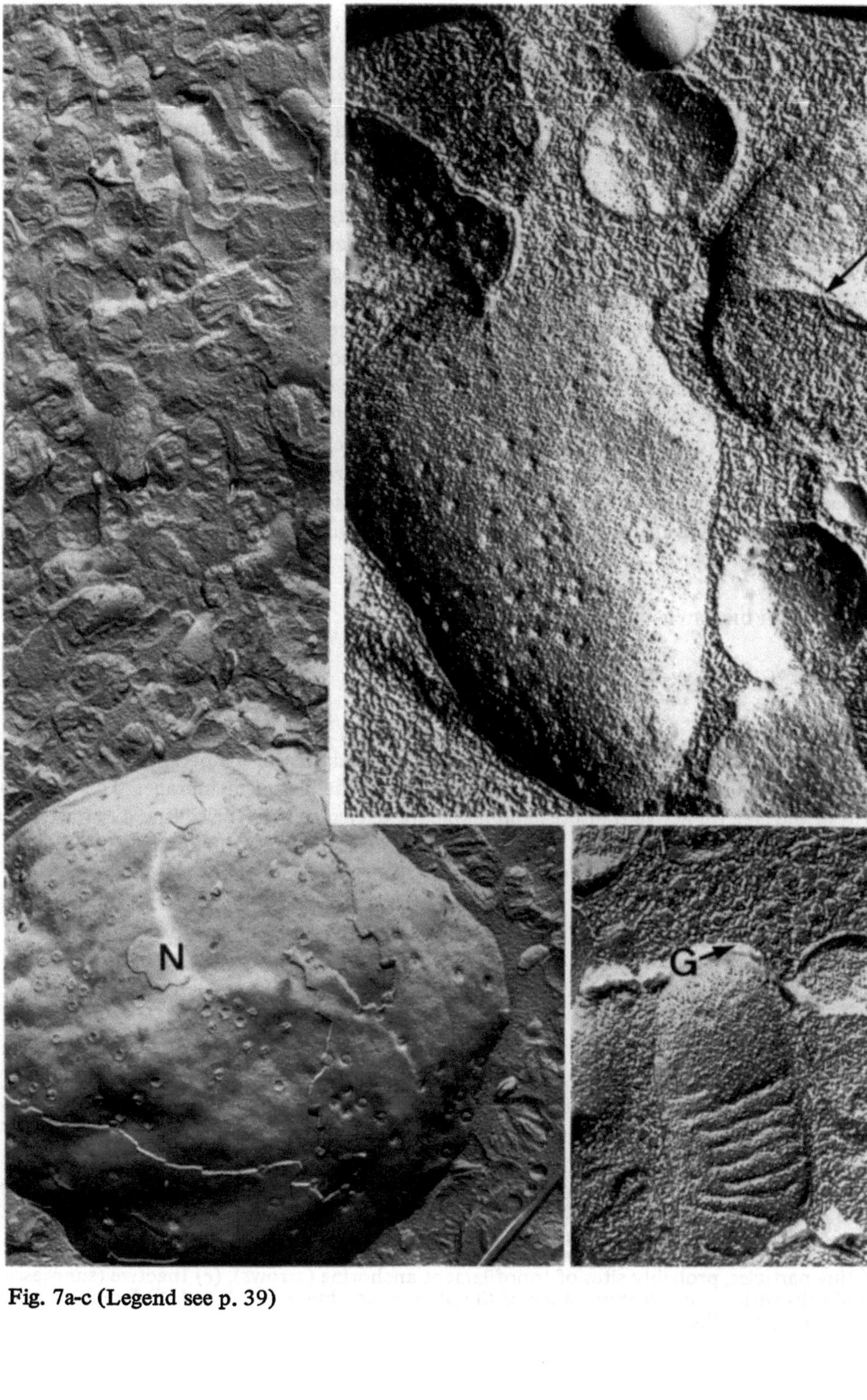

a b c

Fig. 7a-c (Legend see p. 39)

d) Oxyphil Cells

Oxyphil cells are characterized by a cytoplasm densely packed with numerous mitochondria (Fig. 6a). This abnormally high content of mitochondria is responsible for the acidophilic granulation in light microscopy, and similarly applies to the other so-called oncocytes of various organs (review by *Roth* and *Capen*, 1974). In the human parathyroids oxyphil cells of the normal glands differ from those of the adenomatous and hyperplastic parathyroids by not displaying the organelles connected with protein synthesis (compare Figs. 6a, c with Fig. 7a). On the other hand, in secondary hyperplastic glands, transitional forms between active chief cells and oxyphil cells can be frequently recognized. These transitional oxyphil cells have an increased amount of mitochondria but still retain a Golgi apparatus with associated secretory granules, rough-surfaced endoplasmic reticulum, glycogen, and polysomes. In consequence, active endocrine oxyphilic adenomas associated with primary hyperparathyroidism contain large areas of these transitional forms with numerous mitochondria besides preservation of the parathormone-producing organelles, and would therefore be more correctly interpretated as chief cell adenomas of mixed cell type (*Faccini*, 1970;*Heimann* et al., 1971). Freeze-fracture of a normal human parathyroid gland (Fig. 7a) confirms the well known fine structure of the oxyphil cell, but may also contribute towards a greater insight into the derangement of the mitochondrial structure (see later section).

2. Analysis of the Parenchyma Cell Constituents

a) Plasma Membrane

As shown in many experiments in vitro (*Roth* and *Raisz*, 1964, 1966) and in vivo (reviews by *Capen* and *Roth*, 1973;*Roth* and *Capen*, 1974) stimulation of the parathyroid cells leads to a gradual and reversible increase in the tortuosity of the plasma membranes. This enlargement of the area for active transport and metabolic exchange between cells and extracellular space is directly correlated to the ionized calcium concentration (*Roth* and *Raisz*, 1966), and results in an increased cellular uptake (*Raisz*, 1969), particularly of amino acids built into the polypeptide chain of the parathormone (*Hamilton* and *Cohn*, 1969). Consequently the degree of membrane infolding is generally thought to present one of the most reliable and important indicators for endocrine activity. In thin sections the increase in cellular surface is only documented by extensive invaginations of the plasma membranes (Fig. 1b), whereas freeze-fracture allows a direct en-face view of the split membranes.

The stimulated chief cell has a surface which may be compared in its three-dimensional apperance with a mountain range, with several depressions on the "B-face" corresponding to secretory granule extrusion (Fig. 8a). The nonactive chief cell, on the other hand, ex-

Fig. 8a-c. Freeze-fracture replicas with en-face views of the plasma membranes. (a) Active chief cell with highly undulating plasma membranes ("B-face") displaying, several depressions suggestive of secretory granules extrusion (arrows) and an area with groupings of small particles corresponding to a desmosome *(D)*. (b) Two desmosomes with assemblies of tiny particles, probably sites of tonofilament anchoring (arrows). (c) Inactive (suppressed) chief cells with a smooth appearance of the plasma membrane ("A-" and "B-faces"). a and c x 21,500; b x 40,000

a

b

c

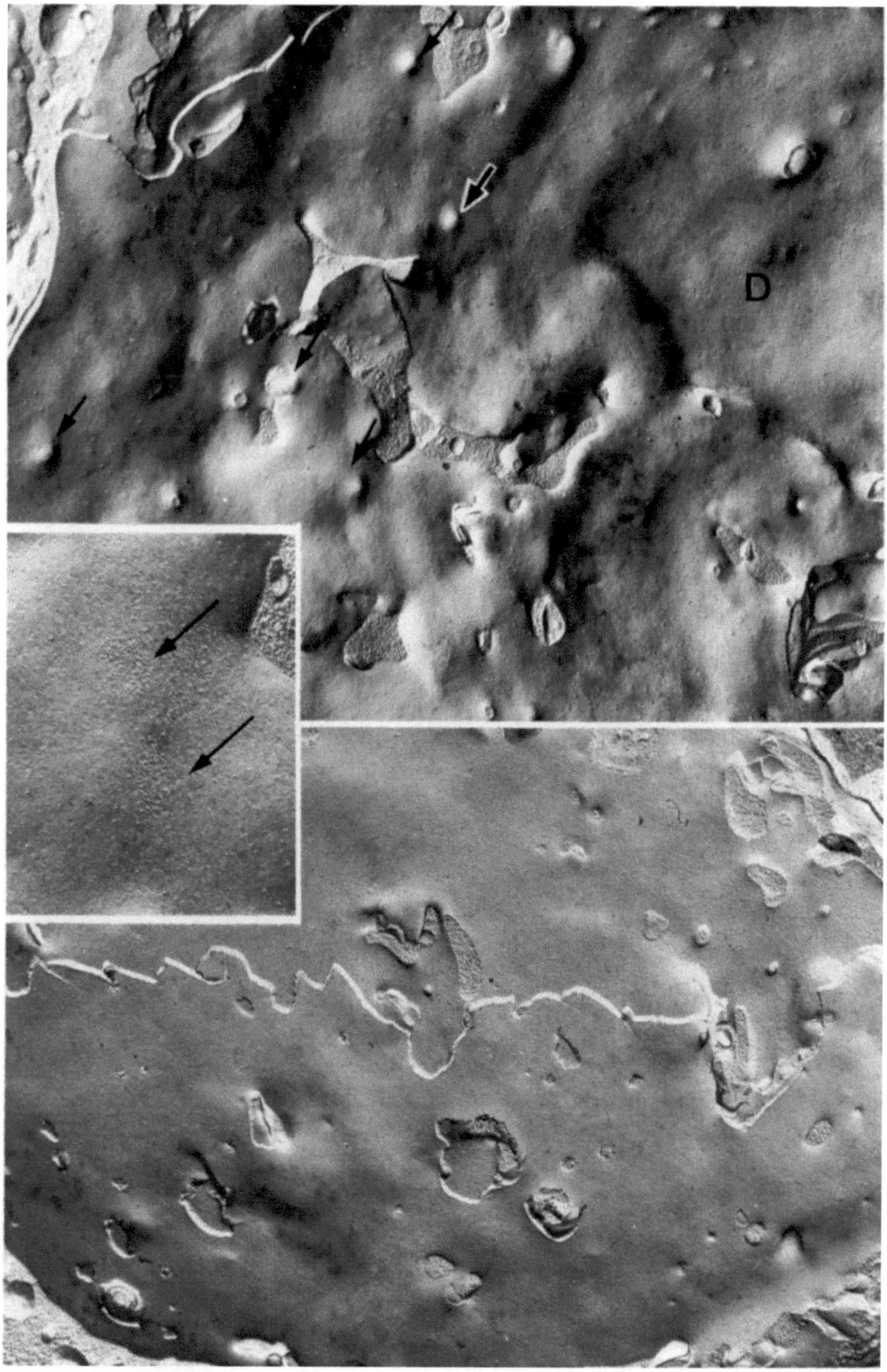

Fig. 8a-c (Legend see p. 44)

hibits an almost smooth surface (Fig. 8c). In transverse fracture planes the infoldings are cleaved into ridges and appear similar to thin sections (compare Fig. 1b with Fig. 2c). Moreover, freeze-fracture confirms that numerous small desmosomes are the only junctions between parathyroid cells. They appear as assemblies of very small particles, possibly the anchoring sites of the tonofilaments (Fig. 8b). As well as often being encountered in thin sections (Figs. 1b, 15a), they also connect chief cells and oxyphil cells, probably indicating a common origin of these two cell types (Fig. 6b). The absence of other kinds of junctions (e.g. gap junctions) with their special function between adjacent cells of the parathyroid gland supports the assumption of an independent secretory cycle in each cell (*Thiele* et al., 1974).

These findings of an apparently deficient structural coupling between parathyroid chief cells contrast sharply with the specialized junctions, gap junctions as well as tight junctions, observed by *Orci* et al. (1972a, 1975) in pancreatic islet cells. In some chief cells, pairs of cilia with central filaments and well developed rootlets at their base were observed (Fig. 9a, b). Increased numbers of cilia and derangement of the central filaments have been noticed by several authors (review by *Polyzonis*, 1970) especially in cells of parathyroid adenomas.

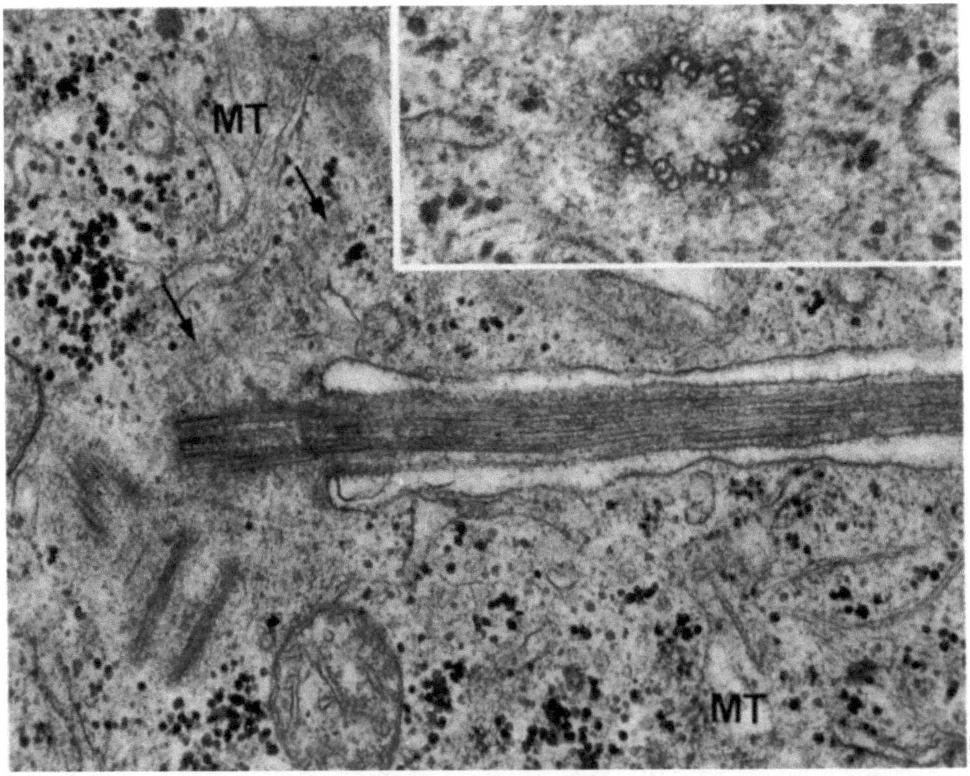

a

b

Fig. 9a and b. Cilia of chief cells. (a) A long cilium showing axoneme, basal bodies and a cross striated rootlet (arrows). Cytoplasm with several microtubules *(MT)*. (b) A cross-sectioned basal body at high magnification. a x 42,000; b x 84,000

b) Nucleus

Freeze-fracture replicas demonstrate the ovoid, sometimes slightly indented structure of the nuclei of parathyroid cells and reveal many pores of the nuclear envelope (Figs. 2a, 5b, 7a). On gross assessment the number of nuclear pores can probably be related to endocrine activity (*Thiele* and *Wermbter*, 1974): in highly stimulated chief cells there are up to 18 pores per μm^2, whereas in water-clear cells and in inactive chief cells there are about 10-12 pores per μm^2 (compare Fig. 2a with Fig. 5a), but the number of pores and their mean distance apart vary considerably from cell to cell. Comparison of this somewhat rough estimate with the figures calculated by *Maul* et al. (1971) by subtle mathematical methods for the cells of the rat kidney and stimulated lymphocytes, shows that the frequency of nuclear pores is quite high. In the human parathyroid gland this suggests a close nuclear-cytoplasmic exchange, particularly in the active chief cells in the course of parathormone synthesis. The split outer and inner membranes of the nuclear envelope show a different distribution of small particles intermingled with irregular smooth areas (Fig. 2a), as described by *Breathnach* et al. (1972) in the nuclei of mouse liver cells. This is similar to the concentrations of particles observed in the cleaved membranes of the rough-surfaced endoplasmic reticulum and mitochondria (see later section). The nucleoli have a spongy structure, which is especially well demonstrated in serial sections, in keeping with the findings of *Thoenes* et al. (1972) in other cells. The nucleoli are remarkable for their large size (about 2-3 μm in diameter) and their almost constant location at the periphery of the nucleus, with an extensive area of close contact to the nuclear envelope (Fig. 1a, 4a).

This appearance, which occurs in highly stimulated parathyroid cells of adenomas, carcinomas, and secondary hyperplasias (*Thiele* et al., 1973a and b; *Thiele* and *Wermbter*, 1974), suggests an increased function of this organelle. This is not surprising when the alterations found due to experimental changes of hormone synthesis in the exocrine pancreas of animals are taken into consideration (*Altmann*, 1952; *Bannasch* and *Thoenes*, 1965). Around the nucleus a dense arrangement of microfilaments is often noticed (Fig. 4b). These extend to the plasma membrane and surround cytoplasmic organelles as well as secretory granules (Figs. 17a, b).

c) Endoplasmic Reticulum

The amount of the rough-surfaced endoplasmic reticulum in the parathyroid cells is a good indicator of endocrine activity, since polypeptide hormone synthesis is dependent on this organelle, as shown in various endocrine glands (*Fawcett* et al., 1969). The active chief cell contains large, cup-shaped arrangements of cisternae with membranes studded with polysomes (Fig. 10a). In freeze-fracture replicas with an extensive exposition of internal aspects of cisternal membranes, a few round to oval depressions about 60-70 nm in diameter on the "A-face" and corresponding slight elevations on the "B-face" can sometimes be observed (Figs. 5b, 10b).

These structures are consistent with the cisternal pores described by *Orci* et al. (1972b) in the exocrine pancreas. The "B-face" shows only a few scattered small particles, whereas the "A-face" exhibits a finely particulated appearance (Figs. 5b, 10b). Sometimes smooth circular areas are to be seen on the "B-face," which are completely devoid of these particles (Figs. 2a, 10c) and demonstrate a mosaic pattern revealed only in more extensively exposed

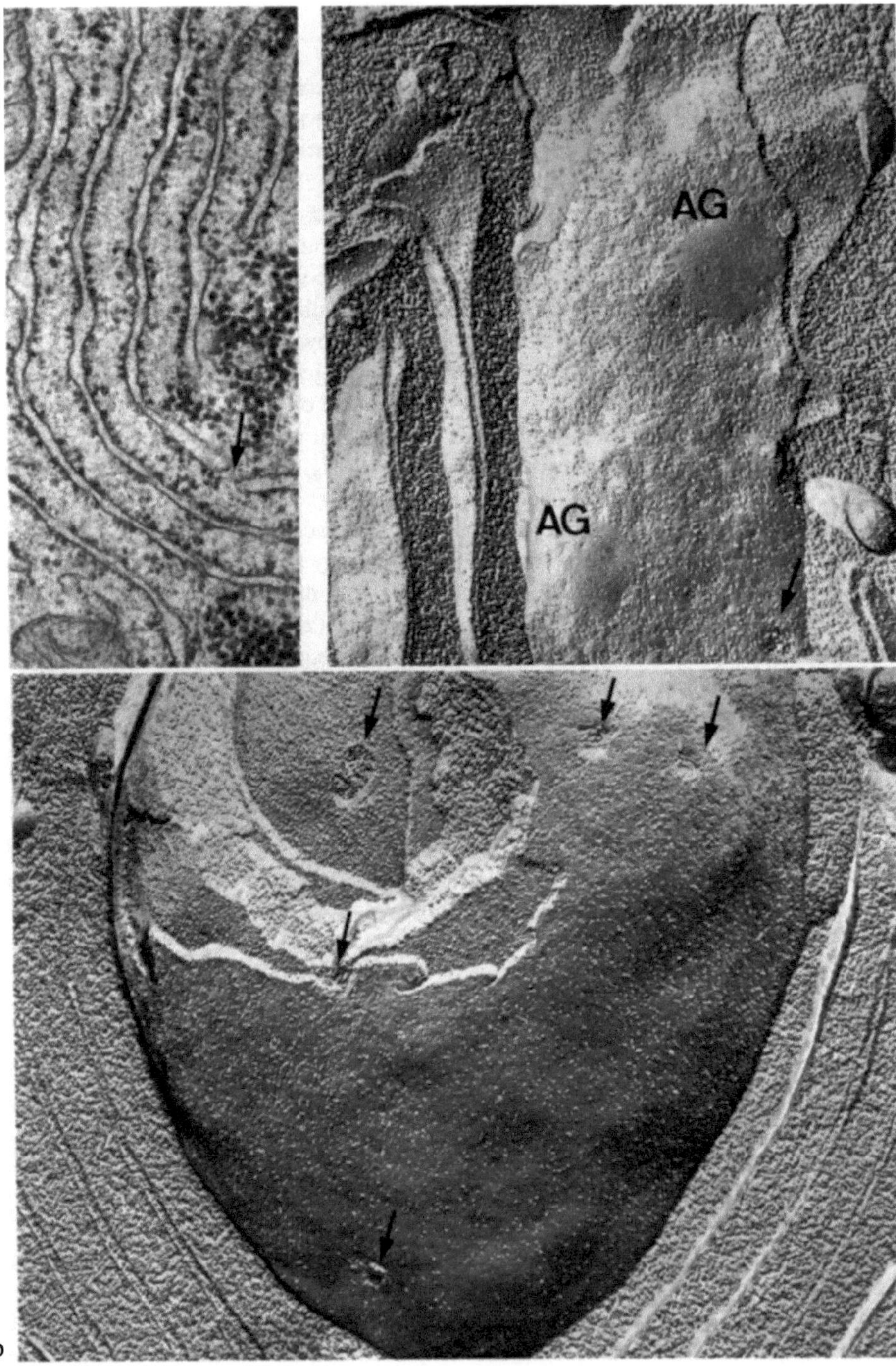

a c b

Fig. 10a-c (Legend see p. 49)

areas (Fig. 10c). A similar distribution of particles in cleaved plasma membranes was seen by *Breathnach* et al. (1972) in mouse liver cells. This arrangement possibly displays areas of different internal membrane structure, but the significance is not known.

In highly active chief cells a remarkably regular arrangement of elongated mitochondria and cisternae of the rough-surfaced endoplasmic reticulum is found (Fig. 22a). There is also a close relationship to large areas of β-glycogen particles and solitary lipid droplets, which probably have a functional as well as a morphological significance (*Nunez* et al., 1972). Several authors report annulate lamellae in parathyroid cells (*Elliott* and *Arhelger*, 1966; *Marshall* et al., 1967; *Boquist*, 1970; *Altenähr*, 1972), which were only found in a few cells of one adenoma in our series. The possibility of their being due to accelerated cell proliferation in tumors is under discussion, as they are hardly ever demonstrated in normal chief cells of the human parathyroid gland.

d) Golgi Apparatus

The fine structure of the Golgi apparatus is best studied in the active (stimulated) chief cell of secondary hyperplastic parathyroid glands at the peak of their secretory cycle. As already discussed in several detailed reviews (*Beams* and *Kessel*, 1968; *Favard*, 1969; *Morré* et al., 1971; *Cook*, 1973; *Northcote*, 1973; *Fineran*, 1973) mostly dealing with plant or animal cells, this organelle is composed of stacks of disc-shaped, slightly curved saccules which display an obvious polarity (*Mollenhauer* and *Whaley*, 1963). Transition elements (*Zeigel* and *Dalton*, 1962) have been observed between the cisternae of the rough-surfaced endoplasmic reticulum and the outer saccules, the convex or forming surface of the Golgi complex (*Mollenhauer* and *Whaley*, 1963). The interior of the Golgi apparatus, the concave or maturing surface (*Mollenhauer* and *Whaley*, 1963), shows vesicles and granules of different size and electron density.

In the human parathyroid gland the stacks consist of 5-6 flattened saccules (Figs. 11a, b, 12) exhibiting small nonperforated portions, probably the so-called cisternal part (Fig. 11b), and in the periphery an increased amount of pores, as demonstrated in freeze-fracture replicas (Figs. 11b, 12). Besides the pores there are several small pits or protrusions (Fig. 11a, b), probably corresponding to the shuttle transport vesicles from the rough-surfaced endoplasmic reticulum (transition elements); this is consistent with findings of *Akert* et al., (1971) in the Golgi apparatus of animals. The pores in the outer saccules become gradually larger, with less regular circumferences as they reach the edges, until saccules are transformed almost into an anastomosing tubular system (Fig. 12). The tubular polygonal structures at the edges of the dictyosomes actually form a continuous convoluted network, as observed by *Rambourg* et al. (1973 and 1974) in nerve cells of the rat following osmium impregnation of thick sections; these workers made use of high-voltage electron microscopy, thus demonstrating the "appareil rêticulaire interne" described by *Golgi* (1898a and b). From the outer aspect to the interior of the stack the number and, especially, the diameter of

---

Fig. 10a-c. Rough-surfaced endoplasmic reticulum of a chief cell. (a) Thin section showing one cisterna with an interruption (arrow). (b) Freeze-fracture replica of a corresponding cup-like arrangement of cisternae, exposting "A-" and "B-faces" of cleaved membranes and several pores (arrows). (c) "B-face" of split cisternal membrane, displaying an irregular, almost mosaic-like pattern of intramembranous particle distribution with smooth polyhedral areas *(AG)*. Cisternal pore (arrow). a x 38,000; b x 44,000; c x 40,000

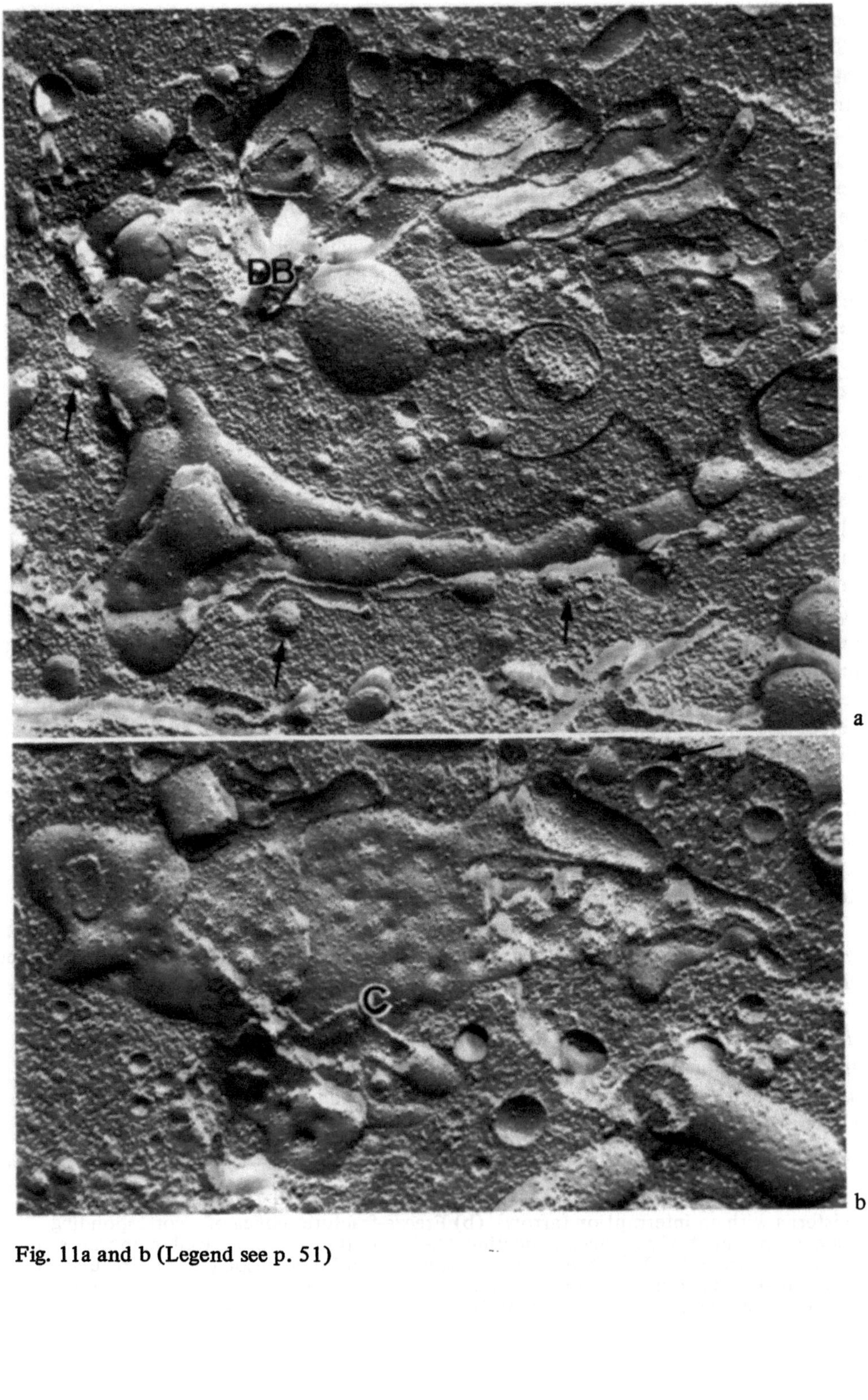

Fig. 11a and b (Legend see p. 51)

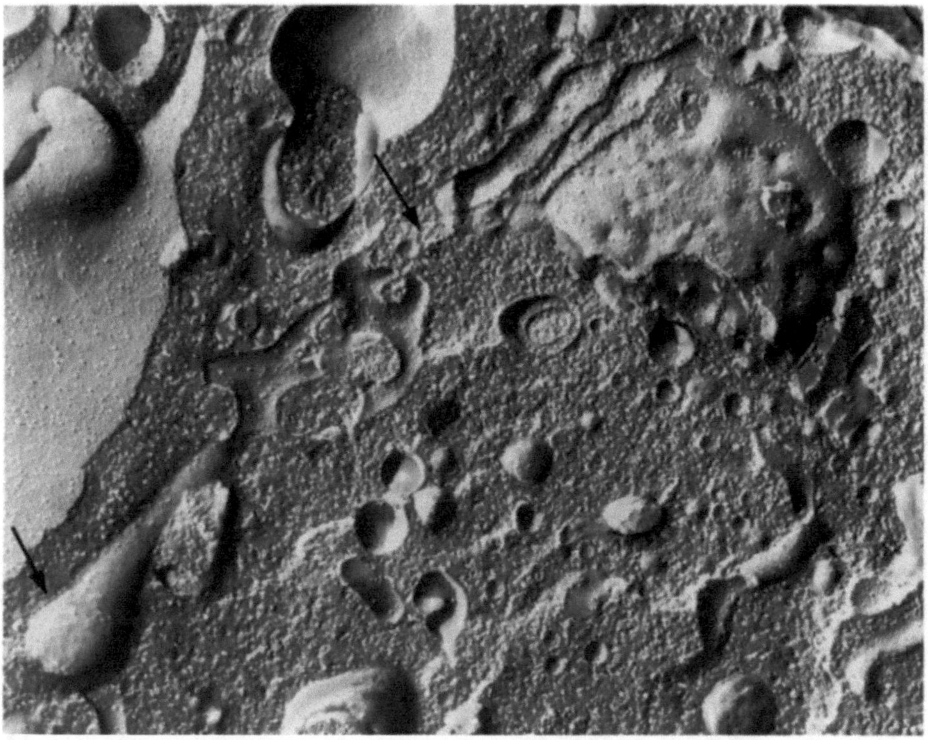

Fig. 12. Freeze-fracture of the Golgi apparatus in an activated chief cell. Inner saccules of the Golgi stack with several very small pores. Outer sacculus with pores of irregular size and large diameter forming an anastomosing tubular system (arrows). x 45,000

the pores decrease with every saccule (from about 60-70 nm for the first saccule to about 20 nm for the innermost saccule). In conclusion, freeze-fracture of the human Golgi complex generally confirms the dictoyosomal structures as containing perforated saccules, a result obtained in numerous animals cells (*Reale* and *Luciano*, 1964; *Flickinger*, 1969; *Rambourg* and *Chretien*, 1970), especially following isolation of the stacks with further morphological and functional analysis of the saccule membranes (*Fleischer* et al., 1969; *Ehrenreich* et al., 1973; *Hodson* and *Brenchley*, 1976) and in plant cells (*Cunningham* et al., 1966; *Fineran*, 1973).

A general function of the Golgi apparatus is the formation and packing of material for export from the cells across the plasma membrane by a process of reverse pinocytosis (exo-

---

Fig. 11a and b. Freeze-fracture of the Golgi apparatus in an activated chief cell. (a) Transverse and longitudinal cleavage planes with saccules of a different width and a few pores. In the interior large spherical body *(DB)*, probably corresponding to condensing vacuole (progranula?). Arrows point towards small vesicles close to the outer saccules and compatible with transition elements. (b) En-face view of several saccules displaying "A-" and "B-faces" of the split membranes showing many pores. A central portion of the stack is exposed as devoid of pores *(C)*. A few small spherical bodies consistent with transition elements at the periphery of the stack (arrow). a x 52,000; b x 45,000

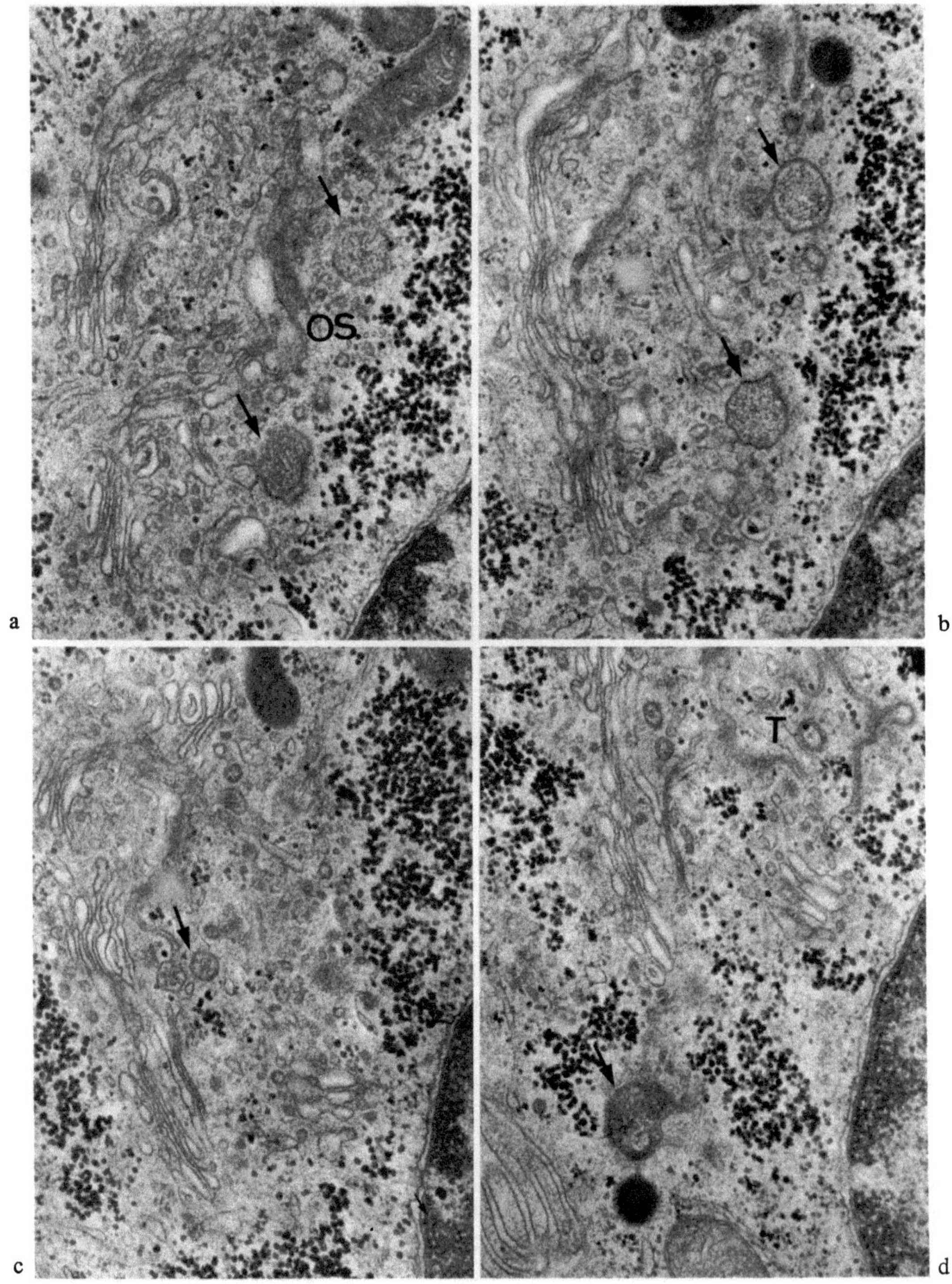

Fig. 13a-d (Legend see p. 53)

a 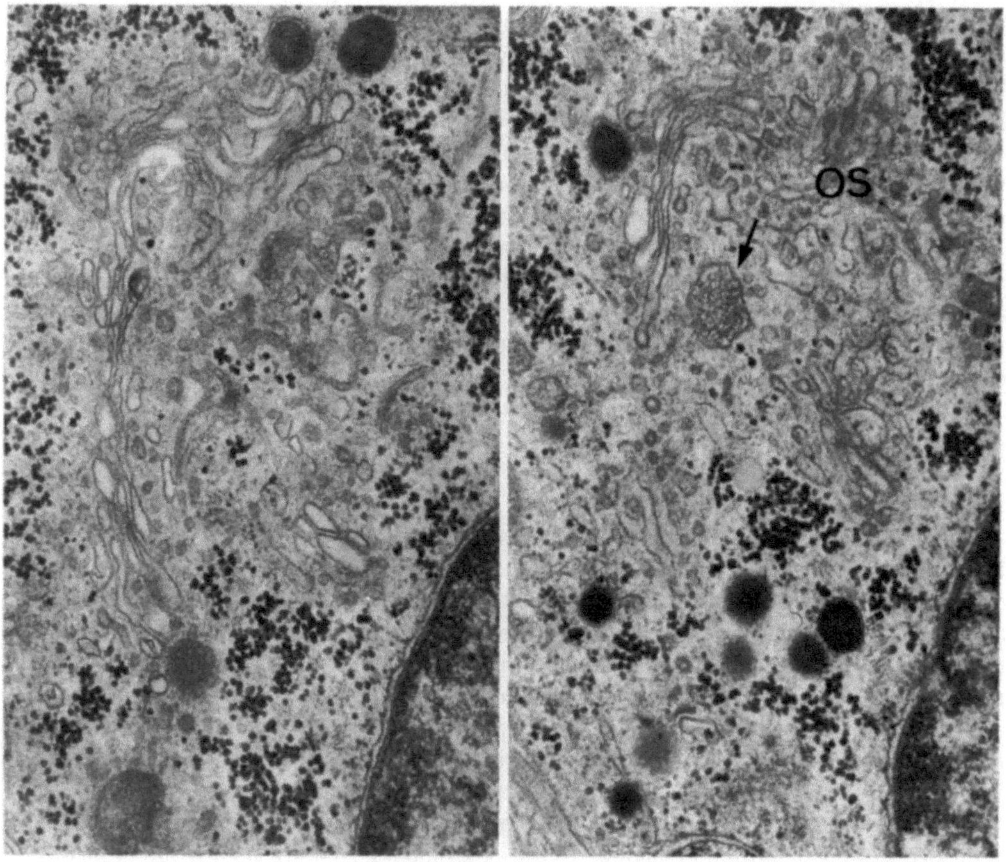 b

Fig. 14a and b. Serial sections of a Golgi apparatus in an activated chief cell, continuation of Fig. 13a-d. (Parallel sections with section levels about 50-100 nm apart). (a) Dense reticulum in the interior of the Golgi apparatus in grazing section corresponding to the GERL, in close connection to small dense bodies and coated vesicles. (b) Large condensing vacuole in the interior of the Golgi stack (arrow). Outer saccules *(OS)* with large pores especially at the periphery of this section. a and b x 30,000

cytosis or emiocytosis). The studies of *Palade* and co-workers (*Caro* and *Palade*, 1964; *Jamieson* and *Palade*, 1967a, b), dealing with the synthesis of digestive enzymes in the guinea-pig exocrine pancreas, clearly demonstrate that precursors of the proteohormone are manufactured in the polysomes of the rough-surfaced endoplasmic reticulum. These

---

Fig. 13a-d. Serial sections of a Golgi apparatus in an activated chief cell. (Parallel sections with section levels about 50-100 nm apart). (a) Golgi stack with slightly undulating saccules exposing outer saccules with pores in grazing sections *(OS)*. Two condensing vacuoles (prosecretory granules?) with a flocculent content (arrows). (b) Fully exposed condensing vacuoles (arrows) partially connected with a dense body (upper vacuole). (c) Interior of the Golgi apparatus with a dense tubular structure in connection with a small dense body (early condensing vacuole, prosecretory granule?) indicated by an arrow. (d) A region of the Golgi apparatus with a dense tubular reticulum in the interior *(T)* and a large dense body with connection to a secretory granule (arrow). a-d x 30,000

precursor proteins enter the lumen of the cisternae and move towards the Golgi apparatus. Transportation to the Golgi stack is mediated by transition elements (*Zeigel* and *Dalton*, 1962) or portions of the smooth-surfaced endoplasmic reticulum (reviews by *Smith* and *Farquhar*, 1966; *Fawcett* et al., 1969). This process is apparently facilitated by microtubules which, according to experimental findings in bovine parathyroid glands, seem to transport pro-parathyroid hormone to the Golgi complex (*Kemper* et al., 1975). Here pro-parathyroid hormone fractions appear to be transported through the saccules of the stacks by vesicles. Later on they are recognizable as "condensing vacuoles" at the inner (concave) surface, where "condensation" or packing occurs and sometimes interaction between the protein and other components such as polysaccharides. At this stage pro-parathyroid hormone is thought to be converted into parathyroid hormone, also by the interaction of microtubules (review by *Malaisse*, 1976). An almost identical course of polypeptide synthesis has been shown in the rat parathyroid gland by *Nakagami* et al. (1971), using autoradiographic methods. These authors established that a tracer (^{3}H-tyrosine) and labelled galactose were built into the secretory product, the last probably as part of the glycoprotein component of the secretory granule membrane.

Morphological analysis of parathormone synthesis is limited to the tracing of secretory granule formation in the interior of the Golgi stacks. Examination of thin sections and freeze-fracture replicas reveals that the so-called maturing surface (*Mollenhauer* and *Whaley*, 1963) is filled with vesicles and tubules, varying in size and electron density but without obvious structural relation to each other. Serial sectioning (Figs. 13a-d, 14a, b) shows a continuous convoluted and dense tubular network in different planes (Figs. 13c, d, 14a). These tubular structures are best recognized in completely tangential sections (Figs. 14a, 15a), where they are often connected to large dense bodies generally referred to as "condensing vacuoles" or "pro-secretory granules" in the pertinent literature (Figs. 13c, 15b).

The tubular network, and particularly the dense bodies, are probably the sites of protein packing or condensation in analogy to the experimental findings already mentioned. Further support of this assumption is given by the fact that in some planes secretory granules are observed budding off from the "condensing vacuoles" (Figs. 13d, 15b). This tortuous tubular system is either very closely related or possibly, identical to the so-called GERL of *Holtzman* et al. (1967) and *Novikoff* et al. (1971). We were, however, unable to show a definite interconnection of this system with the endoplasmic reticulum. Consequently this dense reticulum or GERL has to be regarded as a part of the Golgi complex for both functional and morphological reasons, as already suggested by *Whaley* et al. (1971). Instead of the term GERL (*G*olgi associated *ER* from which *L*ysosomes are thought to arise), an abbreviation such as CRG (*C*ondensing *R*eticulum of the *G*olgi complex) would probably be more appropriate, as this would not imply lysosome formation alone. This avoids a functional limitation which further investigations may have to be correct.

In the activated hormone-releasing human parathyroid chief cell microtubules are noticed only infrequently (Figs. 9a, 15a), in contrast to microfilaments (Figs. 17a, b). This is remarkable in the context of experimentally found conversion and transportion of parathormone precursor compounds mediated by microtubules (see above).

e) Secretory Granules and Exocytosis

In chief cells of normal, hyperplastic, and adenomatous parathyroid glands there are round, sometimes slightly elongated dense bodies (diameter ranging from 150-500 nm), which have been called secretory granules (Figs. 16, 17a). This was generally accepted by reason of their

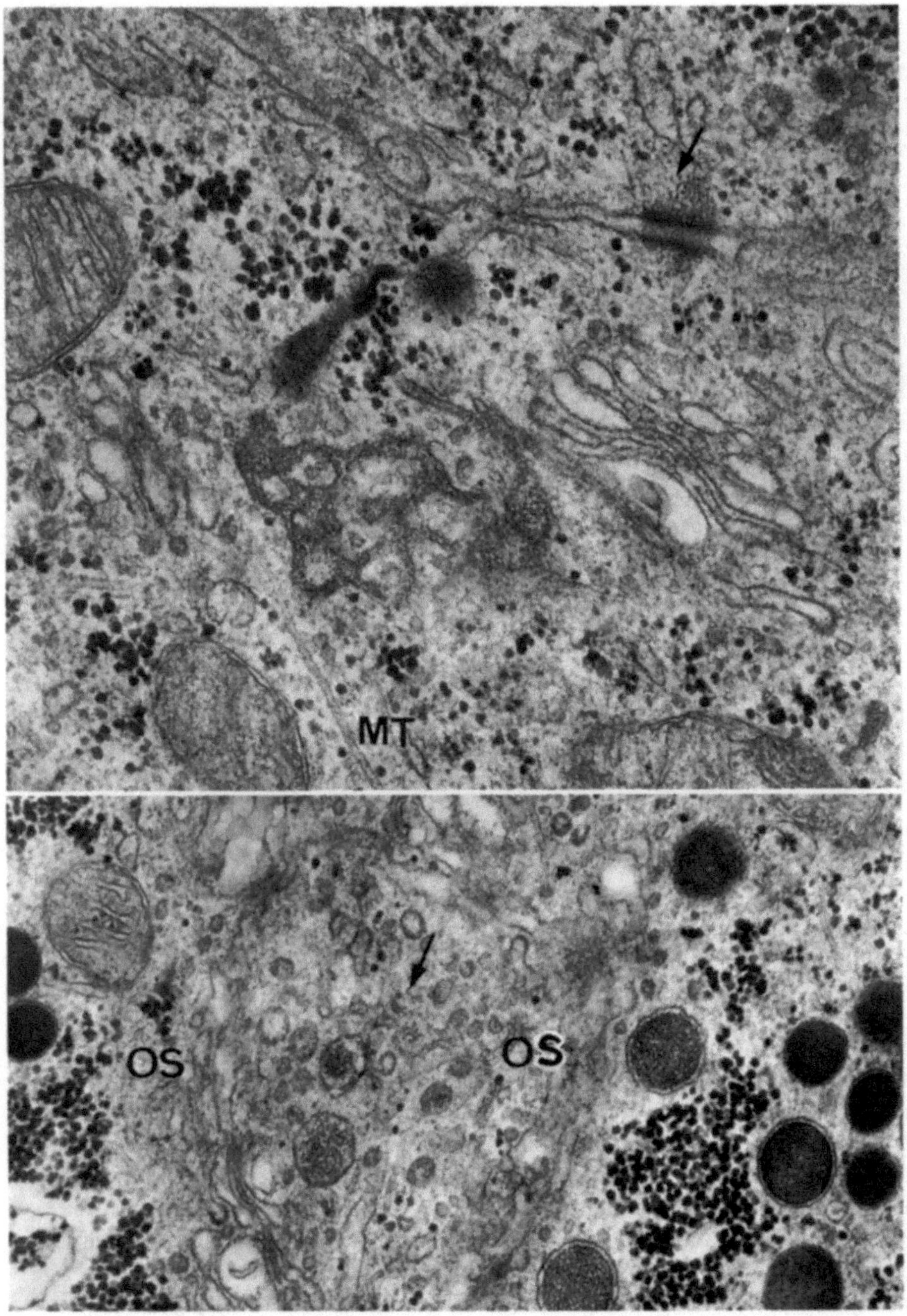

a

b

Fig. 15a and b. Grazing sections of the interior of the Golgi apparatus. (a) Dense tubular reticulum in connection with small and large dense bodies (condensing vacuoles?) in grazing sections. Small desmosomes with bundles of tonofilaments (arrow) and a few microtubules *(MT)*. (b) Interior of another Golgi apparatus embraced by the outer saccules *(OS)*, showing small segments of tubular structures with budding off of condensing vacuoles or prosecretory granules (arrow). a x 50,000; b x 36,000

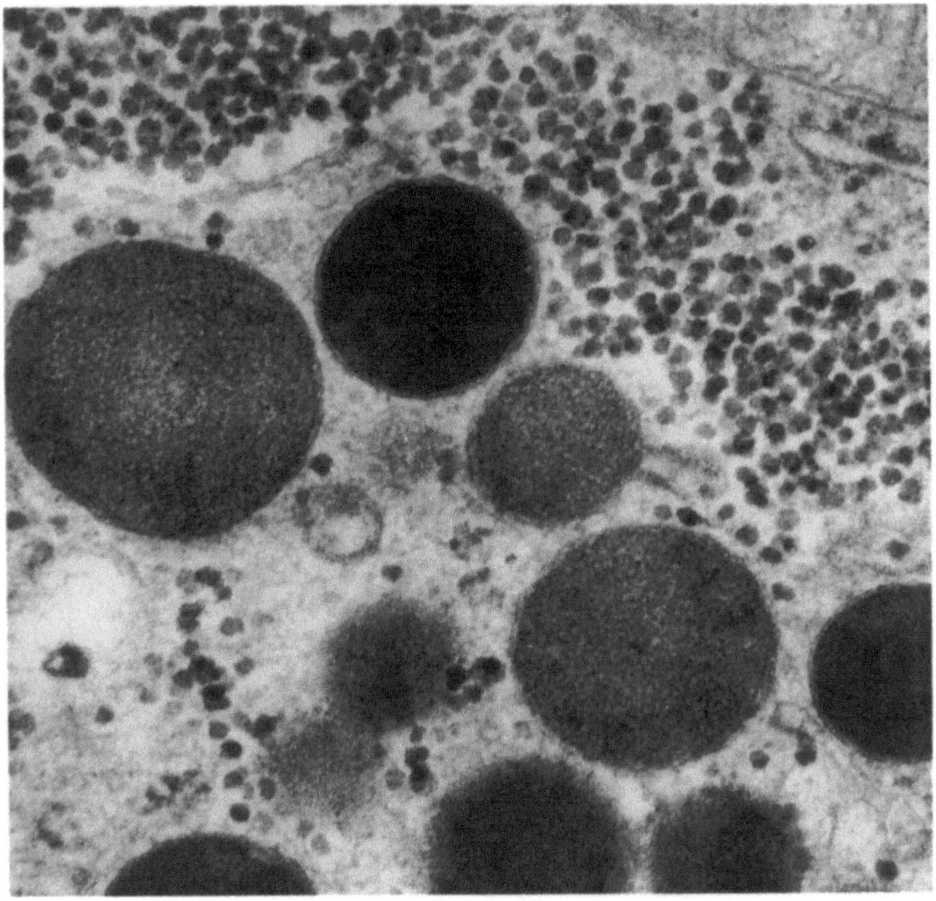

Fig. 16. Secretory granules. Granules with a finely particulated and partially dense homogeneous content surrounded by crowded β-glycogen granules. x 88,000

relationships to the maturing surface of the Golgi apparatus (see above), their modification in various animal experiments, and the demonstration of exocytosis. The assumption that these dense bodies represent secretory granules was further supported by their morphological similarity to the polypeptide hormone containing granules of the anterior lobe of the pituitary gland and the islet cells of the pancreas. Although previously there has been no definite proof that these granules actually represent the storage sites of parathormone or possible precursors (see above), this has been generally assumed on the basis of findings in many animal experiments and of observations made in human glands in patients with clinical symptoms of parathyroid disease. After aldehyde fixation, human secretory granules show

---

Fig. 17a and b. Secretory granules. (a) Thin section of granules embraced by a felt-like arrangement of microfilaments. (b) Freeze-fracture of a corresponding area with small bundles of microfilaments between spherical bodies consistent with secretory granules. a and b x 52,000

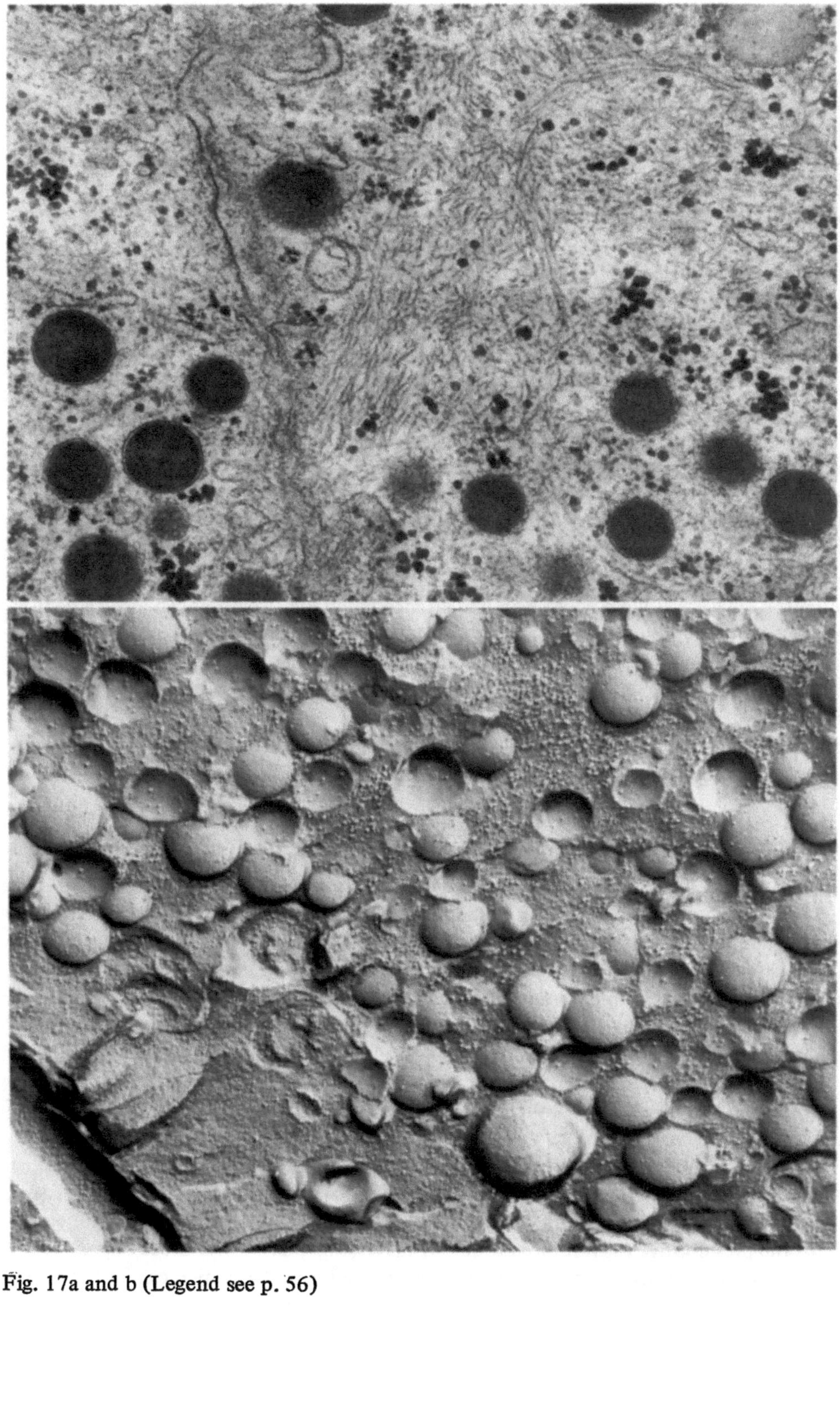

a

b

Fig. 17a and b (Legend see p. 56)

an electron-dense, completely homogeneous interior, but sometimes, they have a finely particulated content (Fig. 16) similar to that in the granules found in bovine parathyroid glands (*Capen* and *Roth*, 1973). However, we suspect that this variation in the appearance of human granules may be attributable to different stages of maturity and consequent different fluid content. The rare occurrence in freeze-fracture of a cleavage through a granule reveals no special structure, confirming the finding of *Buchheim* and *Welsch* (1972) in secretory granules of different endocrine organs in rats and guinea-pigs.

In human secondary hyperplastic parathyroid glands the secretory granules are often arranged in large clusters between maturing surface of the Golgi apparatus and cellular membrane. These clusters of granules are considered more of an expression of increased parathormone synthesis than of storage (e.g. storage phase of the secretory cycle). Certainly in secondary hyperparathyroidism the level of parathormone measured in the peripheral blood is very high (*Potts* et al., 1969), even higher than in adenomatous cells of primary hyperparathyroidsm (*Berson* and *Yalow*, 1966), and the turnover of the hormone also seems high, as judged from animal experiments (*Potts* et al., 1968; *Nakagami* et al., 1971). The fate of secretory granules is either disintegration or exocytosis. Disintegration means intracellular destruction by lysosomes, as shown in various experiments in several endocrine glands (*Farquhar*, 1961a, 1969; *Rohr* and *Krässig*, 1968) or in human hyperplastic parathyroids in a patient with chronic renal insufficiency as a result of forced hemodialysis (*Thiele* et al., 1974). Movement of the granules toward the plasma membrane and exocytosis are probably influenced by contractile microfilaments (*Spooner* et al., 1972), which are seen surrounding the granules in a dense web-like arrangement (Fig. 17a) and can also be demonstrated in freeze-fracture replicas (Fig. 17b). Microtubules are only rarely to be seen, and unlike the islet cells of the pancreas with their directed granule transport to exocytosis (*Lacy*, 1967; *Lacy* et al., 1968; *Malaisse*, 1976), no attachment to the granule membrane is observed in parathyroid cells.

Exocytosis in human parathyroid cells may be separated into four steps when analyzing the results obtained by comparison of thin sections and freeze-fracture replicas: firstly the granules approach the periphery of the cell and one touches the plasma membrane at a tiny area of its limiting membrane; at this very spot the plasma membrane becomes slightly scalloped (Fig. 18a). Secondly there is a broad fusion between granule and plasma membrane (Fig. 18b). Thirdly the content of the granules is extruded into the extracellular space (Fig. 18c), and finally there remains a residual invagination or scalloping of the cellular membrane marking the place of granule extrusion (Fig. 18d).

In addition, in freeze-fracture replicas the exocytosis of the granule is often preceded by a protrusion of the plasma membrane, a surface phenomenon described by *Daikoku* et al. (1973) and *Dempsey* et al. (1973) in the pituitary gland of rats. Freeze-fracture replicas of the membrane fusion process in transverse cleavage planes display similar results to those seen in thin sections (Fig. 19a, b). Replicas that show "A-" and "B-faces" of the split plasma membrane in en-face views may elucidate the fusion of plasma and granule membrane. Fusion sites appear on "face A" as assemblies of small particles (about 8-10 nm) surrounding a smooth central area. On the complementary "B-face" a circular smooth protuberance is exposed, containing a tiny central depression (Fig. 20b). Completion of membrane fusion is followed by a bulging forward of the granule, showing a small peak which probably represents the presumptive rupture site on the "A-face" (Fig. 20a). These areas of granule protrusion are surrounded by irregular groupings of small particles, which can be compared

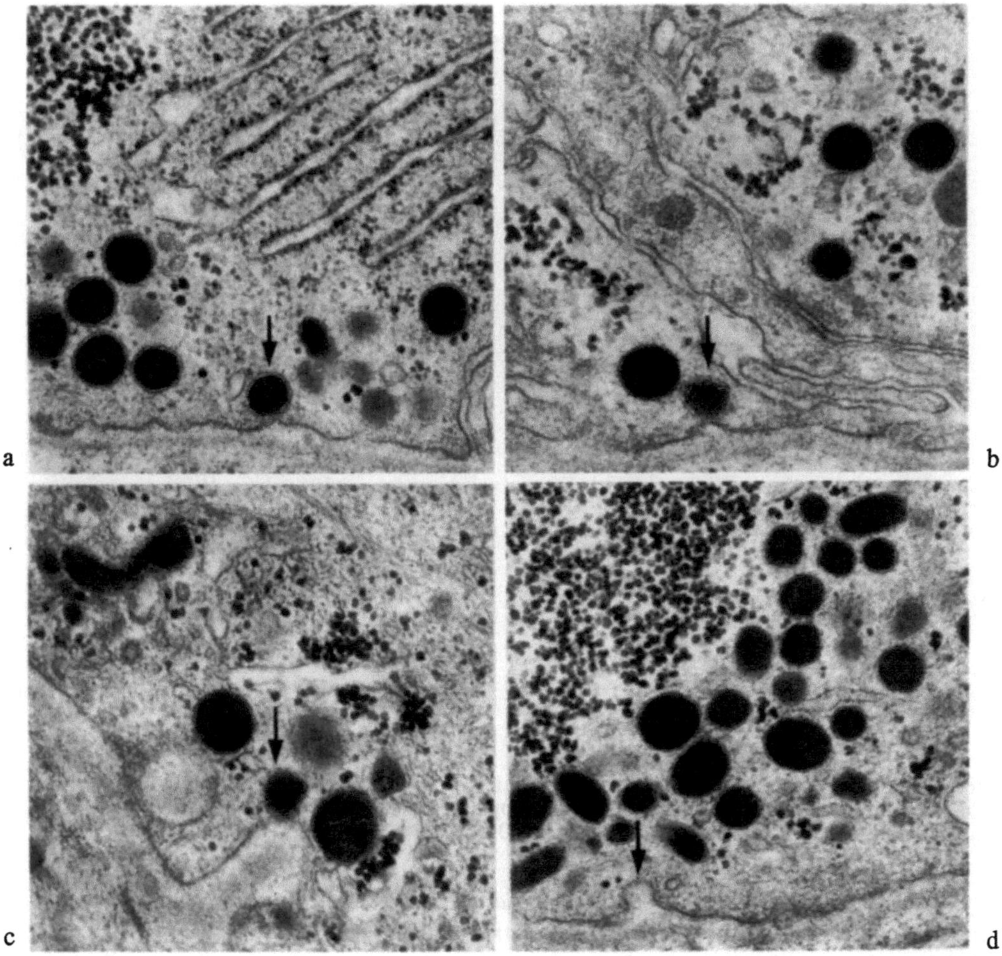

Fig. 18a-d. Exocytosis of secretory granules. Thin sections of the different steps of granule extrusion (arrows always point toward the secretory granules involved). (a) Several granules approach the plasma membrane and one touches the membrane over a tiny area. (b) Fusion between granule and plasma membrane, with a slight invagination at this site (compare with Fig. 19b). (c) Extrusion of the granule content into the extracellular space (compare with Fig. 20a). (d) Site of granule extrusion is marked by a small invagination. a-d x 40,000

to so-called rosette formation (*Satir* et al., 1973). After rupture of the limiting membrane the content of the secretory granule is extruded, and a freeze-fracture replica exhibits circular areas with a coarse surface on the "B-faces" consistent with the cleaved granule content (Fig. 20c). The particles detected on "face A" of the fused granule and plasma membrane are thought to represent proteins or a redistribution of membrane-associated particles that are penetrating into or traversing the split bimolecular lipid layer of the plasma membrane (*Pinto da Silva*, 1972). The smooth central areas should be compatible with the lipid matrix of the plasma membrane (*Deamer* et al., 1970). The findings in human parathyroid

a 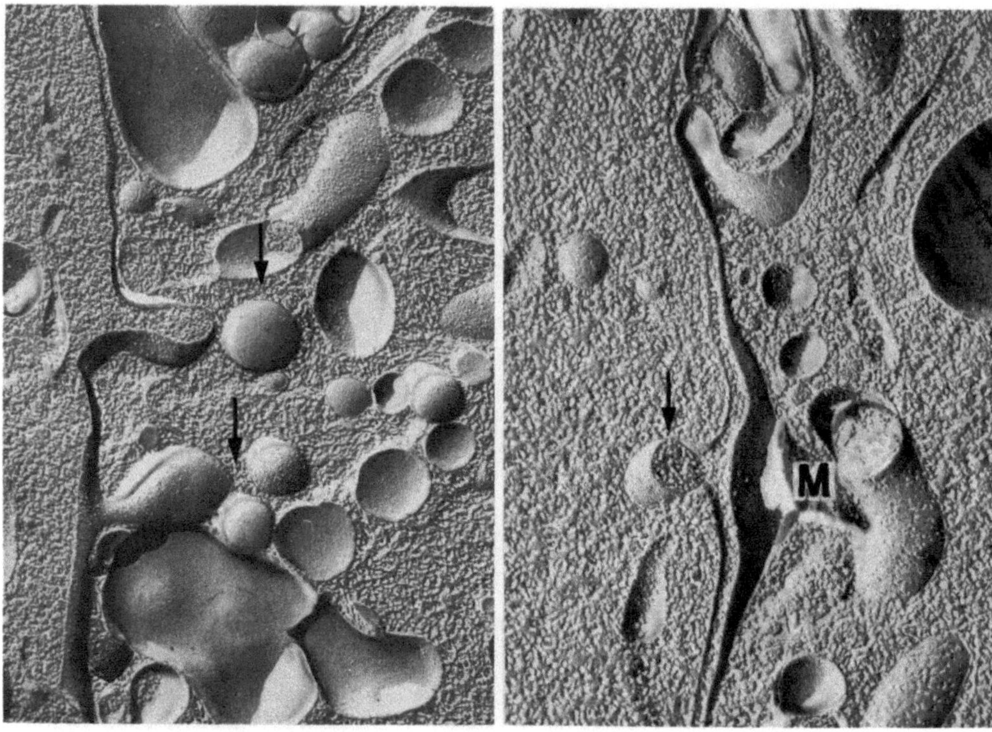 b

Fig. 19a and b. Exocytosis of secretory granules. Freeze-fracture of transversely cleaved plasma membranes with secretory granules approaching the plasma membrane (a) and fusing with it (b); *M* = Mitochondrium. a x 40,000; b x 16,000

cells generally resemble the observations of *Satir* et al. (1973) on the membrane fusion and mucocyst secretion in the protozoon Tetrahymena pyriformis and of *Dreifuss* et al. (1976) in the neurohypophysis of rats; the findings in man are also consistent with those of *Orci* et al. (1973b) and *Berger* et al. (1975) in rodent pancreatic islet cells. In comparison with the very regular rosette formation of *Satir* et al. (1973), however, we were not able to observe such a regular array of particles, this confirming the results of *William* et al.

Fig. 20a-c. Exocytosis of secretory granules. Freeze-fracture replicas with en-face views of the cleaved plasma membranes during exocytosis ("face A," "face B"). (a) "A-face" with small protuberances (arrows) surrounded by assemblies of small particles in irregular array, probably corresponding to the completed fusion between the membranes of secretory granules and plasma membrane. The tiny peaks of these protuberances are compatible with the bulging forward of the granule content and the presumptive rupture sites of the fused membranes. The irregular aggregates of particles are probably comparable with the rosette formations (*Satir* et al., 1973). An area of a deeper level of cleavage reveals crowded spherical bodies consistent with secretory granules approaching the plasma membrane *(S)*, comparable to Fig. 18a. (b) "B-face" of the split plasma membrane at an early fusion site. Smooth protuberance with a tiny central depression corresponding to the central particle of the particle aggregates on the "A-face" at the beginning of the fusion process; compare with Figs. 18a and 19b. (c) "B-face" with rupture of the fused membranes and extrusion of granule content, comparable with Fig. 18c. Fracture plane runs through the particulated content of granules. a x 50,000; b x 70,000; c x 65,000

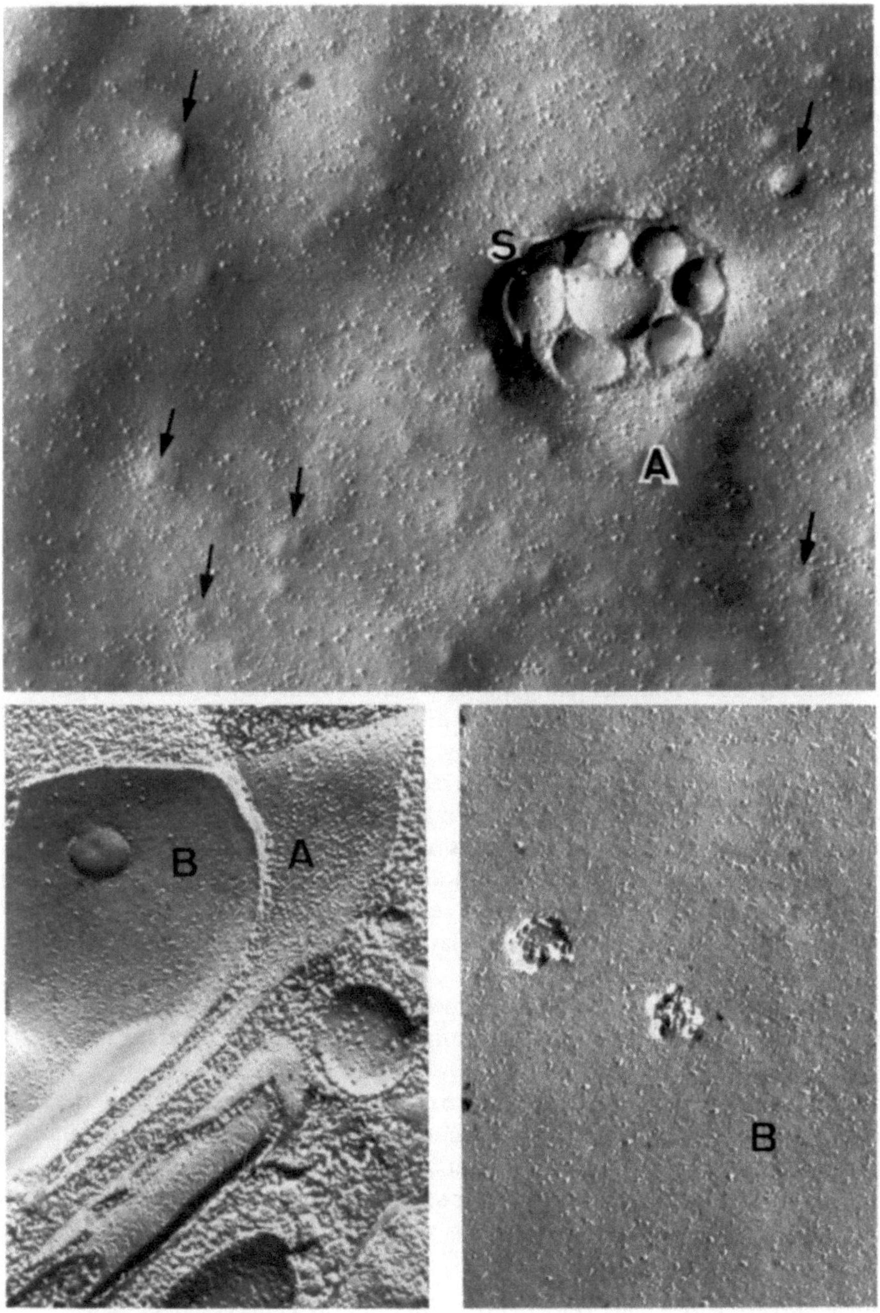

a b c

Fig. 20a-c (Legend see p. 60)

(1976). These protein particles seen in the lipid layer of the split plasma membrane may provide channels or pathways for the exchange of ions and fluids between the fused membranes, thus displaying functions generally attributed to the gap junction particles (*McNutt* and *Weinstein*, 1973). In view of calcium-mediated release of parathormone, it is intriguing to speculate that by this mechanism of coupling, the ionized calcium concentration of the extracellular space may directly influence the extrusion of the content of the secretory granules.

In summary, the mechanism of secretion is generally similar to that of other endocrine glands (*Kurosumi*, 1961). Fusion of the granule and plasma membrane has already been observed in thin sections of the parathyroids of cows (*Capen* and *Roth*, 1973) and an identical procedure has been suggested by *Altenähr* (1972) in man. *Perkin* et al. (1968), using a highly purified antigen and immunofluorescent methods, localized parathormone in the extracellular space in bovine parathyroid glands, thus implicating exocytosis.

As in the glucose-stimulated beta cell of the pancreatic islet exocytosis may be coupled with a compensatory movement of Golgi-derived membranous material (remnants of the secretory granule membrane) initially incorporated in the plasma membrane at the time and site of exocytosis, which is by this procedure restituted to the cytoplasmic compartment (*Orci* et al., 1973a).

f) Mitochondria

Number, size, and shape of the mitochondria are found to be extremely variable in different pathological parathyroid conditions, possibly depending on endocrine activity. This is particularly well demonstrated in adenomatous cells of patients with severe hyperparathyroidism, where the increase in mitochondrial number is often accompanied by a bizarre shape (*Thiele* et al., 1973a). In highly stimulated chief cells of secondary hyperplastic glands there are giant, roughly cup-shaped mitochondria displaying invagination of cisternae of the rough-surfaced endoplasmic reticulum (Fig. 21a). Another frequent finding is elongation and parallel arrangement to cisternae of the rough-surfaced endoplasmic reticulum (Fig. 22a). Mitochondria of patients with primary hyperparathyroidism (due to an adenoma, carcinoma, or primary hyperplasia) exhibit giant electron-dense round inclusions in their matrix (*Thiele* et al., 1973a, b; *Thiele* and *Pichlmayr*, 1974). The experiments of *Peachey* (1964) and *Weinbach* and *von Brand* (1967), concerning the accumulation of divalent cations in mitochondria of different animal cells, show that calcium may be stored in large dense bodies. These bodies are almost identical to the inclusions observed in mitochondria of human parathyroid tumor cells (Fig. 21b), or in severe hypercalcemic hyperparathyroidism, and it is therefore also suspected that they may contain calcium deposits.

The mitochondria of the oxyphil and transitional oxyphil cells, mostly found in secondary hyperplasias and adenomas of the mixed cell type, display an enormous increase in number and size, as well as a bizarre shape and arrangement of their densly packed cristae (Fig. 6b, c). Freeze-fracture replicas of these large mitochondria exhibit irregularly dispersed small granules on the "A-" and "B-faces" of the inner mitochondrial membrane (Figs. 7b,c,

---

Fig. 21a-c. Mitochondria of active chief cells and oxyphil cells. (a) Thin section of giant cup-shaped mitochondrium with invaginated cisternae of the rough-surfaced endoplasmic reticulum. Most cristae follow an apparently circular course. (b) Mitochondrium in the chief cell of a highly active parathyroid adenoma with large electron-dense inclusion of the matrix entirely displacing the cristae; only outer and inner mitochondrial membranes are recognizable. (c) Freeze-fracture replica of a cup-shaped giant mitochondrium of an oxyphil cell almost identical to Fig. 21a. "A-" and "B-faces" with tiny intramembranous particles (arrow). a x 44,000; b x 42,000; c x 46,000

a

b

c

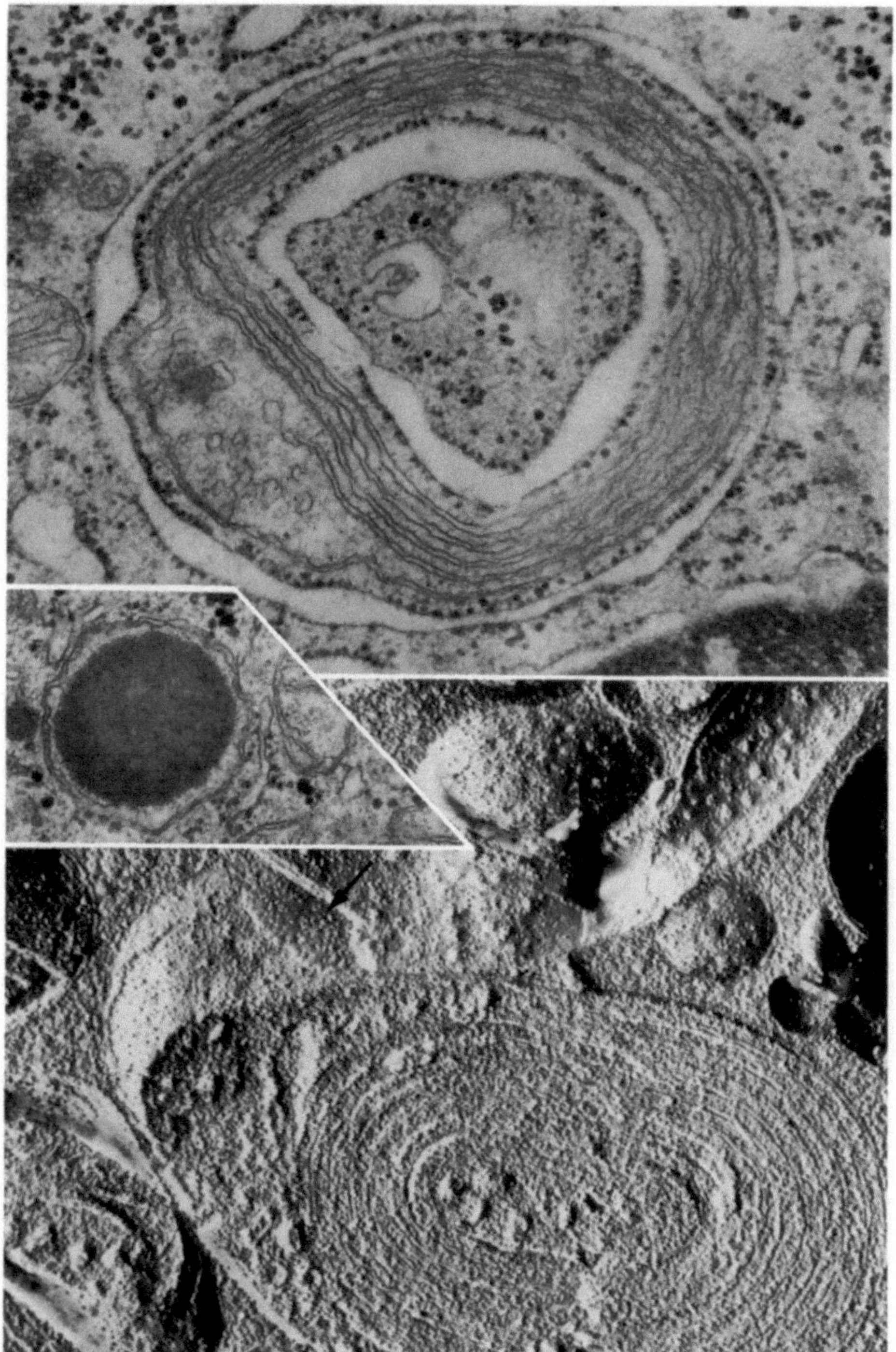

Fig. 21a-c (Legend see p. 62)

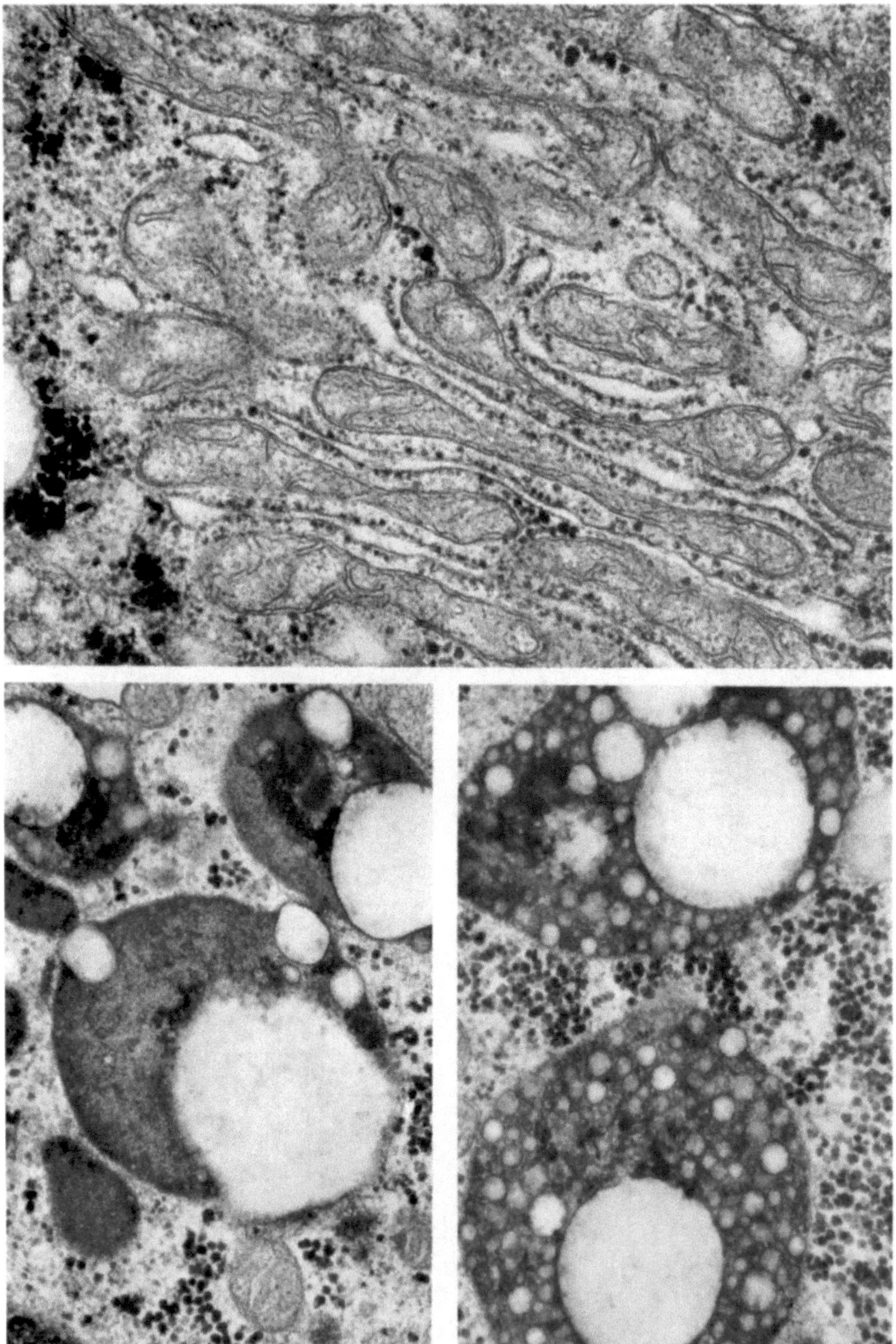
a b c

Fig. 22a-c (Legend see p. 65)

21c). These particulated components of the membrane structure have been shown to be most prominent in non-chemically fixed material, as described by *Wrigglesworth* et al. (1970) and *Breathnach* et al. (1972) in rodent heart and liver mitochondria. These tiny granules may be compared with similar particles observed in the cisternal membranes of the rough-surfaced endoplasmic reticulum (*Breathnach* et al., 1972). These common structural components of organelle membranes are regarded as protein particles that probably contain enzymes; in the inner mitochondrial membrane there are enzymatic proteins of the respiratory chain (review by *Wrigglesworth* et al., 1970). In addition, "face A" of the inner mitochondrial membrane displays small depressions which might suggest *pediculi cristae* as observed in liver parenchymal cells (*Daems* and *Wisse*, 1966). There are also giant mitochondria with a circular and parallel appearance of their cristae similar to that in chief cells (Fig. 21c) and to that of organelles found in the oxyphil cells of experimental tumors (*Gusek*, 1975).

g) Dense Bodies

In chief cells of the normal and inactive parathyroids, especially in patients with an endocrine-active adenoma or carcinoma, large, complex dense bodies are seen in the cytoplasm of the remaining hormonally suppressed glands. In thin sections these bodies are shown to be composed either of clusters of numerous translucent vacuoles of different sizes, sometimes containing dense round bodies (Fig. 22b, c), or of a particulated material and several membrane-bound vacuoles. In freeze-fracture replicas the content is demonstrated to consist of lipids, mainly cholesterin compounds, by reason of the very smooth cleavage plane (Fig. 3a, b); this is borne out by the experimental findings of *Ruska* et al. (1972). These bodies exhibit lipopigment granules and are closely related to the so-called wear- and-tear pigment, lipofuscin, and may therefore be identical to the residual bodies of lysosomal origin (review by *de Duve* and *Wattiaux*, 1966). These complex dense bodies are produced by the disintegration of excess secretory granules and other cytoplasmic debris by autophagosomes as shown in other endocrine cells (*Farquhar*, 1961a; *Smith* and *Farquhar*, 1966; *Farquhar*, 1969). This is supported by the fact that particularly in normal glands of elderly patients and in the inactive (e.g. resting or suppressed) parathyroids removed concomitantly with a highly active adenoma, large inclusion bodies are found in high concentrations.

Dense bodies of a smaller size (but larger than secretory granules) are often encountered in close relation to the Golgi apparatus and are thought to be lysosomes. Small, solitary lipid droplets in the active chief cells and the water-clear cell are to be differentiated from the complex lipid bodies of the inactive cells mentioned above. These lipid vacuoles are always closely related to glycogen (Fig. 4a), mitochondria, rough-surfaced endoplasmic reticulum, and Golgi apparatus (Fig. 1a). According to *Nunez* et al. (1972) the cyclic changes of parathyroid fine structure of the hibernating bat show that these lipid droplets, together with glycogen, may serve as a source of energy for parathormone synthesis.

Fig. 22a-c. Mitochondria and dense bodies. (a) Elongated mitochondria alternating in parallel arrangement with cisternae of the rough-surfaced endoplasmic reticulum. (b and c) Dense bodies containing translucent areas of different sizes corresponding to freeze-fracture replica of Fig. 3b. a x 42,000; b and c x 40,000

h) Glycogen

In the chief cells of human parathyroid glands the amount of glycogen is quite variable and probably dependent upon changes in endocrine activity. In the extreme case of a patient with a prolonged hyperparathyroid crisis the highly activated cells of the adenoma did not show any glycogen or lipid droplets (*Thiele*, unpubl.). On the other hand, the chronically stimulated gland of secondary hyperparathyroidism due to renal insufficiency exhibits under light microscopy clusters of so-called small water-clear cells (or highly vacuolated cells) which are almost completely filled with large accumulations of β-glycogen granules closely associated with lipid droplets (Figs. 4a, 5a). In the cyclic secreting chief cells the concentration of glycogen granules varies with the grade of activity. It is high (up to a certain degree) in resting (inactive) and low in active (stimulated) cells (*Roth* and *Raisz*, 1966).

The glycogen accumulations of the parathyroid cells consist of densely packed spheroidal granules so-called, β-particles (*Drochmans*, 1962; *Biava*, 1963). Following lead citrate staining of thin sections these particles appear almost homogeneous (Figs. 16, 23a). Negative staining of β-glycogen in various animal tissues (*Drochmans*, 1962; *Wanson* and *Tielemans*, 1971) and the human parathyroid gland (*Biava*, 1963) discloses very small subunits composing each β-particle. The use of special staining methods, e.g. thiocarbohydrazine with silverproteinate (*Thiery*, 1967, 1969) (Fig. 23b) or the periodic acid-alkaline bismuth procedure (*Ainsworth* et al., 1972) (Fig. 23c) allows confirmation of the presence of these small subunits. Freeze-fracture replicas reveal a finely, almost regularly particulated surface of the single cleaved β-particle (Fig. 23d). In conclusion, all these findings made by very different methods of tissue preparation suggest the presence of γ-subunits composing each human β-glycogen particle, as already postulated by *Drochmans* and co-workers (*Drochmans*, 1962; *Wanson* and *Tielemans*, 1971).

Freeze-fracture replicas show the β-particles to possess a polygonal, sometimes even an almost pentagonal shape and to be about 50 nm in diameter (Fig. 23d). This contrasts with the size measured in thin sections and negative-stained preparations, where the β-particle of the human parathyroid chief cell has a diameter of only 30 nm (*Biava*, 1963). The latter size also agrees with our findings in thin sections (Figs. 16, 23a). This difference in the size of human particulate glycogen is easily explained if the small halo of lower electron density surrounding every particle is taken into consideration. This almost translucent area around the β-granule is not taken into consideration when measuring the diameter of an individual particle in thin sections. In the light of biochemical evidence of enzymes bound to glycogen this translucent halo may be due to a protein moiety, possibly of enzymatic nature (*Leloir* and *Goldemberg*, 1960; *Luck*, 1961). In freeze-fracture replicas however, polysaccharide and protein components of each β-glycogen particle are both cleaved and replicated, but not differentiated, so that the individual particle seems larger.

Fig. 23a-d. β-Glycogen granules in different preparations: a-c thin section, d freeze-fracture. (a) Lead-citrate staining with almost homogeneous dense particles surrounded by a tiny translucent halo. (b) Silver proteinate method displays smaller subunits composing a β-particle consistent with γ-particles. (c) Alkaline bismuth procedure confirms the presence of smaller particles (γ-subunits) composing a β-glycogen granule. (d) Freeze-fracture with a polygonal almost pentagonal cleavage plane of the single β-particle with a finely particulated surface in en-face view. a, b and d x 80,000; c x 160,000

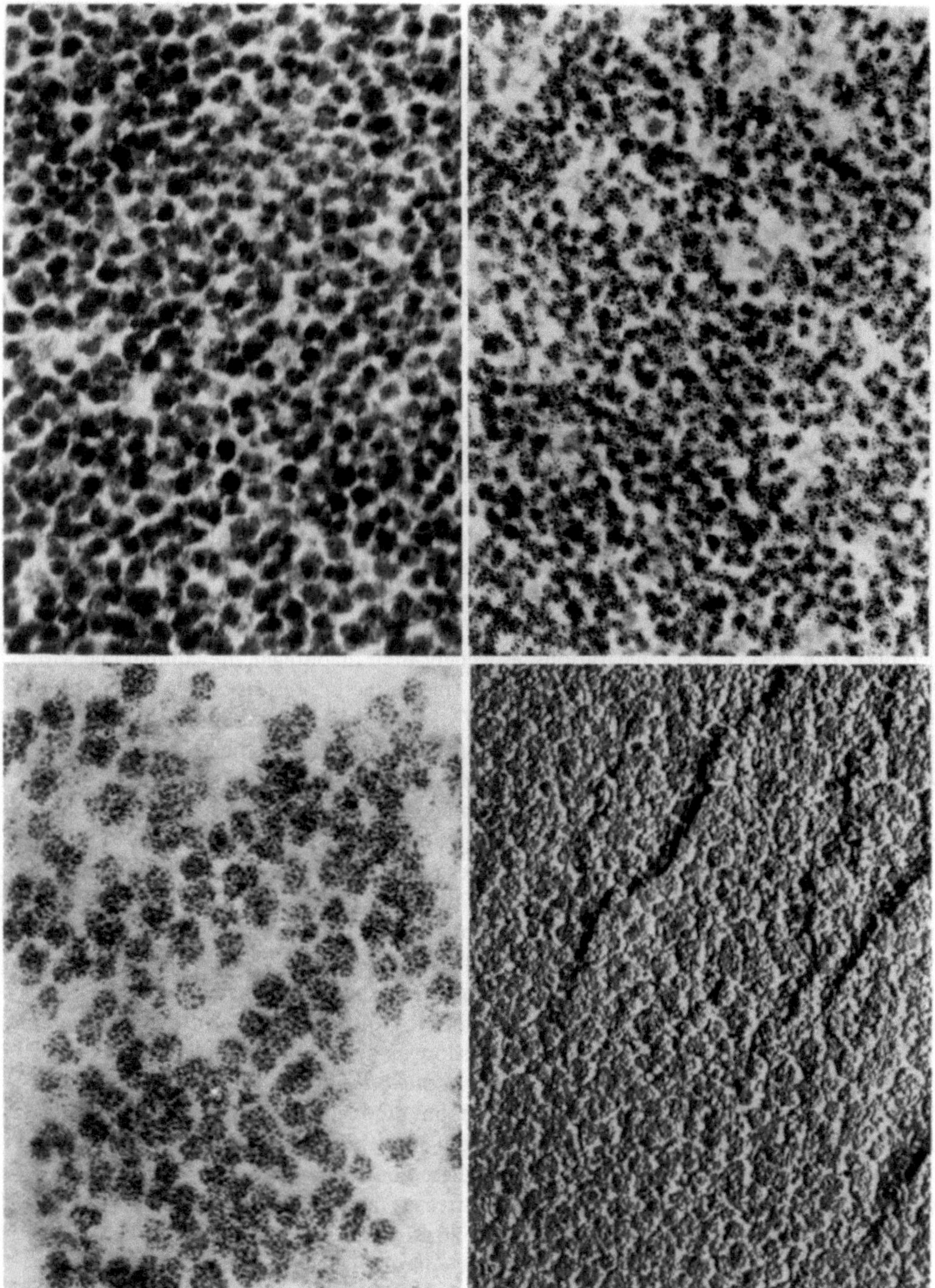

a b c d

Fig. 23a-d (Legend see p. 66)

V. Interstitium

1. Vessels

The most prominent feature of the interstitial space of the parathyroid gland is the large number of vessels, most of which are capillaries closely attached with their basement membranes to those of the chief cells. The endothelial cells lining the small capillary basement membranes are extremely thin, with slightly bulging nuclei and many pores in their cytoplasm (Fig. 24a). In thin sections these openings or pores of the endothelium show a dense particle in their center (Fig. 25a) and have a regular diameter of about 50 nm. From freeze-fracture replicas it is evident that these pores are actually fenestrations, since they are spanned by a diaphragm with a central thickening or knob (Fig. 24b). In addition, by presenting en-face views of the basal plasma membrane of the endothelial layer, freeze-fracture demonstrates crowded pinocytic vesicles of different sizes and random distribution (Fig. 24c).

The fine structure of human parathyroid vessels has previously been only briefly described by *Elliott* and *Arhelger* (1966), who mentioned many pores of the endothelial cells. In animals, however, there are several extensive reports, in particular one by *Trier* (1958; review by *Capen* and *Roth*, 1973). Our observations show that the fine structure of the human parathyroid vessels follows the general scheme of construction found in other endocrine organs, e.g. in the anterior lobe of the pituitary gland, and in tumors originating from this organ (*Farquhar*, 1961b; *Hirano* et al., 1972), and in the adrenal medulla (*Elfin*, 1965). The fenestrations, especially their diaphragm, are comparable with the thin-section findings of *Rhodin* (1962) and freeze-fracture results of *Friederici* (1968, 1969), *Maul* (1971), and *Yamamoto* et al. (1976), obtained in different animal tissues. The large numbers of pinocytic vesicles are similar to those described e.g. by *Nickel* and *Grieshaber* (1969), *Leak* (1971), and *Simionescu* et al. (1974), mostly in heart and skeletal muscle cells of rodents. In addition to normal organelles and structures, such as the rough-surfaced endoplasmic reticulum, Golgi apparatus, mitochondria, and polysomes, all endothelial cells contain multiple rod-like bodies up to 3 μm in length and 150 nm in width, densely packed with tubular structures (Fig. 25b). These bodies have been described in the endothelial cells of a variety of endocrine tumors, including those of the parathyroid gland (*Elliott* and *Arhelger*, 1966; *Tomiyasu* et al., 1973) and are called Weibel-Palade granules (*Weibel* and *Palade*, 1964). These granules can generally be seen in the endothelium of different organs and are thought to be derived from the Golgi apparatus (*Matsuda* and *Sugiura*, 1970; *Sengel* and *Stoebner*, 1970). Since they show no acid phosphatase activity they do not belong into any group of lysosomal bodies (*Lemeunier* et al., 1969). The functional significance of these structures remains obscure, but a possible role in the blood coagulation system is discussed by several authors (*Fuchs* and *Weibel*, 1966; *Burri* and *Weibel*, 1968). Thin sections confirm the structure of these bodies in man to be closely associated with bundles of microfilaments (Fig. 25b) and freeze-fracture demonstrates the rod-like appearance in transversely cleaved bodies (Fig. 26a, b).

In thin sections, extensive overlapping of the endothelial cells is noticeable. *Zonulae occludentes* (tight junctions) between the adjacent cells show small areas of localized attachments of two cellular plasma membranes. In freeze-fracture replicas these areas of close membranous attachments are consistent with a network of anastomosing discontinuous strands on "face A" (Fig. 27a) and corresponding grooves on "face B." Because the sutures between these cells are very tortuous their extension is quite short, and evaluation

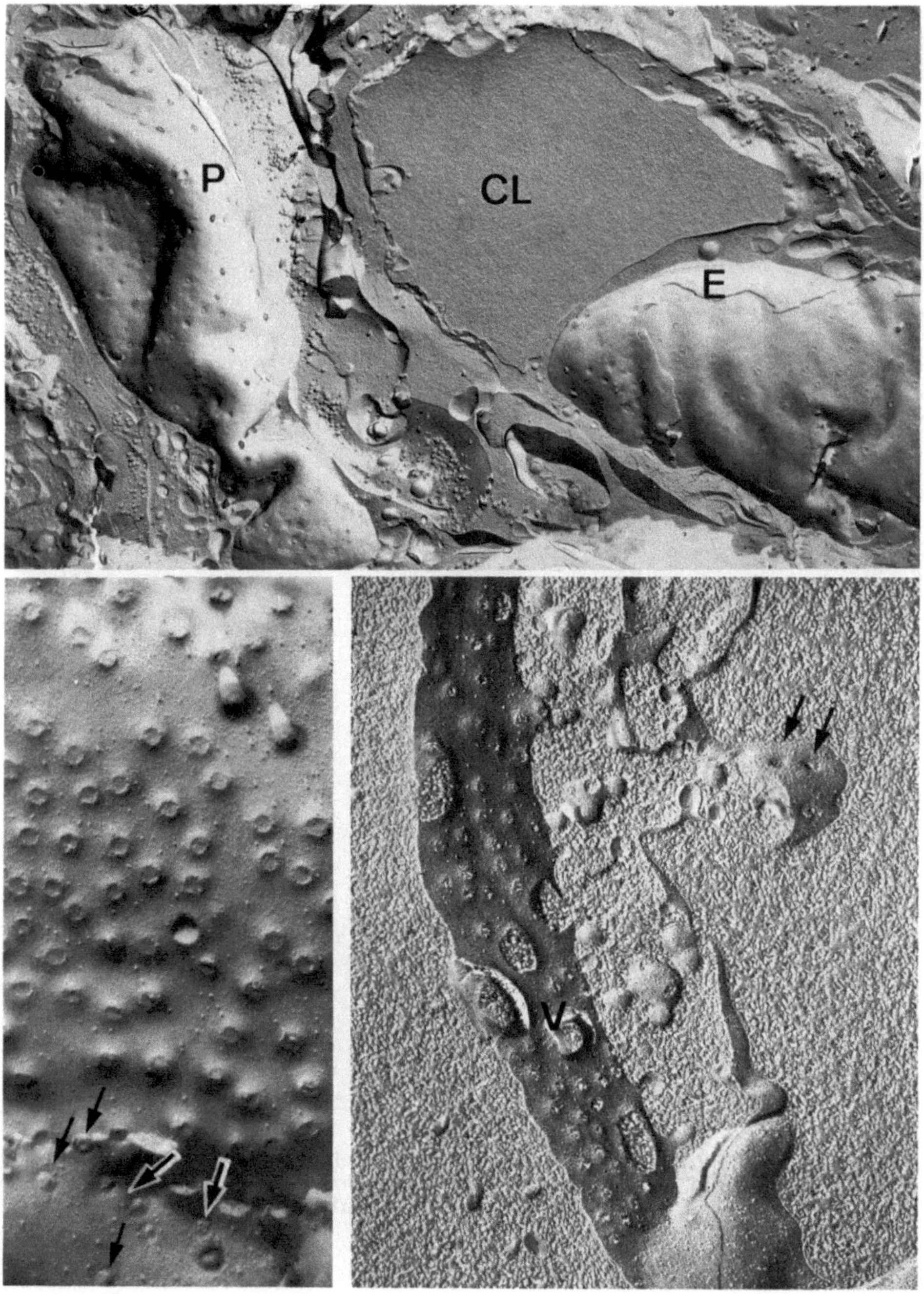

Fig. 24a-c. Freeze-fracture of parathyroid vessels. (a) Survey with endothelial cell *(E)* and capillary lumen *(CL)*. An adventitial cell *(P)* with undulating nucleus adjacent to the capillary. (b) En-face view of the endothelial layer with many fenestrations. Several display a diaphragm with a central knob (arrows) in favorable cleavage planes. (c) Transverse and longitudinal cleavage of an endothelial cell with openings of pinocytic vesicles at the luminal surface of the plasma membrane (arrows) and in en-face view of the basal membrane *(V)*. a x 9,000; b x 42,000; c x 40,000

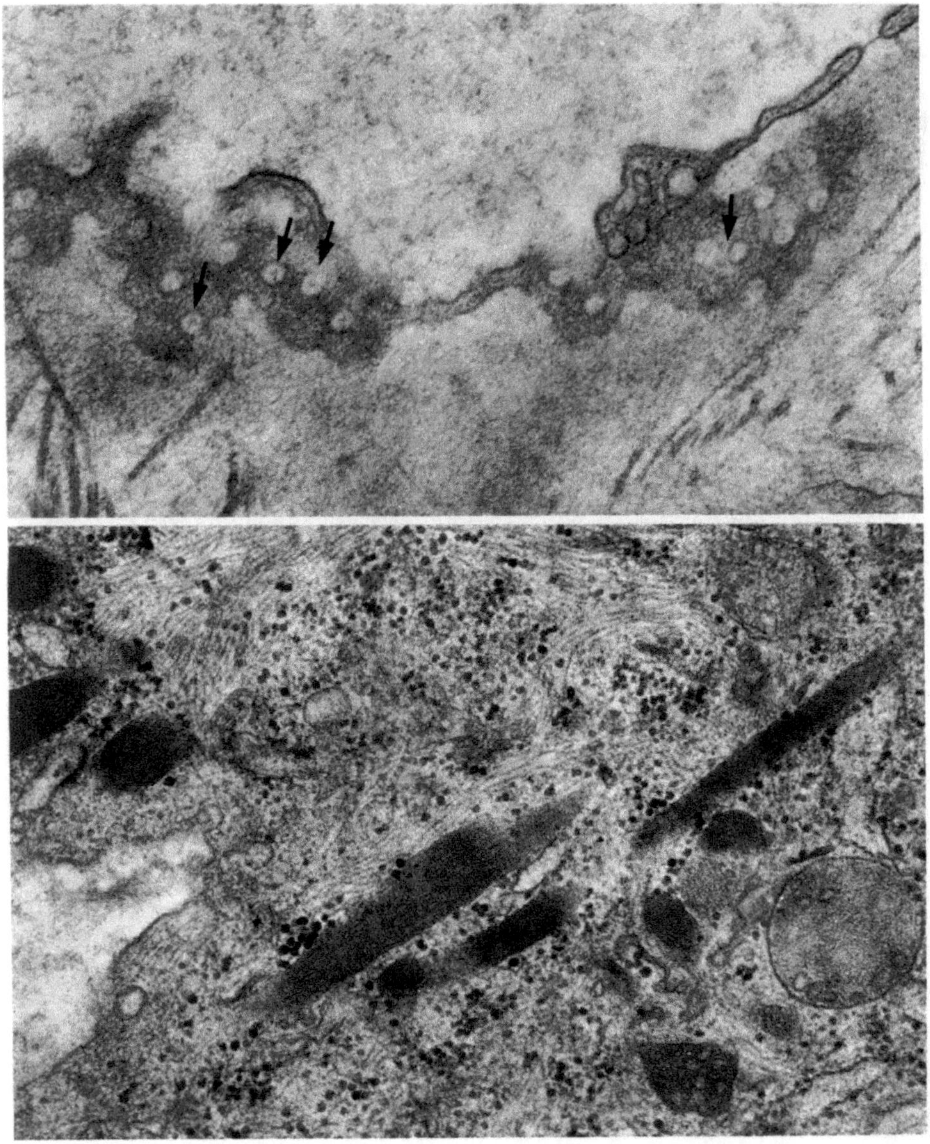

a

b

Fig. 25a and b. Thin sections of parathyroid endothelial cells. (a) Fenestrations of the endothelium in grazing section with dense central knobs (arrows) comparable to Fig. 24b. (b) Large rod-like Weibel-Palade granules packed with tubular-fibrilar structures and surrounded by a web of microfilaments. a x 48,000; b x 42,000

is limited to the small areas properly exposed, exhibiting at least 3-4 interrupted strands. A segmental differentiation of cell junctions such as is postulated by *Simionescu* et al. (1975, 1976) is therefore impossible to assess. The *zonula occludens*-like junctions actually represent a *fascia occludens* for their discontinuity. The strands are punctate in nature, composed of intermembranous individual particles arranged in a linear deployment and surrounded by

a

b

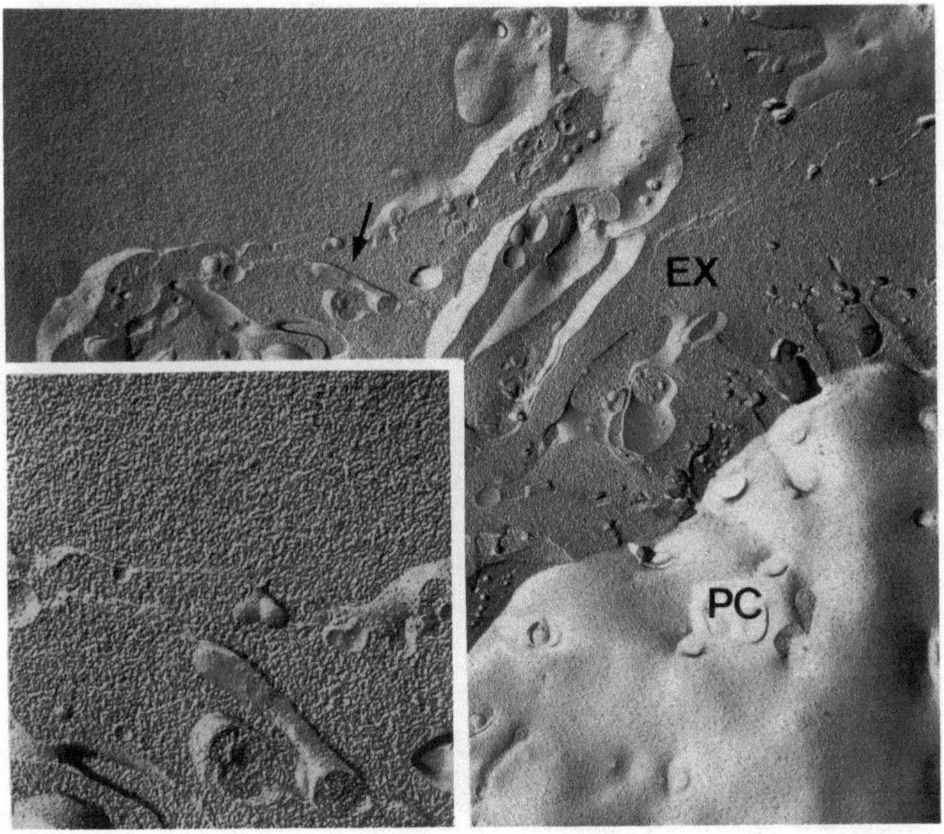

Fig. 26a and b. Freeze-fracture of Weibel-Palade granules. (a) Survey with endothelial cell containing elongated bodies (arrow) corresponding to Weibel-Palade granules. Extracellular space *(EX)*, en-face view of plasma membrane of parathyroid cell *(PC)*. (b) High magnification of the Weibel-Palade granules with a particulated cleavage plane running through the interior of the granules. a x 20,000; b x 40,000

other isolated particles (Fig. 27b), as described by *Yee* and *Revel* (1975) and *Staehelin* (1975) in different vessels of animal specimens. Similar structures have been reported in capillaries of the brain, the myocardium (review by *McNutt* and *Weinstein*, 1973), the kidney (*Kühn* et al., 1975), choroidal vessels of the human eye (*Spitznas* and *Reale*, 1975) and the thyroid gland (*Thiele* et al., 1977). The physiological function of these junctions is to maintain some kind of barrier between two adjacent cells, probably impairing bypass diffusion of certain molecules. From experimental findings, the permeability of these junctions is related to the number and continuity of strands (*Claude* and *Goodenough*, 1973). Thus transepithelial resistance increases in indirect proportion to the number of strands and the molecular weight. These close correlations between physiology and morphology of *zonulae occludentes* were demonstrated in the follicular cells of the human and rodent thyroid gland and their vessels (*Thiele* et al., 1976, 1977; *Thiele* and *Reale*, 1976), and by *Clementi* and *Palade* (1969) in the intestinal capillaries, using horseradish peroxidase and ferritin as tracer molecules. These authors found that horseradish peroxidase (molecular weight 40,000; molecular diameter

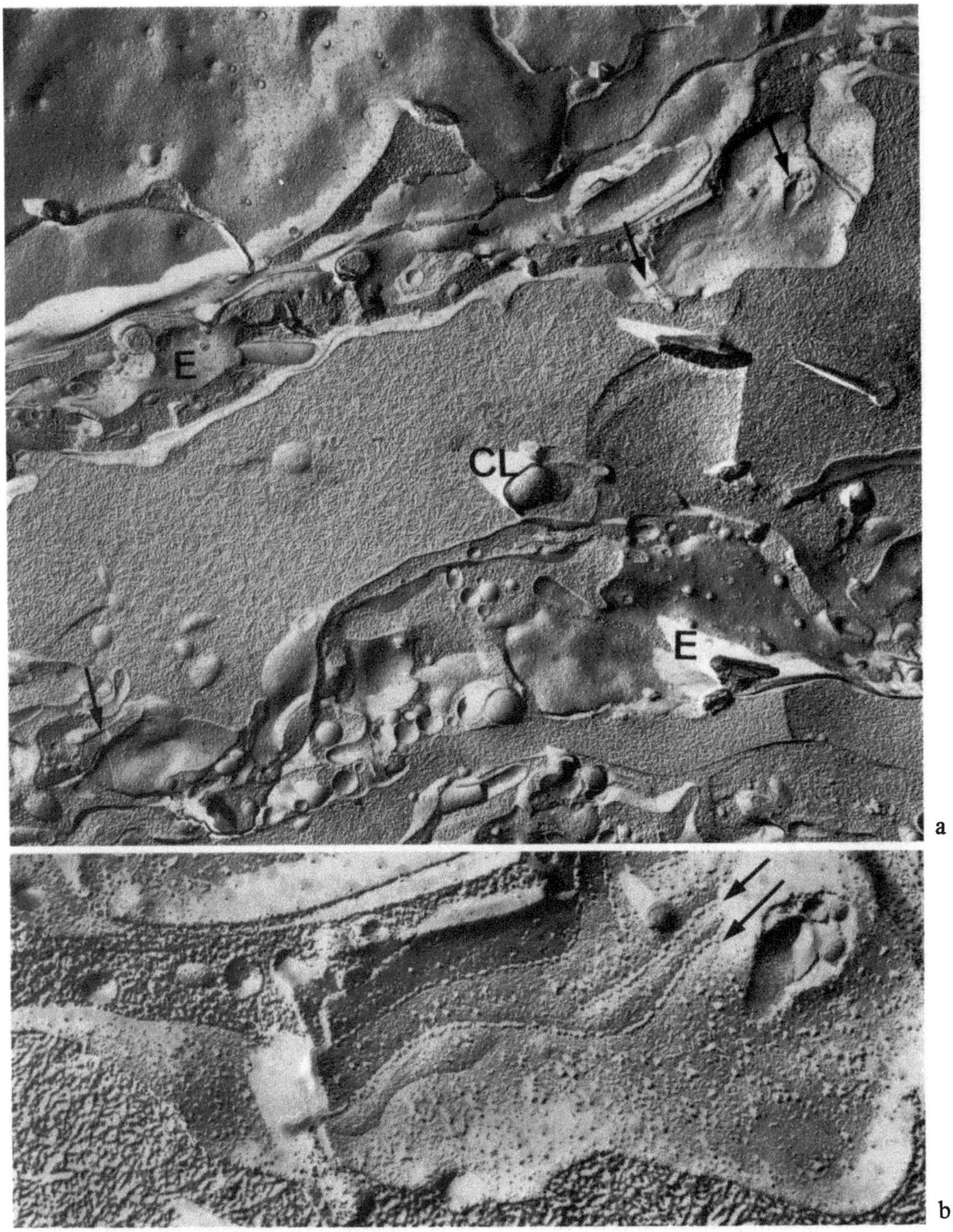

Fig. 27a and b. Freeze-fracture of the junctional complexes of the endothelial cells. (a) Lumen of a small vessel, probably a capillary *(CL)* with overlapping endothelial cells *(E)* exposing discontinuous strands of *zonula occludens*-like junctions (arrows). (b) High magnification of the "A-face" shows these junctions to be composed of interrupted strands (arrows) consisting of a linear deployment of particles and surrounded by numerous isolated particles. a x 20,000; b x 65,000

about 5 nm) did not pass through these intercellular junctions of the intestinal vessels. Since its transport by pinocytic vesicles seemed to be negligible, outflow through the fenestrations was considered the main route of high molecular diffusion. In further experiments (*Simionescu* et al., 1974) it was concluded that the areas of discontinuity of the strands of the *zonula occludentes* could be the morphological equivalents of the small pore or slit system postulated by physiologists, as well as the large pore system (review by *Landis* and *Pappenheimer*, 1963). Our demonstration of *zonulae occludentes* in the endothelial cells of the human parathyorid gland displaying interrupted strands, and therefore belonging to the "leaky" type of cellular junctions (*Claude* and *Goodenough*, 1973), supports this assumption. On the other hand, the fenestrations are the best candidates for the structural substrate of the large pore system (*Simionescu* et al., 1974). On the analogy of these experiments, the passage of the relatively large parathormone molecule (molecular weight about 7,000) into circulation could possibly be through these endothelial fenestrations.

2. Interstitial Cells

The interstitial space is bordered by the basement membranes of both the chief cells and the capillaries. It is filled by a fluffy, electron-dense material containing numerous bundles of collagen and occasional elastic fibers. Among these fibers are a variety of cells, predominantly fibroblasts with extensive spider-like cytoplasmic processes that are always closely associated with collagen. There are also many pericytes that accompany the vessels (Fig. 24a), but it is the mast cell that is most remarkable. The mast cells contain large amounts of electron-dense granules, which almost completely fill the cytoplasm. In addition, a few monocytic cells and lymphocytes can be identified. Numerous unmyelinated nerve fibers partially enclosed by Schwann cells run parallel to the small arteries and their smooth muscle cells, and show clusters of microvesicles in the axons, as described in the parathyroid glands of the dog (*Yeghiayan* et al., 1972). However, axon bundles next to the parathyroid chief cells or their basement membrane, as mentioned by *Altenähr* (1971), with the functional implication of a direct innervation of the chief cell by autonomic nerves, have not been observed.

VI. Summary

Freeze-fracture morphology of the human parathyroid gland adds considerably to the information obtained by conventional thin sections. A critical examination of the cellular surface is made possible by a direct en-face view, thus allowing an exact assessment of the expansion following changes in endocrine activity. Moreover, the obvious lack of special cell junctions shows that the secretory cycle involves cells individually. The number of nuclear pores acts as an indicator of functional activity and the fine structure of the nucleolus and its changes during protein synthesis supports earlier experimental findings. The presence of few large pores in the cisternae of the rough-surfaced endoplasmic reticulum and areas of changing cisternal membrane structure are likewise confirmed. The bizarre shape of the mitochondria and their increase in number are attributed to energy requirements that follow excessive hormone synthesis in the highly stimulated cells. Study of the fine structure of the Golgi apparatus using extensive serial sectioning in combination with freeze-fracture lends support to the proposal of a dictyosomal arrangement for the saccules, their web-like anastomosing formations in the cells and most important of all, presents evidence of a GERL-like system in the interior or the maturing surface as the source of secretory granule formation and package. The exact course of granule exocytosis is demonstrated by comparison of thin sections and freeze-fracture replicas to take place in several defined steps. Freeze-fracture in particular reveals the exact course of membrane fusion preceding exocytosis.

Large complex bodies in inactive chief cells are shown to consist predominantly of cholesterin compounds, and in addition freeze-fracture suggest γ-subunits in the β-particle of glycogen granules. Evidence of fenestrations in the endothelial cells of the interstitial vessels is demonstrated in both thin sections and freeze-fracture replicas by showing the diaphragm and its central knob. Between endothelial cells discontinuous *zonulae occludentes* are shown, compatible with intercellular junctions of the leaky type. By deduction from experimental observations it is concluded that the transport of the high-molecular-weight parathormone from the extracellular space into the capillary lumen is most likely to occur via the numerous fenestrations of the endothelial layer, thus equating morphologically with the large pore system.

Acknowledgements: We are indebted to Professor *R. Pichlmayr*, Clinic for Abdominal and Transplantation Surgery, Medical School Hanover, for providing the surgical specimens and the clinical data on the patients. We have to thank Professor *E. Reale*, Laboratory of Electron Microscopy, Department of Anatomy, Medical School Hanover, for his encouraging support during the work and his critical review of the manuscript. The excellent technical assistance of Mrs. *M. Rissmann* (thin sections) and Mrs. *G. Voss-Wermbter* and Mr. *H. Heidrich* (freeze-fracture replicas) is gratefully acknowledged.

Note Added in Proof

Recently *Chu* et al. (1977) confirmed that pro-parathormone is transferred from the rough-surfaced endoplasmic reticulum to the Golgi region where its conversion to parathormone occurs. These authors found that this transfer process is independent of the synthesis of the prohormone and its conversion to the final hormone. Moreover this translocation appears to require metabolic energy and is probably mediated by microtubules [Chu, L.L.H., MacGregor, R.R., Cohn, D.V.: Energy-dependent intracellular translocation of proparathormone. J. Cell Biol. **72**, 1-10 (1977)]. A further role for the microtubules in the intracellular movement of secretory granules was shown by *Sherline* et al. (1977) who bound in vitro assembled microtubules to purified porcine pituitary secretory granules and isolated granule membranes [Sherline, P., Lee, Y.-C., Jacobs, L.S.: Binding of microtubules to pituitary secretory granules and secretory granule membranes. J. Cell Biol. **72**, 380-389 (1977)]. Molecular events occurring during the membrane fusion process were studied in the exocytosis of the granules of the rat peritoneal mast cells by *Lawson* et al. (1977). Their results indicate that membrane proteins are displaced laterally into adjacent membrane areas before the fusion process and that membrane fusion occurs between protein-depleted lipid layers [Lawson, D., Raff, M.C., Gomperts, B., Fewtrell, C., Gilula, N.B.: Molecular events during membrane fusion. J. Cell Biol. **72**, 242-259 (1977)]. In a most recent freeze-fracture study *Ravazzola* and *Orci* (1977) describe tight and gap junctions between chief cells of the parathyroid gland in rats [Ravazzola, M., Orci, L.: Intercellular junctions in the rat parathyroid gland: a freeze-fracture study. Biol. Cellulaire **28**, 137-144 (1977)]. The finding of gap junctions strongly suggests an intercellular communication which should probably be interpretated in the light of the somewhat different ultrastructure of the rat parathyroid gland as compared with man (review by *Roth* and *Capen*, 1974).

References

Ainsworth, S.K., Ito, S., Karnovsky, M.J.: Alkaline bismuth reagent for high resolution ultrastructural demonstration of periodate-reactive sites. J. Histochem. Cytochem. 2, 995-1005 (1972).

Akert, K., Moor, H., Pfenninger, K.: Synaptic fine structure. Adv. in Cytopharmacol. 1, 273-289 (1971).

Altenähr, E.: Electron microscopical evidence for innervation of chief cells in human parathyroid gland. Experientia 27, 1077 (1971).

Altenähr, E.: Ultrastructural pathology of parathyroid glands. Curr. Top. Path. 56, 1-54 (1972).

Altmann, H.-W.: Über den Funktionsformwechsel des Kernes im exokrinen Pankreas. Z. Krebsforsch. 58, 632-645 (1952).

Arnaud, C.D.: Immunochemical heterogeneity of circulating parathyroid hormone in man: sequal to an original observation by Berson and Yalow. Mount Sinai J. Med. 40, 422-433 (1973).

Arnaud, C.D., Sizemore, G.W., Oldham, S.B., Fischer, J.A., Tsao, H.S., Littledike, E.T.: Human parathyroid hormone: glandular and secreted molecular species. Amer. J. Med. 50, 630-638 (1971).

Aurbach, G.D., Potts, J.T., Jr., Chase, L.R., Melson, G.L.: Polypeptide hormones and calcium metabolism. NIH clinical staff conference. Ann. Intern. Med. 70, 1243-1265 (1969).

Bannasch, P., Thoenes, W.: Zum Problem der nucleolären Stoffabgabe. Elektronenmikroskopische Untersuchungen am Pankreas der weißen Maus. Z. Zellforsch. 67, 674-692 (1965).

Beams, H.W., Kessel, R.G.: The Golgi apparatus: structure and function. Int. Rev. Cytol. 23, 209-276 (1968).

Berger, W., Dahl, G., Meissner, H.P.: Structural and functional alterations in fused membranes of secretory granules during exocytosis in pancreatic islet cells of the mouse. Cytobiol. 12, 119-139 (1975).

Berson, S.A., Yalow, R.S.: Parathyroid hormone in plasma in adenomatous hyperparathyroidism, uremia, and bronchiogenic carcinoma. Science 154, 907-909 (1966).

Biava, C.: Identification and structural forms of human particulate glycogen. Lab. Invest. 12, 1179-1197 (1963).

Black, W.C.: Correlative light and electron microscopy in primary hyperparathyroidism. Arch. Path. 88, 225-241 (1969).

Boquist, L.: Annulate lamellae in human parathyroid adenoma. Virchows Arch. Abt. B 6, 234-246 (1970).

Branton, D.: Fracture faces of frozen membranes. Proc. nat. Acad. Sci. (Wash.) 55, 1048-1056 (1966).

Breathnach, A.S., Stolinski, C., Gross, M.: Freeze-fracture replication of rough endoplasmic reticulum of mouse liver cells. J. Cell Sci. 2, 477-489 (1972).

Buchheim, W., Welsch, U.: Die Feinstruktur gefriergebrochener Hormongranula. Z. Zellforsch. 131, 429-436 (1972).

Burri, P.H., Weibel, E.R.: Beeinflussung einer spezifischen cytoplasmatischen Organelle von Endothelzellen durch Adrenalin. Z. Zellforsch. 88, 426-440 (1968).

Capen, C.C., Roth, S.I.: Ultrastructural and functional relationships of normal and pathologic parathyroid cells. Pathobiol. Annu. 3, 129-175 (1973).

Caro, L.G., Palade, G.E.: Protein synthesis, storage, and discharge in the pancreatic exocrine cell. An autoradiographic study. J. Cell Biol. 20, 473-495 (1964).

Chalcroft, J.P., Bullivant, S.: An interpretation of liver cell membrane and junction structure based on observation of freeze-fracture replicas of both sides of the fracture. J. Cell Biol. 47, 49-60 (1970).

Claude, P., Goodenough, D.A.: Fracture faces of zonulae occludentes from "tight" and "leaky" epithelia. J. Cell Biol. 58, 390-400 (1973).

Clementi, F., Palade, G.E.: Intestinal capillaries. I. Permeability to peroxidase and ferritin. J. Cell Biol. 41, 33-58 (1969).

Cook, G.M.: The Golgi apparatus: Form and function. In: Lysosomes in Biology and Pathology. J.R. Dingle (ed.). Amsterdam–London: North Holland 1973, pp. 237-277.

Cotran, R.S., Karnovsky, M.J.: Ultrastructural studies on the permeability of the mesothelium to horseradish peroxidase. J. Cell Biol. 37, 123-137 (1968).

Cunningham, W.P., Morré, D.J., Mollenhauer, H.H.: Structure of isolated plant Golgi apparatus revealed by negative staining. J. Cell Biol. 28, 169-179 (1966).

Daems, W.T., Wisse, E.: Shape and attachment of the cristae mitochondriales in mouse hepatic cell mitochondria. J. Ultrastruct. Res. 16, 123-140 (1966).
Daikoku, S., Takahashi, T., Kojimoto, H., Watanabe, Y.G.: Secretory surface phenomena in freeze-etched preparations of the adenohypophysial cells and neurosecretory fibers. Z. Zellforsch. 136, 207-214 (1973).
Deamer, D.W., Leonhard, R., Tardieu, A., Branton, D.: Lamellar and hexogonal lipid phases visualized by freeze-etching. Biochim. biophys. Acta 219, 47-60 (1970).
De Duve, C., Wattiaux, R.: Functions of lysosomes. Ann. Rev. Phys. 28, 453-492 (1966).
Dempsey, G.P., Bullivant, S., Watkin, W.B.: Ultrastructure of the rat posterior pituitary gland and evidence of hormone release by exocytosis as revealed by freeze fracturing. Z. Zellforsch. 143, 465-484 (1973).
Dowell, W.C.T.: Die Entwicklung geeigneter Folien für elektronenmikroskopische Präparationsträger großen Durchlaßbereiches und ihre Verwendung zur Untersuchung von Kristallen. Optik 21, 47-58 (1964).
Dreifuss, J.J., Akert, K., Sandri, C., Moor, H.: Specific arrangements of membrane particles at sites of exo-endocytosis in the freeze-etched neurohypophysis. Cell Tiss. Res. 165, 317-325 (1976).
Drochmans, P.: Morphologie du glycogén: etude au microscope electronique de colorations négatives du glycogén particulaire. J. Ultrastruct. Res. 6, 141-163 (1962).
Eger, W., Lessen, H. van: Beiträge zu einer funktionellen Deutung der Zelltypen menschlicher Epithelkörperchen mit Wertung ihres Verhaltens bei einzelnen Krankheitszuständen. Beitr. path. Anat. 114, 323-354 (1954).
Ehrenreich, J.H., Bergeron, J.J.M., Siekevitz, P., Palade, G.E.: Golgi fraction prepared from rat liver homogenate. I. Isolation procedure and morphological characterization. J. Cell Biol. 59, 45-72 (1973).
Elfin, L.-G.: The ultrastructure of the capillary fenestrae in the adrenal medulla of the rat. J. Ultrastruct. Res. 12, 687-704 (1965).
Elliott, R.L., Arhelger, R.B.: Fine structure of parathyroid adenomas; with special reference to annulate lamellae and septate desmosomes. Arch. Path. 81, 200-212 (1966).
Faccini, J.M.: The ultrastructure of parathyroid glands removed from patients with primary hyperparathyroidism: a report of 40 cases, including four carcinomata. J. Path. 102, 189-199 (1970).
Farquhar, M.G.: Origin and fate of secretory granules in cells of the anterior pituitary gland. Trans. N.Y. Acad. Sci. 23, 346-351 (1961a).
Farquhar, M.G.: Fine structure and function in capillaries of the anterior pituitary gland. Angiology 12, 270-292 (1961b).
Farquhar, M.G.: Lysosome function in regulation secretion: disposal of secretory granules in cells of the anterior pituitary gland. In: Lysosomes in Biology and Pathology. J.T. Dingle, H.B. Fell (eds.). Amsterdam-London: North Holland 1969, pp. 462-482.
Favard, P.: The Golgi apparatus. In: Handbook of Molecular Cytology, Lime-de-Faria, A. (ed.). Amsterdam-London: North Holland 1969, pp. 1130-1155.
Fawcett, D.W., Long, J.A., Jones, A.L.: The ultrastructure of endocrine glands. Recent Progr. Hormone Res. 25, 315-368 (1969).
Fineran, B.A.: Organization of the Golgi apparatus in frozen-etched root tips. Cytobiol. 8, 175-183 (1973).
Fleischer, B., Fleischer, S., Ozawa, H.: Isolation and characterization of Golgi membranes from bovine liver. J. Cell Biol. 43, 59-79 (1969).
Flickinger, C.J.: Fenestrated cisternae in the Golgi apparatus of the epididymis. Anat. Rec. 163, 39-54 (1969).
Friederici, H.H.R.: The tridimensional ultrastructure of fenestrated capillaries. J. Ultrastruct. Res. 23, 444-456 (1968).
Friederici, H.H.R.: On the diaphragm across fenestrae of capillary endothelium. J. Ultrastruct. Res. 27, 373-375 (1969).
Fuchs, A., Weibel, E.R.: Morphometrische Untersuchung der Verteilung einer spezifischen cytoplasmatischen Organelle in Endothelzellen der Ratte. Z. Zellforsch. 73, 1-9 (1966).
Golgi, C.: Sur la structure des cellules nerveuses. Arch. Ital. Biol. 30, 60-71 (1898a).
Golgi, C.: Sur la structure des cellules nerveuses des ganglions spinaux. Arch. Ital. Biol. 30, 278-286 (1898b).
Gusek, W.: Die Ultrastruktur Cycasin-induzierter Nierenadenome. Virchows Arch. Abt. A 365, 221-237 (1975).
Habener, J.F., Powell, D., Murray, T.M., Mayer, G.P., Potts, J.T., Jr.: Parathyroid hormone: secretion and metabolism in vivo. Proc. nat. Acad. Sci. (Wash.) 68, 2986-2991 (1971).

Hamilton, J.W., Cohn, D.W.: Studies on the biosynthesis in vitro of parathyroid hormone. J. biol. Chem. 244, 5421-5429 (1969).
Heimann, P., Hansson, G., Nilsson, O.: Primary hyperparathyroidism in a case of oxyphilic adenoma. Acta path. microbiol. scand. A 79, 10-14 (1971).
Hesch, R.D., McIntosh, C.H.S., Woodhead, J.S.: New aspects of radioimmunochemical measurement of human parathyroid hormone using the labelled antibody technique. Horm. Metab. Res. 7, 347-352 (1975).
Hirano, A., Tomiyasu, U., Zimmerman, H.M.: The fine structure of blood vessels in chromophobe adenoma. Acta neuropath. (Berl.) 22, 200-207 (1972).
Hodson, S., Brenchley, G.: Similarities of the Golgi apparatus membrane and the plasma membrane in rat liver cells. J. Cell Sci. 20, 167-182 (1976).
Holtzman, E., Novikoff, A.B., Villaverde, H.: Lysosomes and GERL in normal and chromatolytic neurons of the rat ganglion nodosum. J. Cell Biol. 33, 419-435 (1967).
Jacobs, J.W., Kemper, B., Niall, H.D., Habener, J.F., Potts, J.T., Jr.: Structural analysis of human proparathyroid hormone by a new microsequencing approach. Nature 249, 155-157 (1974).
Jamieson, J.D., Palade, G.E.: Intercellular transport by secretory proteins in the pancreatic exocrine cell. I. Role of the peripheral elements of the Golgi complex. J.Cell Biol. 34, 577-596 (1967a).
Jamieson, J.D., Palade, G.E.: Intercellular transport of secretory proteins in the pancreatic exocrine cell. II. Transport to condensing vacuoles and zymogen granules. J. Cell Biol. 34, 597-615 (1967b).
Kemper, B., Habener, J.F., Potts, J.T., Jr., Rich, A.: Pro-parathyroid hormone: identification of a biosynthetic precursor to parathyroid hormone. Proc. nat. Acad. Sci. (Wash.) 69, 643-647 (1972).
Kemper, B., Habener, J.F., Rich, A., Potts, J.T., Jr.: Microtubules and the intracellular conversion of proparathyroid hormone to parathyroid hormone. Endocrinology 96, 903-912 (1975).
Kühn, K., Reale, E., Wermbter, G.: The glomeruli of the human and the rat kidney studied by freeze-fracturing. Cell Tiss. Res. 160, 177-191 (1975).
Kurosumi, K.: Electron microscopic analysis of the secretion mechanism. Int. Rev. Cytol. 2, 1-124 (1961).
Lacy, P.E.: The pancreatic beta cell: structure and function. New Engl. J. Med. 276, 187-195 (1967).
Lacy, P.E., Howell, S.L., Young, D.A., Fink, C.J.: New hypothesis of insulin secretion. Nature 219, 1177-1179 (1968).
Landis, E.M., Pappenheimer, J.R.: Exchange of substances through the capillary walls. In: Handbook of Physiology, Section 2: Circulation (Hamilton, D.C., Dow, P., eds.). Washington, D.C.: American Physiology Society 1963, Vol. 2, pp. 1013-1034.
Leak, L.V.: Frozen-fractured images of blood capillaries in heart tissue. J. Ultrastruct. Res. 35, 127-146 (1971).
Leloir, L.F., Goldemberg, S.H.: Synthesis of glycogen from uridine diphosphate glucose in the liver. J. biol. Chem. 235, 919-923 (1960).
Lemeunier, A., Burri, P.H., Weibel, E.R.: Absence of acid phosphatase activity in specific endothelial organelles. Histochemie 20, 143-149 (1969).
Liddle, G.W., Hardman, J.G.: Cyclic adenosine monophosphate as a mediator of hormone action. N. Engl. J. Med. 285, 560-566 (1971).
Luck, D.J.L.: Glycogen synthesis from uridine diphosphate glucose. The distribution of the enzyme in liver cell fractions. J. biophys. biochem. Cytol. 10, 195-209 (1961).
Luft, J.H.: Improvements in epoxy resin embedding methods. J. biophys. biochem. Cytol. 9, 409-414 (1961).
Malaisse, W.J.: Role of microtubules in hormone biosynthesis. V. Internat. Congr. Endocrinology, Hamburg, July 18-24 (1976).
Marshall, R.B., Roberts, D.K., Turner, R.A.: Adenomas of the human parathyroid. Light and electron microscopy study following selenium 75 methionine scan. Cancer 20, 512-524 (1967).
Matsuda, H., Sugiura, S.: Ultrastructure of "tubular body" in the endothelial cells of the ocular blood vessels. Invest. Ophthalmol. 9, 919-925 (1970).
Maul, G.: Structure and formation of pores in fenestrated capillaries. J. Ultrastruct. Res. 36, 768-782 (1971).
Maul, G.G., Price, J.W., Liebermann, M.W.: Formation and distribution of nuclear pore complexes in interphase. J. Cell Biol. 51, 405-418 (1971).

McNutt, N.S., Weinstein, R.S.: The ultrastructure of the nexus. A correlated thin-section and freeze-cleave study. J. Cell Biol. 47, 666-688 (1970).

McNutt, N.S., Weinstein, R.S.: Membrane ultrastructure at mammalian intercellular junctions. Progr. Biophys. mol. Biol. 26, 45-101 (1973).

Millonig, G.: Advantages of a phosphate buffer for OsO_4 solutions in fixation. J. appl. Phys. 32, 1637 (1961).

Mollenhauer, H.H., Whaley, W.G.: An observation on the functioning of the Golgi apparatus. J. Cell Biol. 17, 222-225 (1963).

Moor, H., Mühlethaler, K.: Fine structure in frozen-etched yeast cells. J. Cell Biol. 17, 609-628 (1963).

Morré, D.J., Mollenhauer, H.H., Bracker, C.E.: Origin and continuity of Golgi apparatus. In: Origin and Continuity of Cell Organelles (Reinert, J., Ursprung, H., eds.). Berlin-Heidelberg-New York: Springer 1971.

Munger, B.L., Roth, S.I.: The cytology of the normal parathyroid glands of man and Virginia deer. A light and electron microscopy study with morphological evidence of secretory activity. J. Cell Biol. 16, 379-400 (1963).

Nakagami, K., Warshawsky, H., Leblond, C.P.: The elaboration of protein and carbohydrate by rat parathyroid cells as revealed by electron microscope radioautography. J. Cell Biol. 51, 596-610 (1971).

Nickel, E., Grieshaber, E.: Elektronenmikroskopische Darstellung der Muskelkapillaren im Gefrierätzbild. Z. Zellforsch. 95, 445-461 (1969).

Northcote, D.H.: The Golgi complex. In: Cell Biology in Medicine (Bittar, E.E., ed.). New York-London-Sydney-Toronto: Wiley 1973, pp. 197-214.

Novikoff, P.M., Novikoff, A.B., Quintana, N., Hauw, J.-J.: Golgi apparatus, GERL, and lysosomes of neurons in rat dorsal root ganglia, studied by thick section and thin section cytochemistry. J. Cell Biol. 50, 859-886 (1971).

Nunez, E.A., Whalen, J.P., Krook, L.: An ultrastructural study of the natural secretory cycle of the parathyroid gland of the bat. Amer. J. Anat. 134, 459-480 (1972).

Orci, L., Unger, R.H., Renold, A.E.: Structural coupling between pancreatic islet cells. Experimentia 29, 1015-1018 (1972a).

Orci, L., Perrelet, A., Like, A.A.: Fenestrae in the rough endoplasmic reticulum of the exocrine pancreatic cells. J. Cell Biol. 55, 245-249 (1972b).

Orci, L., Malaisse-Lagae, F., Ravazzola, M., Amherdt, M.: Exocytosis-endocytosis coupling in the pancreatic beta cell. Science 181, 561-562 (1973a).

Orci, L., Amherdt, M., Malaisse-Lagae, F., Rouiller, C., Renold, A.E.: Insulin release by emiocytosis: demonstration with freeze-etching technique. Science 179, 82-84 (1973b).

Orci, L., Malaisse-Lagae, F., Amherdt, M., Ravazzola, M., Weisswange, A., Dobbs, R., Perrelet, A., Unger, R.: Cell contacts in human islets of Langerhans. J. clin. Endocrinol. Metab. 41, 841-844 (1975).

O'Riordan, J.L.H., Potts, J.T., Jr., Aurbach, G.D.: Isolation of human parathyroid hormone. Endocrinology 89, 234-239 (1971).

Palade, G.E.: Structure and function at the cellular level. J. Amer. med. Ass. 198, 815-825 (1966).

Peachey, L.D.: Electron microscopic observations on the accumulation of divalent cations in intramitochondrial granules. J. Cell Biol. 20, 95-109 (1964).

Perkin, A.B., Bader, H.J., Tashgian, A.H., Jr., Goldhaber, P.: Immunofluorescent localization of parathyroid hormone in extracellular spaces of the bovine parathyroid gland. Proc. Soc. exp. Biol. Med. (N.Y.) 128, 218-221 (1968).

Pinto da Silva, P.: Translational mobility of the membrane intercalated particles of human erythrocyte ghosts: pH-dependent, reversible aggregation. J. Cell Biol. 53, 777-787 (1972).

Polyzonis, M.B.: Ultrastructural study of human parathyroid adenoma and the occurrence of abnormal cilia in the adenoma cells. Path. europ. 5, 454-469 (1970).

Potts, J.T., Jr., Buckle, R.M., Sherwood, L.M., Ramberg, C.F., Jr., Mayer, C.P., Kronfeld, D.S., Deftos, L.J., Care, A.D., Aurbach, G.D.: Control of secretion of parathyroid hormone. In: Parathyroid Hormone and Thyrocalcitonin (Calcitonin) (Talmage, R.V., Belanger, L.F., eds.). Amsterdam: Excerpta Med. Found. 1968, pp. 407-416.

Potts, J.T., Jr., Reitz, R.E., Deftos, L.J., Kaye, M.B., Richardson, J.A., Buckle, R.M., Aurbach, G.D.: Secondary hyperparathyroidism in chronic renal disease. Arch. intern. Med. 124, 408-412 (1969).

Rambourg, A., Chretien, M.: L'appareil de Golgi: examen en microscopie électronique de coupes épaisses (0,5-1 μ), après impregnation des tissues par la tétroxyde d'osmium. C.R. Acad. Sci. Paris 270, 981-983 (1970).

Rambourg, A., Marraud, A., Chretien, M.: Tri-dimensional structure of the forming face of the Golgi apparatus as seen in the high voltage electron microscope after osmium impregnation of the small nerve cells in the semilunar ganglion of the trigeminal nerve. J. Microscopy (Oxf.) 97, 49-57 (1973).
Rambourg, A., Marraud, A., Clermount, Y.: Three-dimensional aspects of the forming face of the Golgi apparatus as seen in the high voltage electron microscope after osmium impregnation. Proceedings of the 3rd International Congress on High Voltage Electron Microscopy, Oxford, 1974, pp. 419-422.
Raisz, L.G.: Parathyroid gland metabolism. Arch. intern. Med. 124, 389-396 (1969).
Reale, E., Luciano, L.: Beobachtungen an parallel zur Lage der Sacculi des Golgiapparates geführten Schnitten. J. Microscopie 3, 545-550 (1964).
Reynolds, E.S.: The use of lead citrate at high pH as an electron-opaque stain in electron microscopy. J. Cell Biol. 17, 208-212 (1963).
Rhodin, J.A.G.: The diaphragm of capillary endothelial fenestrations. J. Ultrastruct. Res. 6, 171-185 (1962).
Rohr, H.P., Krässig, B.: Elektronenmikroskopische Untersuchungen über den Sekretionsmodus des Parathormons. Beitrag zu einer lysosomalen Mitbeteiligung bei Sekretionsvorgängen in endokrinen Drüsen. Z. Zellforsch. 85, 271-290 (1968).
Roth, S.I., Capen, C.C.: Ultrastructural and functional correlations of the parathyroid gland. Int. Rev. exp. Path. 14, 161-221 (1974).
Roth, S.I., Munger, B.L.: The cytology of the adenomatous, atrophic, and hyperplastic parathyroid glands of man. A light- and electron-microscopic study. Virchows Arch. Abt. A 335, 389-410 (1962).
Roth, S.I., Raisz, L.G.: Effect of calcium concentration on the ultrastructure of rat parathyroid in organ culture. Lab. Invest. 13, 331-345 (1964).
Roth, S.I., Raisz, L.G.: The course and reversibility of the calicum effect on the ultrastructure of the rat parathyroid gland in organ culture. Lab. Invest. 15, 1187-1211 (1966).
Ruska, H., Ruska, C., Meyer-Delpho, W.: Das Gefrierätzbild von Lipidablagerungen in der Aortenintima cholesteringefütterter Kaninchen. Virchows Arch. Abt. B 11, 279-283 (1972).
Satir, B., Schooley, C., Satir, P.: Membrane fusion in a model system. Mucocyst secretion in Tetrahymena. J. Cell Biol. 56, 153-176 (1973).
Sengel, A., Stoebner, P.: Golgi origin of tubular inclusions in endothelial cells. J. Cell Biol. 44, 223-226 (1970).
Silverman, R., Yalow, R.S.: Heterogeneity of parathyroid hormone. J. clin. Invest. 52, 1958-1971 (1973).
Simionescu, M., Simionescu, N., Palade, G.E.: Morphometric data on the endothelium of blood capillaries. J. Cell Biol. 60, 128-152 (1974).
Simionescu, M., Simionescu, N., Palade, G.E.: Segmental differentiations of cell junctions in the vascular endothelium. The microvasculature. J. Cell Biol. 67, 863-885 (1975).
Simionescu, M., Simionescu, N., Palade, G.E.: Segmental differentiatons of cell junctions in the vascular endothelium. Arteries and veins. J. Cell. Biol. 68, 705-723 (1976).
Smith, R.E., Farquhar, M.G.: Lysosome function in the regulation of the secretory process in cells of the anterior pituitary gland. J. Cell Biol. 31, 319-347 (1966).
Spitznas, M., Reale, E.: Fracture faces of fenestrations and junctions of endothelial cells in human choroidal vessels. Invest. Ophthalmol. 14, 98-107 (1975).
Spooner, B.S., Yamada, K., Wessels, N.K.: Microfilaments and cell locomotion. J. Cell Biol. 49, 595-613 (1972).
Staehelin, L.A.: Structure and function of intercellular junctions. Int. Rev. Cytol. 39, 191-283 (1974).
Staehelin, L.A.: A new occludens-like junction linking endothelial cells of small capillaries (probably venules) of rat jejunum. J. Cell Biol. 18, 545-551 (1975).
Thiele, J., Georgii, A., Reale, E.: Über Unterschiede in der cellulären Feinstruktur von Nebenschilddrüsen bei schweren und leichten Formen des sekundären Hyperparathyreoidismus. Klin. Wschr. 52, 444-450 (1974).
Thiele, J., Hehrmann, R., Reale, E.: Freeze-fracture of the thyroid follicle cells under different functional conditions. In: Biochemical Basis of Thyroid Stimulation and Thyroid Hormone Action (Mühlen, A. v. zur, Schleusener, H., eds.). Stuttgart: Thieme 1976, pp. 101-114.
Thiele, J., Pichlmayr, R.: Der akute Hyperparathyreoidismus bei primärer Wasserheller-Zellen-Hyperplasie. Klin. Wschr. 52, 1063-1069 (1974).

Thiele, J., Reale, E.: Freeze-fracture study of the junctional complexes of human and rabbit thyroid follicles. Cell Tiss. Res. **168**, 133-140 (1976).
Thiele, J., Reale, E., Georgii, A.: Elektronenmikroskopische Befunde an Epithelkörperadenomen unterschiedlicher endokriner Aktivität. Virchows Arch. Abt. B **12**, 168-188 (1973a).
Thiele, J., Reale, E., Georgii, A.: Ein Beitrag zur Feinstruktur von endokrin aktiven Epithelkörpercarcinomen. Virchows Arch. Abt. B **13**, 153-168 (1973b).
Thiele, J., Reale, E., Hehrmann, R.: Rodent thyroid gland: a freeze-fracture study under normal and experimental conditions with special reference to parafollicular cells and vessels. Cell Tiss. Res. (submitted) 1977.
Thiele, J., Ries, P., Georgii, A.: Spezielle und funktionelle Pathomorphologie der Epithelkörperchen in einem unausgewählten Obduktionsgut (589 Sektionen). Virchows Arch. Abt. A **367**, 195-208 (1975).
Thiele, J., Wermbter, G.: Die Feinstruktur der aktivierten Hauptzelle der menschlichen Parathyreoidea. Eine Darstellung mit Hilfe der Gefrierätztechnik. Virchows Arch. Abt. B **15**, 251-265 (1974).
Thiery, J.-P.: Mise en évidence des polysaccharides sur coupes fines en microscopie électronique. J. Microscopie **6**, 987-1018 (1967).
Thiery, J.-P.: Role de l'appareil de Golgi dans la synthèse des mucopolysaccharides, étude cytochemique. I. Mise en évidence de mucopolysaccharides dans le vésicules de transition entre l'ergastoplasme et l'appareil de Golgi. J. Microscopie **8**, 689-708 (1969).
Thoenes, W., Grossrau, E., Altmann, H.-W.: Untersuchungen zum Feinbau des Nukleolus tierischer Somazellen auf Grund von Modellstudien. Cytobiol. **6**, 150-162 (1972).
Tomiyasu, U., Hirano, A., Zimmermann, H.M.: Fine structure of human pituitary adenoma. Arch. Pathol. **95**, 287-292 (1973).
Trier, J.S.: The fine structure of the parathyroid gland. J. biophys. biochem. Cytol. **4**, 13-22 (1958).
Wanson, J.-C., Tielemans, L.: Morphological and biochemical characteristics of glycogen particles isolated from rabbit polymorphonuclear leucocytes. J. Cell Biol. **49**, 816-829 (1971).
Watson, M.L.: Staining of tissue sections for electron microscopy with heavy metals. J. biophys. biochem. Cytol. **4**, 475-478 (1958).
Weibel, E.R., Palade, G.E.: New cytoplasmic components in arterial endothelia. J. Cell Biol. **23**, 101-112 (1964).
Weinbach, E.C., Brand, Th. von: Formation, isolation and composition of dense granules from mitochondria. Biochem. biophys. Acta (Amst.) **148**, 256-266 (1967).
Whaley, W.G., Dauwalder, M., Kephart, J.E.: Assembly, continuity, and exchange in certain cytoplasmatic membrane systems. In: Origin and Continuity of Cell Organelles (Reinert, J., Ursprung, H., eds.). Berlin-Heidelberg-New York: Springer, 1971, pp. 1-45.
William, H., Fletcher, J., Robertson, J.D., Everett, J.W.: Freeze-fracture studies of membrane specializations in the rat anterior pituitary. V. Internat. Congr. Endocrinology, Hamburg, July 18-24 (1976).
Wrigglesworth, J.M., Packer, L., Branton, D.: Organization of mitochondrial structure as revealed by freeze-etching. Biochim. biophys. Acta **205**, 125-135 (1970).
Yamamoto, K., Fujimoto, S., Takeshige, Y.: The fine structure of endothelial cells in freeze-fracture preparations. J. Ultrastruct. Res. **54**, 22-28 (1976).
Yee, A.G., Revel, J.P.: Endothelial cell junctions. J. Cell Biol. **66**, 200-204 (1975).
Yeghiayan, E., Rojo-Ortega, J.M., Genest, J.: Parathyroid vessels innervation: an ultrastructural study. J. Anat. **112**, 137-142 (1972).
Zeigel, R.F., Dalton, A.J.; Speculations based on the morphology of the Golgi systems in several types of protein-secreting cells. J. Cell Biol. **15**, 45-54 (1962).

Malignant Nephrosclerosis in Patients with Hemolytic Uremic Syndrome (Primary Malignant Nephrosclerosis)

A. BOHLE*, U. HELMCHEN, K.E. GRUND, H.-V. GÄRTNER, D. MEYER, K.D. BOCK, M. BULLA, P. BÜNGER, L. DIEKMANN, U. FROTSCHER, K. HAYDUK, W. KÖSTERS, M. STRAUCH, F. SCHELER and H. CHRIST

Introduction

Schürmann and *MacMahon* (1933) were the first authors to believe that two forms of malignant nephrosclerosis exist. They noted that one form begins insidiously with generalized vasomotor disturbances and gradually develops towards essential hypertension and ends in renal insufficiency. The authors called this form "genuine or endogenous malignant nephrosclerosis." According to their description, the second form begins with acute renal disturbances, hypertension only developing in later stages. *Schürmann* and *MacMahon* chose the term "exogenous or toxic malignant nephrosclerosis" for this form of the disease.

The attention *Schürmann* and *MacMahon*'s study received at that time was limited. It is, therefore, not surprising that a variety of terms has been used in recent years to describe "exogenous malignant nephrosclerosis": "malignant nephrosclerosis in women" (*Scheer* and *Jones*, 1967), "irreversible post partum renal failure. A new syndrome" (*Robson* et al., 1968), "accelerated nephrosclerosis and post partum acute renal failure in normotensive patients" (*Wagoner* et al., 1968), "Renal cortical thrombotic microangiopathy" (*Hammond* et al., 1970), "The haemolytic uremic syndrome in adults" (*Clarkson* et al., 1970), "Post partum renal failure with microangiopathic hemolytic anemia" (*Luke* et al., 1970; *Ponticelli* et al., 1972), "Microangiopathie thrombotique rénale" (*Habib* et al., 1969; *Sraer* et al., 1974), "Oliguric acute renal failure in malignant hypertension" (*Mattern* et al., 1972),

* Supported by the Deutsche Forschungsgemeinschaft.

"Post partum renal failure and haemolytic uremic syndrome" (*Meadows* and *Lawrence*, 1972), "Idiopathic post partum renal failure" (*Sun* et al., 1975), "Malignant nephrosclerosis during pregnancy and in the post partum period (the uremic hemolytic syndrome)" (*Beller* et al., 1976).

From 1969 to 1973 we observed *Schürmann* and *MacMahon*'s "exogenous malignant nephrosclerosis" in 22 patients. Some of these patients were normotensive, others were hypertensive for a short time. We called this form "primary malignant nephrosclerosis" (PMN), as opposed to the "secondary malignant nephrosclerosis" (SMN) which is induced by accelerated hypertension (*Bohle* et al., 1973, 1974; *Bohle* and *Helmchen*, 1975; *Bohle* et al., 1976b).

In the present study we would like to add electron microscopic and immunofluorescent findings in a greater number of patients. Morphological and clinical results of PMN will be discussed and an attempt will be made to differentiate our findings from those found in other renal angiopathies.

II. Material and Methods

The investigations were carried out on kidneys of a total of 84 patients.* Organs other than the kidney (liver, spleen, lung, heart, adrenals and intestine) were studied in 14 of the 84 patients. For light microscopy, paraffin sections 5-8 μm thick were stained with the PAS reaction or according to Goldner-Trichrome respectively, and methacrylate sections 0,5 μm thick were stained by silver impregnation according to *Movat* (1961). Material for electron microscopy was obtained from 19 patients, and material for immunofluorescent microscopy from 21 patients.

III. Results

1. Morphology

a) Light Microscopy

Lesions that are typical of PMN were divided into early and late. Between acute or early stages and chronic or late stages, transitional stages can also be observed.

Typical early lesions of PMN observed in biopsies obtained from patients during the first days or weeks of the disease were a stenosing intimal edema of the interlobular arteries and of the *vasa afferentia* with or without hemorrhage into the vascular wall (Fig. 1), a fibrinoid necrosis of the vascular wall in the same region with or without thrombosis or hemorrhage

---

* For supplying us with clinical data we would like to thank Prof. Dr. H.H. Edel, München-Harlaching, Dr. R. Fischer, Hamburg-Barmbek, Dr. H.K. Fischer, Passau, Prof. Dr. J. Gayer, Bremen, Prof. Dr. D. Harms, Kiel, Prof. Dr. H. Hartert, Kaiserslautern, Prof. Dr. F. Heni, Tübingen, Prof. Dr. W. Künzer, Freiburg, Prof. Dr. H. Losse, Münster, Prof. Dr. H. Otto, Dortmund, Dr. K. Potjan, Bremen, Prof. Dr. E. Quellhorst, Hann.-Münden, Prof. Dr. W. Remmele, Wiesbaden, Prof. Dr. E. Renner, Köln-Merheim, Prof. Dr. D. Renner, Augsburg, Prof. Dr. J. Schirmeister, Karlsruhe, Prof. Dr. P. Schollmeyer, Freiburg, Dr. E. Streicher, Stuttgart.

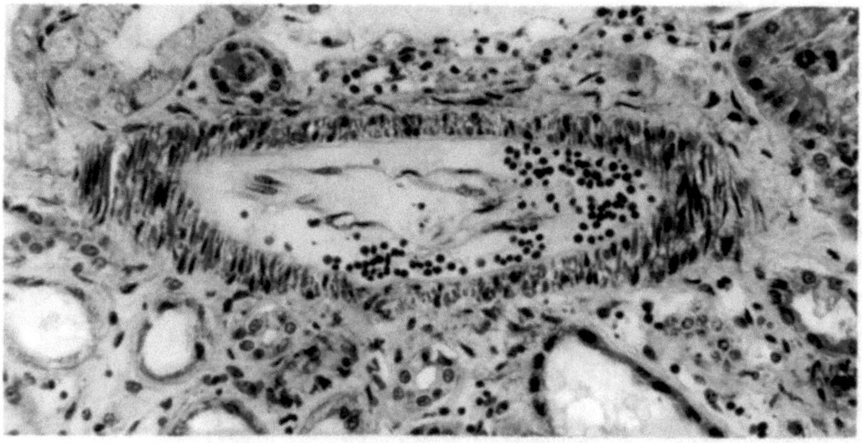

Fig. 1. 361/69, 24 years, female. Primary malignant nephrosclerosis. Stenosing intimal edema with hemorrhage into the intima (erythrocytes and fragmentocytes). (Goldner trichrome 210:1)

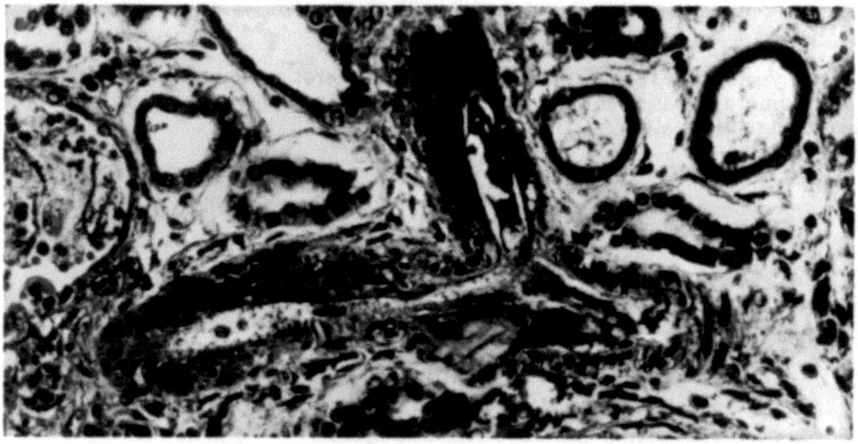

Fig. 2. 361/69, 24 years, female. Fibrinoid necrosis of two afferent arterioles. (Goldner trichrome 285:1)

(Fig. 2), and a usually slight glomerular cell proliferation with swelling or fatty degeneration of the endothelial cells. Furthermore, acute changes such as thickening, wrinkling and focal or diffuse splitting of the glomerular capillary basement membrane were also observed (Fig. 3). Fibrin thrombi in a few capillaries, and fragmentocytes in the capillary convolution occasionally also became apparent (Fig. 4). In the region of the podocytes, hyaline droplets appeared often at this stage. In addition, focal fibrinoid capillary wall necrosis was seen with thrombosis especially in the proximity of the hilus (Fig. 5b).

Tubular lesions similar to those found in biopsies or postmortem examinations of acute renal failure were typical of the early stages of PMN (Fig. 5a, b). The most prominent lesions observed at postmortem examinations were a widening of the lumina of the proximal tubules

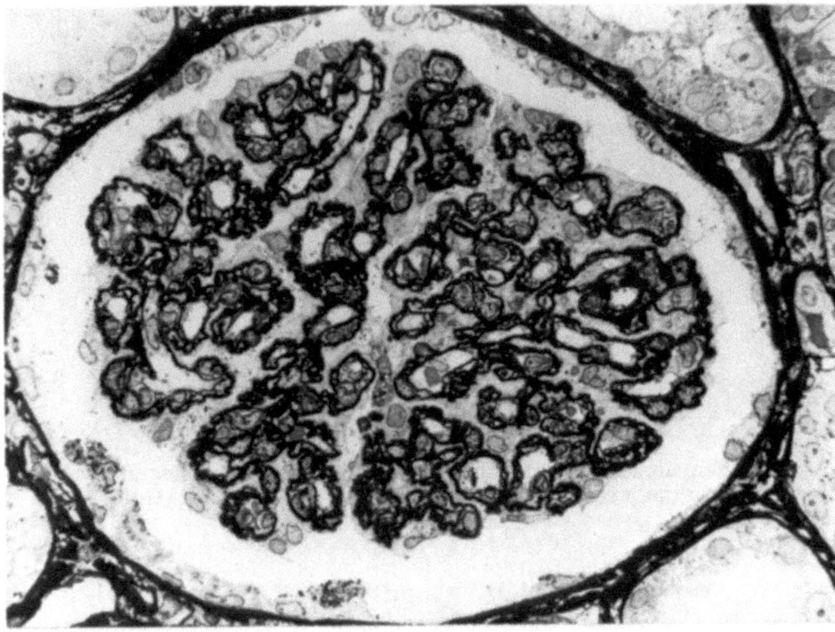

Fig. 3. 7081556, 30 years, male. Primary malignant nephrosclerosis. Slight hypercellularity of cells inside the glomerular basement membrane. Wrinkling and splitting of the basement membrane. (Semithin section, MOVAT silver impregnation, 570:1)

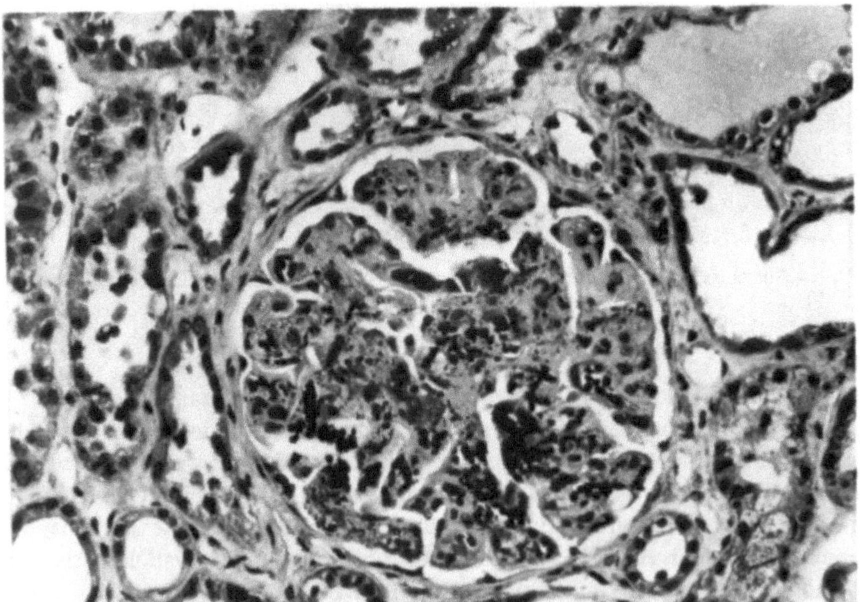

Fig. 4. 7441292, 8 years, male. Primary malignant nephrosclerosis. Numerous fragmentocytes in glomerular capillaries. Sporadic precipitation of fibrin (dark) in narrowed lumina of capillaries. (Goldner trichrome, 225:1)

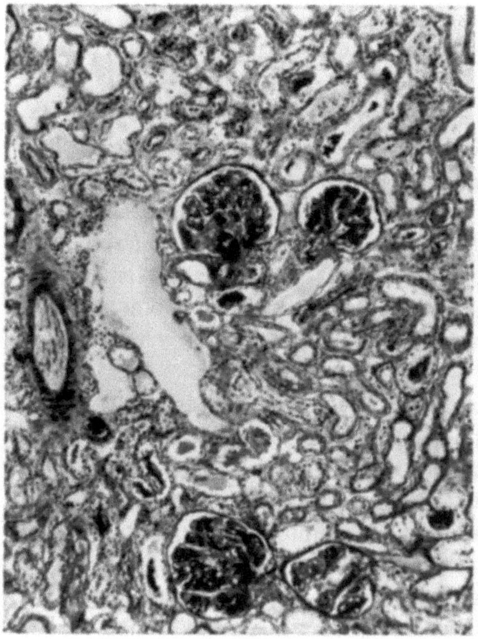

a

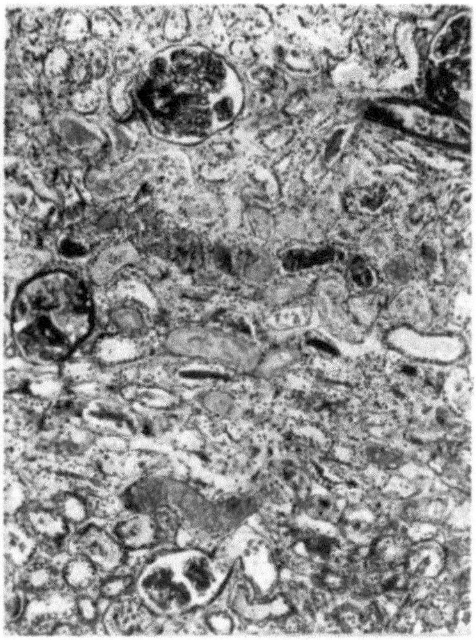

b

Fig. 5a and b. 361/69, 24 years, female. Primary malignant nephrosclerosis. (a) Wide open lumina of proximal tubules, as in acute renal failure (autopsy material). Fibrinoid necroses in the hilar region of glomerula. Stenosing intimal edema of an interlobular artery (left). (b) Focal tubular necroses. Fibrinoid necrosis in the region of the glomerular hilus (above). (Goldner trichrome, 90:1; reduced to 75%)

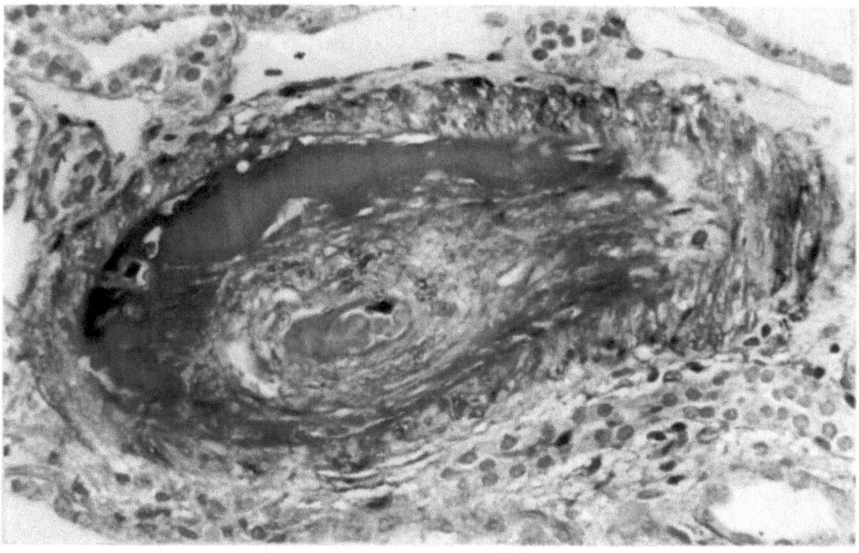

Fig. 6. 721603, 13 years, female. Primary malignant nephrosclerosis (transitional stage). Branch of an interlobular artery with intimal edema in the process of organization. New production of a second wall of the vessel in the subendothelial region of the intimal edema. (Goldner trichrome, 310:1)

and a patchy tubular cell necrosis. In biopsies, however, the commonest findings were epithelial cell swelling, occasional focal tubular necrosis, and tubular regeneration (*Bohle* 1965, 1967; *Bohle* et al., 1964, 1976a).

The transitional stage of PMN was characterized by an organizing process originating from the subendothelial lining of the vessel wall. At this stage new subendothelial wall structures developed and/or signs of obliterating endarteritis with localized persisting edema of the intima became apparent (Fig. 6). Additionally, the glomerular basement membrane was often wrinkled and appeared to be thick when examined by light microscopy. Splitting of the glomerular basement membrane could also be observed. The glomerular basement membrane changes were often absent, however, when severe preglomerular vascular lesions occurred. Slight tubular atrophy and some interstitial fibrosis were also found in the transitional stage (Fig. 7).

In the chronic stage of PMN the most prominent lesions were an obliterating endarteritis and endarteriolitis in the interlobular arteries and *vasa afferentia*, respectively (Fig. 8), with or without hemorrhage into the vascular wall or fibrous vascular occlusions (Fig. 9). At this stage, the glomeruli usually showed distinct thickening and wrinkling of the capillary wall, with shrinking of the capillaries in the vicinity of the hilar region. Focal or diffuse splitting of the glomerular basement membrane was often observed (Fig. 10).

Cells of unknown origin were found between the basement membrane structures that appeared to be split at the periphery of the glomerular capillaries. A small number of segmentally or totally obliterated glomerula likewise appeared in the chronic stage of PMN. Very rarely, similar changes to those seen in hypertensive glomerulopathy were found

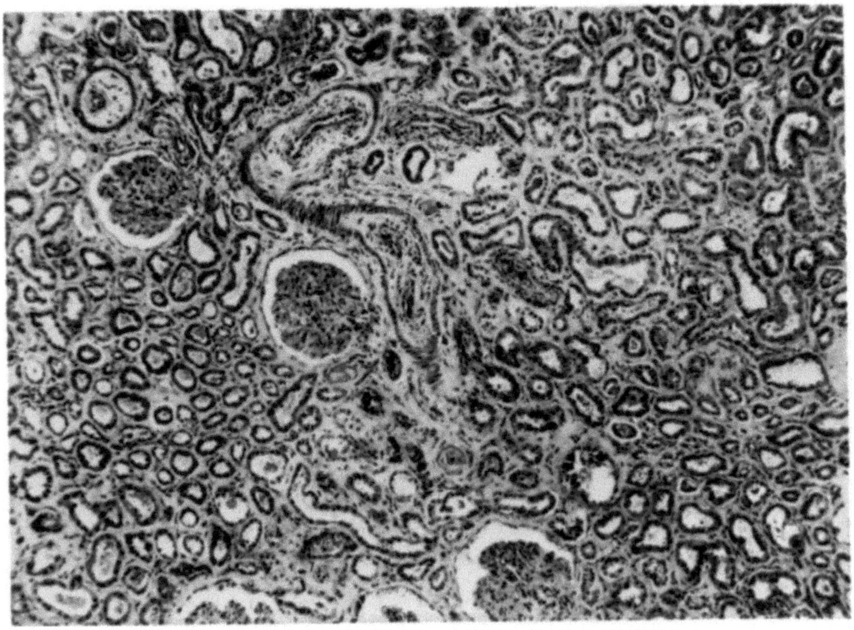

Fig. 7. 69927, 38 years, male. Primary malignant nephrosclerosis (transitional stage). Intimal edema in the process of organization (interlobular artery in the center). Tubular atrophy, diffuse interstitial fibrosis. (Goldner trichrome, 90:1)

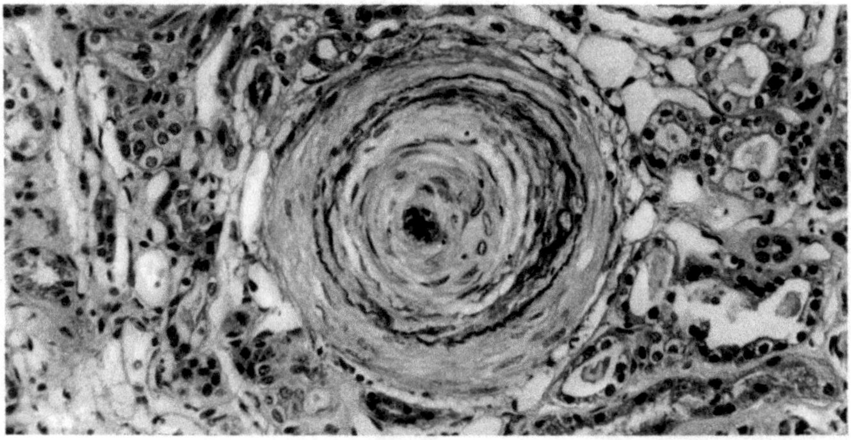

Fig. 8. Primary malignant nephrosclerosis (chronic stage). Interlobular artery with completely organized intimal edema (i.e. obliterating endarteritis). (Goldner trichrome, 210:1)

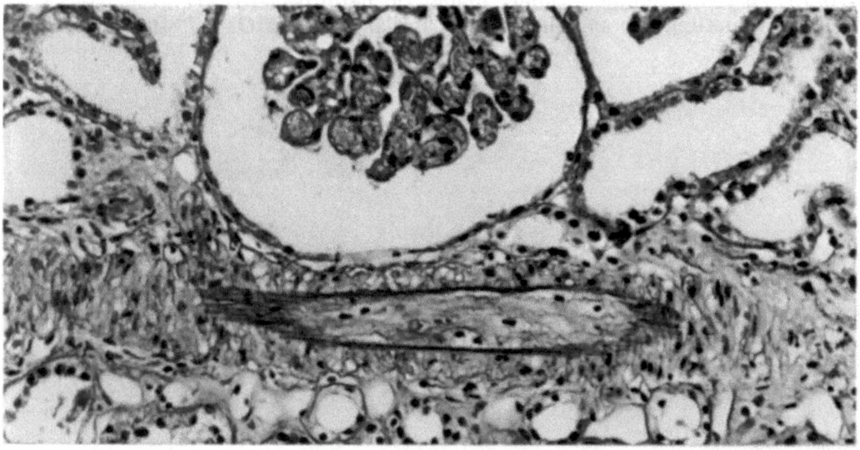

Fig. 9. 707886, 19 years, female. Primary malignant nephrosclerosis (chronic stage). Fibrous obliteration of a branch of an interlobular artery. Splitting and wrinkling of glomerular capillaries, wide open tubules. (Elastica-van Gieson, 210:1)

(Fig. 11) (*Meyer* et al., 1973). Tubular atrophy developed in later stages as a result of the vascular lesions and/or the residual damage caused by the initial acute renal failure. The interstitium was often distinctly widened in the above-mentioned stages.

b) Electron Microscopy

In order to supplement the light microscopy results, electron microscopic studies were carried out on biopsies obtained from 19 patients with PMN two to 10 weeks after hospitalization. They revealed that the pronounced swelling of the endothelial cells (Fig. 12)

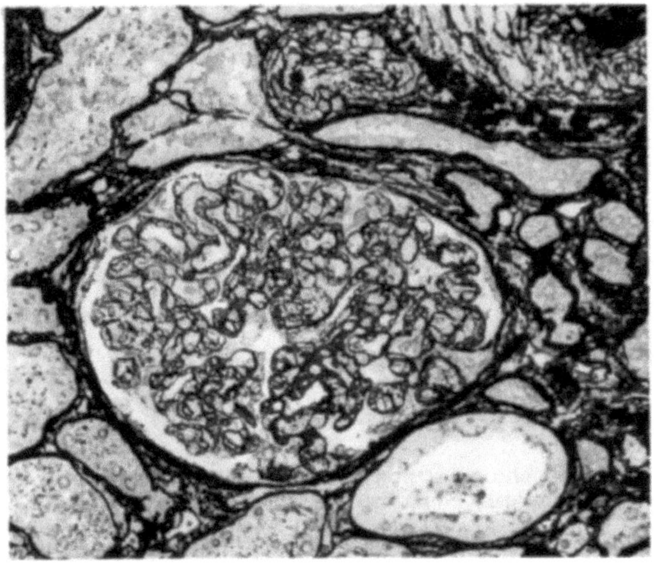

Fig. 10. K 5470/75, 24 years, female. Primary malignant nephrosclerosis (chronic stage). Glomerulus showing wrinkling and splitting of the capillary wall. (MOVAT-silver impregnation, 300:1)

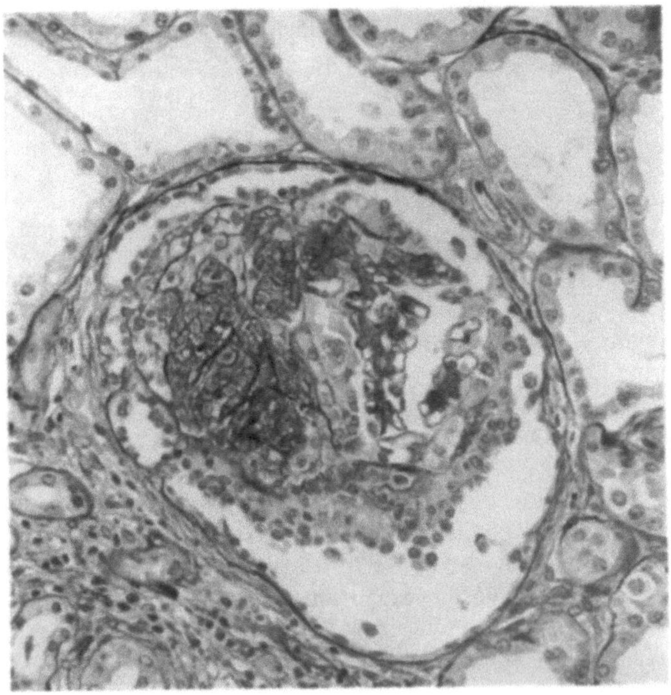

Fig. 11. K 944/72, 21 years, male. Primary malignant nephrosclerosis with hypertensive glomerulopathy: Focal destruction of capillary walls, adhesions between lobules, and formation of pseudotubules in Bowman's space. (PAS reaction, 360:1)

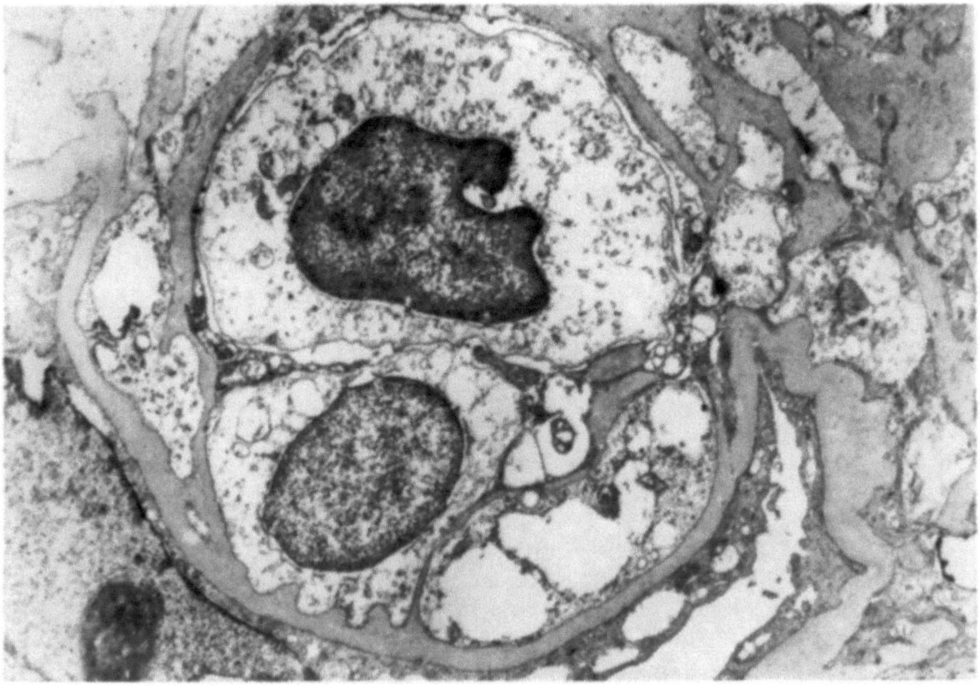

Fig. 12. 75/11/1401. Primary malignant nephrosclerosis. Cross-section of a glomerular capillary with extremely swollen endothelial cells. Between these cells basement membrane-like material (right side of the picture). Splitting of the basement membrane. Between the split structures, parts of cytoplasm of endothelial cells. (Electron microscope 10 000:1; reduced to 75%)

bringing about the considerable narrowing of the capillary lumina was partly the result of water accumulation. On the other hand, endothelial cells showed signs of fatty degeneration as well (Fig. 13). The splitting of the basement membrane was probably due to new production of basement membrane material by endothelial cells when these were detached from the *lamina densa* by subendothelial edema (Fig. 14). Fluid or fibrinous material was also found in the subendothelial area. This fibrinous material was arranged in a periodical pattern similar to that of fibrin. Fibrinous material was also found in the capillary lumina (Fig. 15). Electron microscopy of the glomerula revealed that in the early stages of PMN the endothelial cells produced a basement membrane-like material at their luminal side. These endothelial cells were partly enclosed by basement membrane-like material (Figs. 16 and 17). In such cases it was difficult to distinguish endothelial from mesangial cells.

We did not observe any swelling of the endothelial cells in the chronic stage of PMN, when the capillary lumina were found to be distinctly narrowed. The so-called splitting of the basement membrane could still be detected in circumscribed areas of the glomerula. In other parts of the glomerula only wrinkling and thickening of the basement membrane could be observed. Between the "split" layers of the capillary walls we found cells that were indistinguishable from endothelial cells. These cells were situated in a meshwork of basement membrane material. A new covering layer of endothelial cells was found on the luminal side of this basement membrane material.

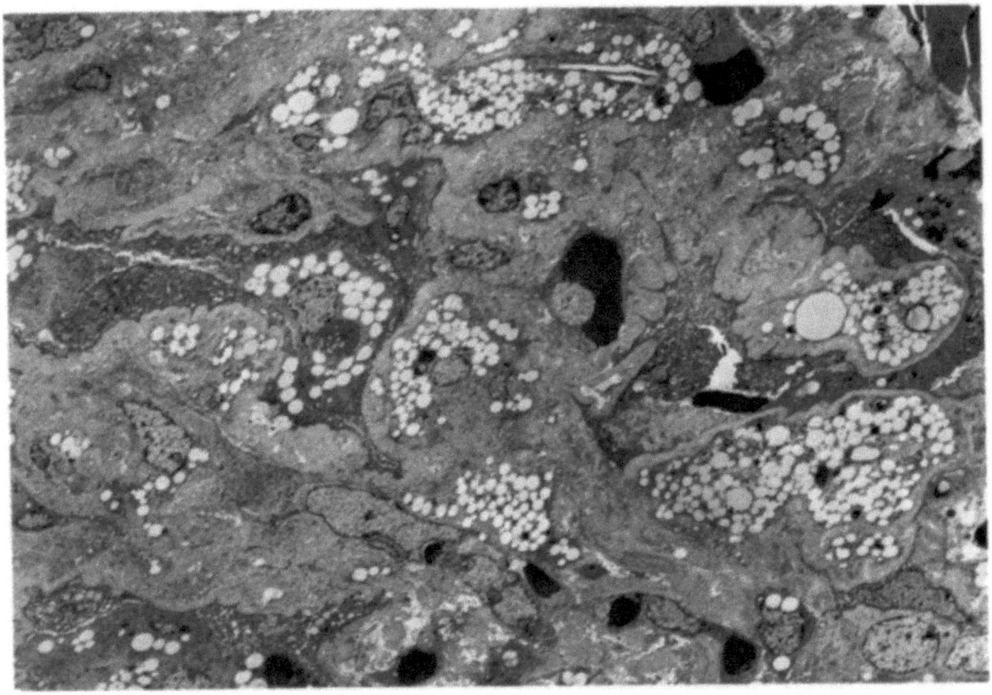

Fig. 13. 74/11/1367. Primary malignant nephrosclerosis. Glomerular detail with pronounced wrinkling and thickening of the basement membrane. Swelling and fatty degeneration of endothelial cells. (Electron microscope 2500:1; reduced to 75%)

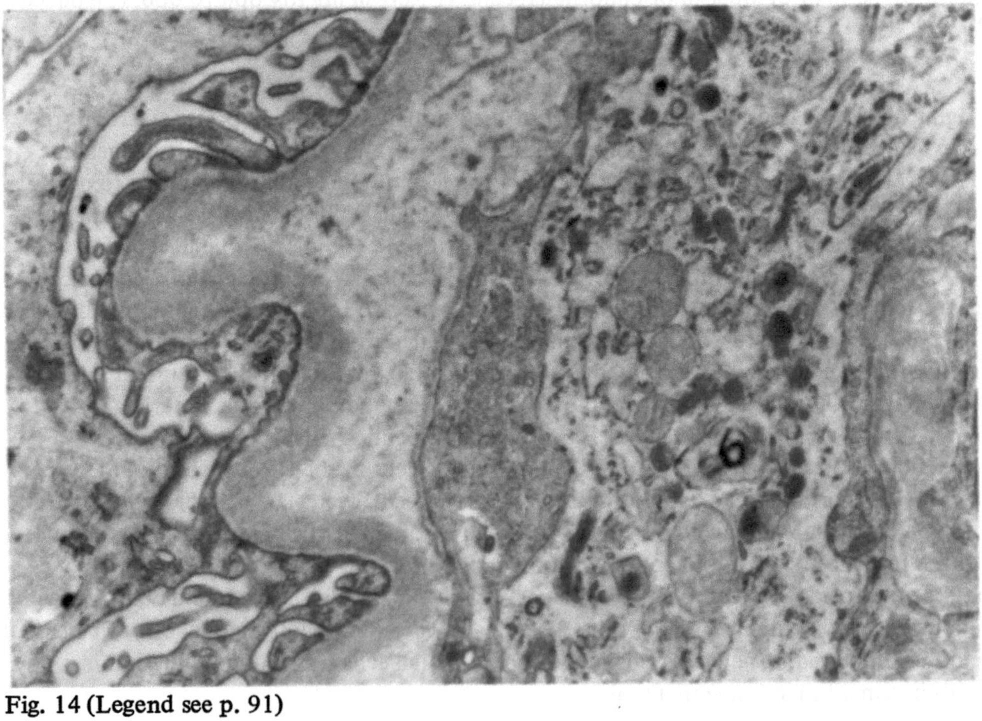

Fig. 14 (Legend see p. 91)

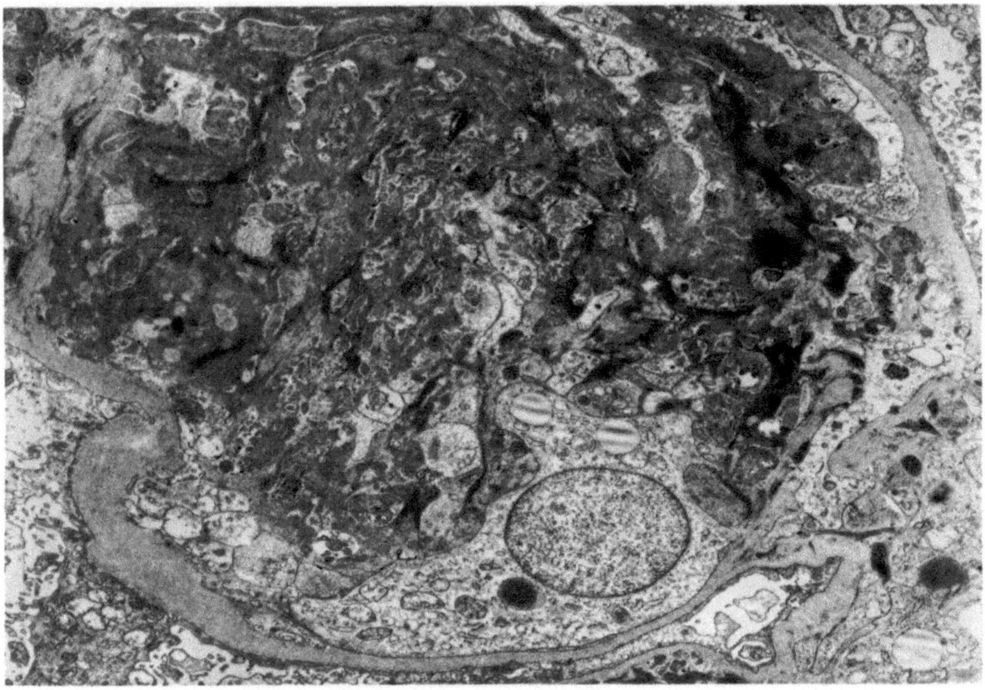

Fig. 15. 75/2/734. Primary malignant nephrosclerosis. Cross-section of a glomerular capillary. In the lumen dense (dark) precipitation of fibrin and platelets. Foot processes of podocytes cannot be seen. (Electron microscope 7500:1; reduced to 75%)

c) Immunofluorescence Microscopy

The results of the immunofluorescent studies carried out on 21 biopsies of 19 patients during the first weeks of the illness and one year after hospitalization were divided into four groups:

α) In five renal biopsies obtained from five patients no positive immunofluorescence findings were obtained in renal vessels or in glomerula.

β) In five renal biopsies, negative results were obtained in the renal vessels, whereas in the glomerula we found C3 in three cases and in two other cases IgG, IgM, C3 and IgA and C3.

γ) In seven cases negative results were obtained in the glomerula, whereas the vessels sometimes showed positive immunohistological reactions. In four cases a deposition of IgM, C3, and $C1_q$ was observed in the vessel walls of the arteries and arterioles, occasionally combined with IgG, IgA and fibrinogen.

δ) Four cases showed positive immunofluorescence findings both in vessels and glomeruli. In three of these four cases IgM, C3, and fibrinogen were found in the walls of arteries and

---

Fig. 14. 74/5/557. Primary malignant nephrosclerosis. Glomerular detail showing subendothelial edema. Endothelium detached from the wrinkled basement membrane. In the interspace a thin subendothelial layer of basement membrane-like material. (Electron microscope 25 000:1; reduced to 75%)

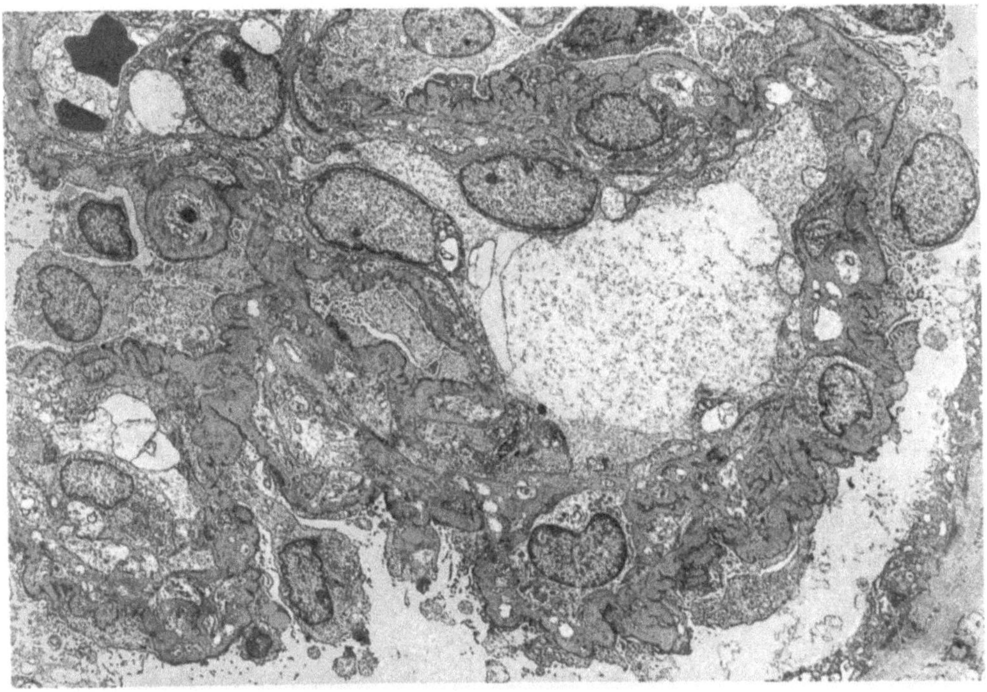

Fig. 16. 75/10/1437. Primary malignant nephrosclerosis. Cross-section of 2 glomerular capillaries. Wrinkled and split basement membrane. In the meshwork of basement membrane-like material some cells, resembling endothelial cells. Newly produced cytoplasm of endothelial cells covering the inner layer of basement membrane. (Electron microscope 3125:1; reduced to 75%)

arterioles. In two of the three cases, the same deposits were detected in the glomeruli as well, whereas in the third case C3 and C4 was found in the glomerular capillary wall. The fourth case showed fibrinogen and IgG deposits in the glomeruli, and IgM, IgG, and fibrinogen in the vessel walls of arteries and arterioles. The pattern of the deposits did not vary. In the intima and media of the vessel walls it was finely or coarsly granular or linear.

In summary, positive immunofluorescence findings in the vessel walls were obtained in 11 out of 21 cases. The findings, however, showed a focal character and could only be established in a few vessels. It is noteworthy that in these cases with positive immunohistological results in the vessel walls, a deposition of IgM ± IgA/IgG and C3 or $C1_q$, often combined with fibrinogen, was observed. There was no correlation between the onset of the disease and the time of biopsy regarding immunofluorescent investigations at the time of biopsy in the four groups.

When immunofluorescent and histological results were compared, light microscopy in three of 10 cases with negative immunofluorescence in the vessel walls revealed neither early lesions (subendothelial edema, fibrinoid necrosis) nor signs of endarteritis and endarteriolitis.

Three further cases showed early lesions in both arteries and arterioles. The four remaining cases revealed either no vessel lesions or only chronic changes (obliterating endarteritis).

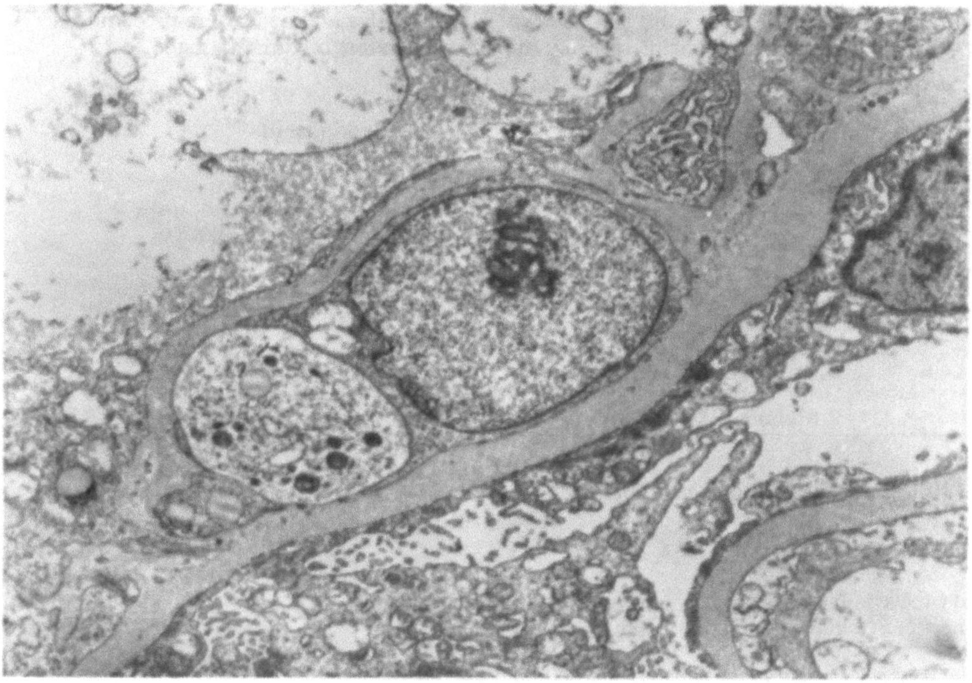

Fig. 17. 75/2/734. Primary malignant nephrosclerosis. Detail of the wall of a glomerular capillary away from mesangium. Endothelial cells covered by basement membrane-like material. A second layer of cytoplasm of endothelial cells is superimposed over the covering basement membrane. (Electron microscope 12 250:1; reduced to 75%)

Out of 11 cases with positive immunofluorescence findings in the vessel walls, nine were shown to have early lesions in either arterioles *or* arteries (5 cases) or in both arterioles *and* arteries (4 cases). In two cases we observed only chronic vessel lesions. Thus, positive immunofluorescent findings were observed more frequently in cases with acute vessel lesions than in those with chronic changes.

2. Clinical Results

Clinically in almost all cases PMN was characterized by an acute onset, often preceded by trivial infections of the gastrointestinal or respiratory tract (35% of the cases). The main symptoms during the first days of illness were severe hemolytic anemia, mostly accompanied by thrombocytopenia, elevated LDH, severe proteinuria, macrohematuria and oliguria or anuria. Some patients had a normal or only slightly elevated blood pressure at this time (Tables 1 and 2). In other patients, however, the blood pressure was distinctly elevated. Of the 20 patients with normal or slightly raised blood pressure, 12 developed hypertension during their stay in hospital.

For example, a 24-year-old woman was admitted to hospital with severe anemia and oliguria. She had been feeling ill and had repeated episodes of vomiting for 3-4 weeks before hospitalization (Fig. 18). On admission she was normotensive and had severe proteinuria. During hospitalization she became severely hypertensive while oliguria persisted.

B.A. 24 years ♀			transfusion	beginning of dialysis
For 3-4 weeks feeling unwell, vomiting	Hb g%	5.9	9.6	9.8
	Retic. %o			
	LDH		1700	
	Platelets		95000	150,000
	Bilirubin mg%	1.87	0.98	0.38
	Creatinine mg%	14.6	15.5	
	BUN mg%	181		
	B.P.	120/80	180/100	210/120
	Urine output	oliguria	oliguria	oliguria
	Proteinuria %o	4.1	12	
		1.	5.	8. day †

Fig. 18. Clinical data of one case with PMN. For details see pp. 93 and 94

Table 1. Patients with Primary Malignant Nephrosclerosis at the time of admission to hospital

	Normotensive n = 20	Hypertensive n = 48
Sex distribution ♂ : ♀	0.33 : 1	0.71 : 1
Age (years)	25 ± 15	33 ± 11
Hypertension (6 months prior to admission)	–	25%

3. Special Patterns

a) The typical clinical symptoms of PMN were also observed in 16 patients (predominantly children) whose renal vasculature showed only patchy fibrinoid necroses and thrombotic material in distal parts of the *vasa afferentia.* The glomerular lesions, however, which were particularly prominent in these cases, corresponded directly to those found in PMN (Fig. 19). The kidneys of these patients also showed lesions typical of acute renal failure with or without patchy tubular necroses such as is found in the early stages of PMN (Fig. 20).

This glomerular variant is considered to be an abortive type of PMN (Table 2; see discussion).

b) Lesions typical for PMN were also seen in kidney transplants (Figs. 21-23). Four of our patients developed PMN in their renal transplants.

Severe hemolysis with thrombocytopenia, oliguria, anuria and hypertension developed three months after successful renal transplantation in an 8-year-old boy (Fig. 21). Glomerula, *vasa afferentia* and the interlobular arteries showed lesions which are typical of early stages of PMN (Fig. 22). The tubular lesions were similar to those found in acute renal failure. We did not observe a cellular interstitial infiltration, as is typical of acute rejection. However,

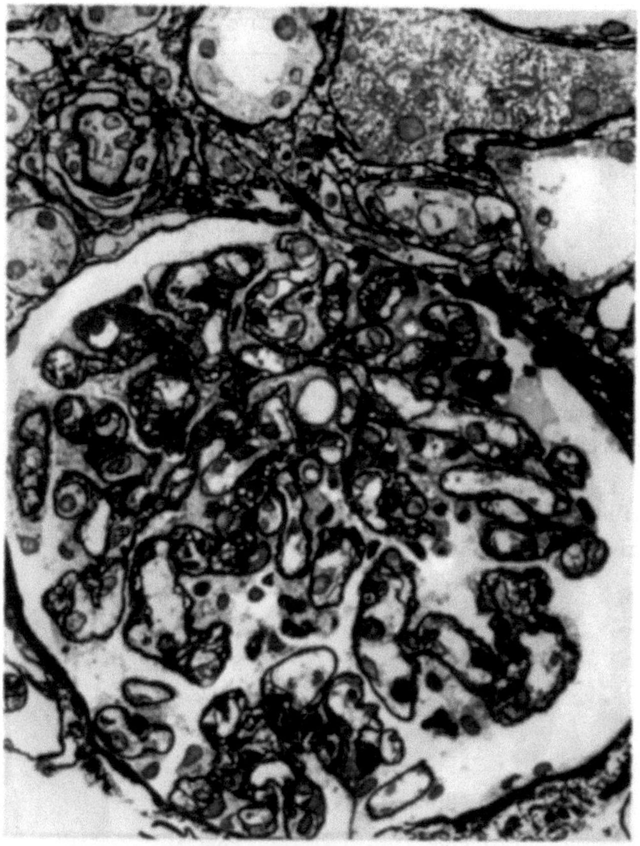

Fig. 19. 73/10/738, 38 years, female. Primary malignant nephrosclerosis, "abortive type". Glomerulus showing slight hypercellulartiy. Wrinkling and splitting of the basement membrane in many regions. Normal appearance of afferent and efferent arterioles. (MOVAT silver impregnation, 480:1)

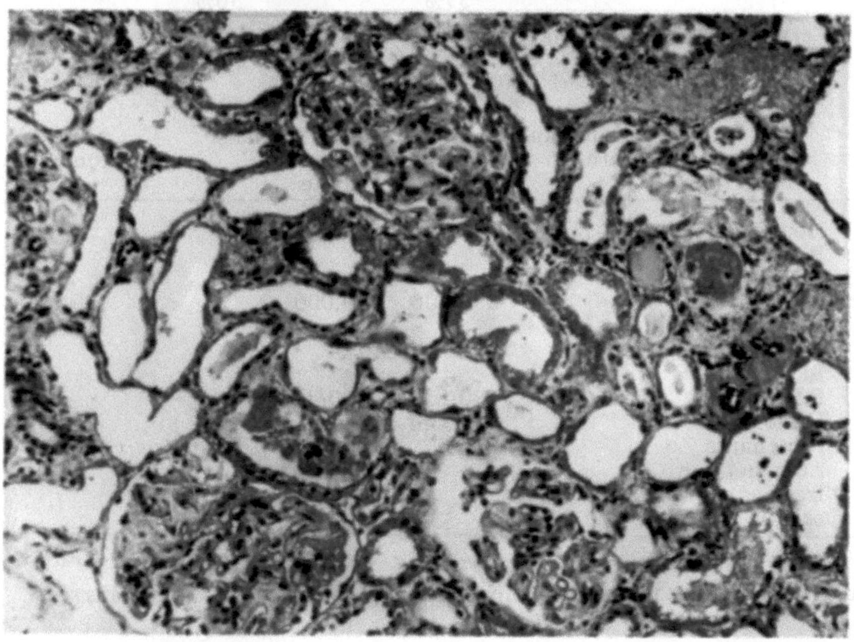

Fig. 20. 73/10/738, 38 years, female. Renal cortex (same patient as Fig. 19). Swollen tubularepithelium, regenerating tubules and focal necrosis of tubules (Goldner trichrome, 144:1)

Table 2. Clinical data of patients with PMN and the so-called "abortive" type.

	Primary malignant nephrosclerosis n = 68	Abortive type n = 16
Sex distribution ♂ : ♀	0.6 : 1	0.3 : 1
Age (years)	30.4 ± 12	22 ± 14 (66% of patients younger than 5 years)
Presenting symptoms:		
Feeling unwell	60%	25%
Edema	42%	17%
Hemorrhage	10%	22%
Vomiting	44%	33%
Infections (within 6 weeks prior to onset)	35%	33%
Hypertension (6 months prior to onset)	17%	6%
No hypertension at admission	28%	10%
Hypertension (developing during illness)	85%	18%
Hemoglobin < 8 g/100 ml at admission	50%	50%
Signs of severe hemolysis	90%	90%
Platelets below 100 000/mm^3	74%	63%
Oligoanuria	86%	87%
Proteinuria > 3 g/d	50%	66%
Macrohematuria	53%	83%
Prognosis:		
Recovery, healing	8%	25%
Permanent dialysis	35%	25%
Dead	57%	50%

Z.A. 8 years ♂		transplantation	on admission	facial edema anaemia icterus		nephrectomy
1969 glom. nephritis	Hb g %		8.7	4.3		
Nov. 1973	Retic. ‰					
haemodialysis	LDH					
	Platelets		359,000	60,000		129,000
	Bilirubin mg%			1.5		
	Creatinine mg%		0.82	7.3		
	BUN mg%					
	B.P.		130/85	180/130		
	Urine output		1150 ml	anuria		
	Proteinuria ‰					
	r.b.c. in urine					
	fragmented cells			+		
		18.1.74	12.3.74	8.4.74	19.4.74	25.4.74

Fig. 21. Clinical data of one patient with PMN in a transplanted kidney. For details see p. 94

the interlobular arteries showed stenosing edema of the intima, while the *vasa afferentia* showed fibrinoid necroses with fragmentocytes (Fig. 23a and b).*

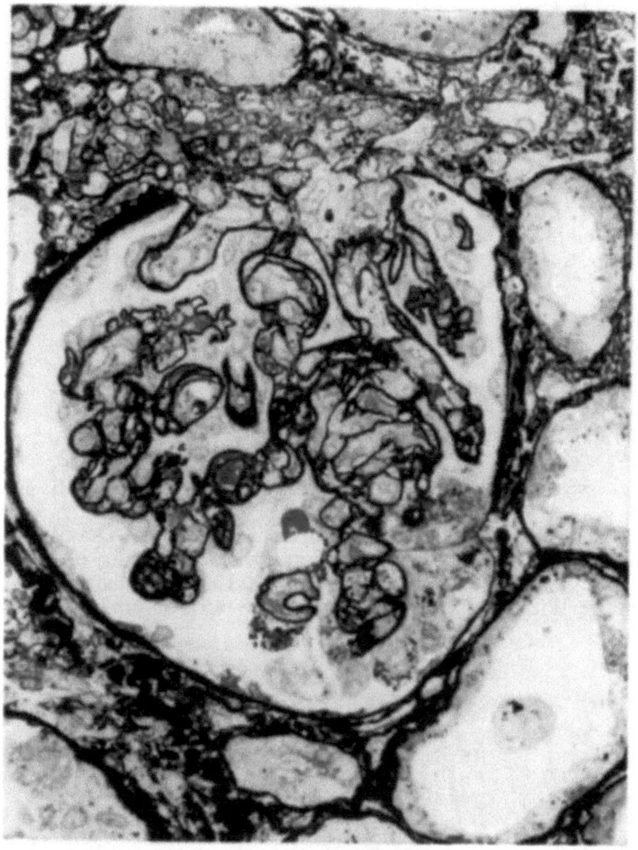

Fig. 22. 74/4/292, 8 years, male. Primary malignant nephrosclerosis in a transplanted renal allograft (see Fig. 21). Distinct splitting and segmental wrinkling of glomerular basement membrane. Hyperplasia of juxtaglomerular apparatus. (MOVAT silver impregnation, 440:1)

c) Possibly PMN has an increased familial incidence.

In our material we observed typical glomerular changes (Fig. 24a and b) and vascular and tubular lesions in biopsy material and postmortem examinations respectively in two sisters. The sisters, who were 21 and 22 years old, developed similar signs and symptoms (severe hemolysis, oliguria, anuria, hypertension) at an interval of 13 months. In addition both showed symptoms of acute renal failure.

---

* We would like to thank Prof. Dr. W. Künzer and Dr. Schindera, Department of Pediatrics, University of Freiburg, for the clinical data.

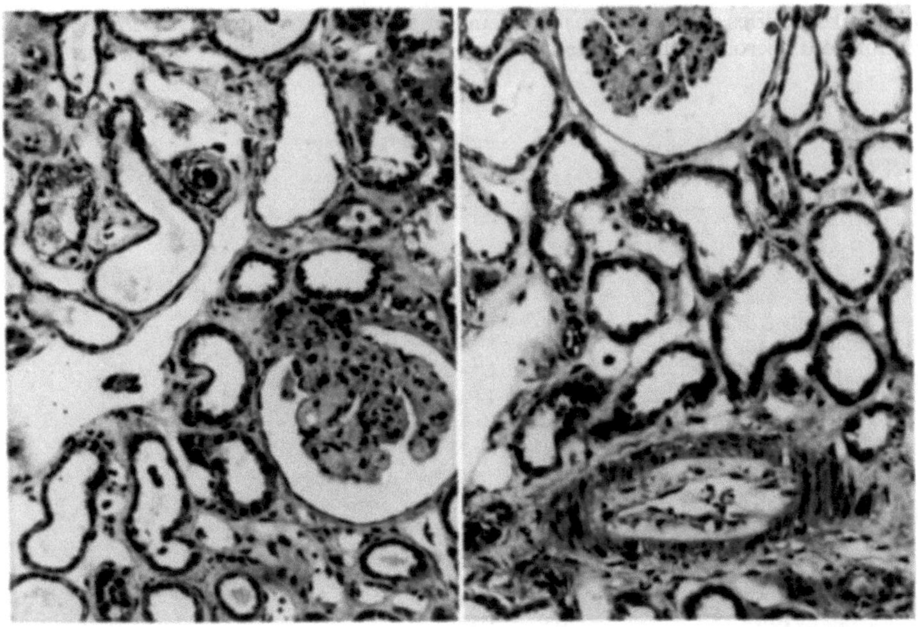

a b

Fig. 23a and b. 74/4/292, 8 years, male. Primary malignant nephrosclerosis: (a) Detail from renal cortex (transplanted renal allograft). Collapse of glomerular capillaries, obliterating arteriolitis with fragmentocytes (upper center); (b) same kidney: stenosing intimal edema of an interlobular artery. Wide open tubules, as in acute renal failure. (Goldner trichrome, 144:1)

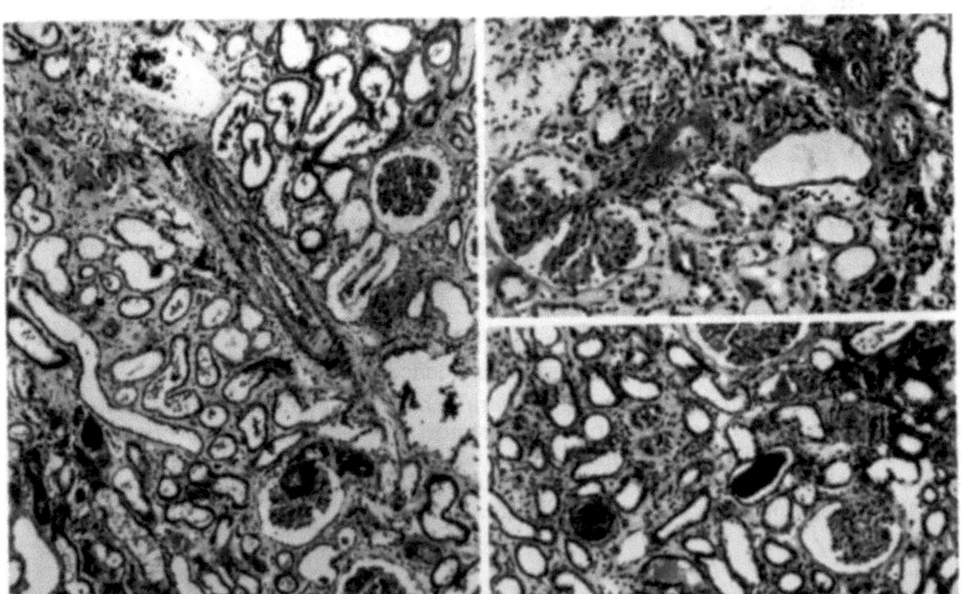

a b

Fig. 24a and b (Legend see p. 99)

IV. Discussion

1. The Term "Malignant Nephrosclerosis"

A review of the results obtained in the present study confirms the concept of *Fahr* (1924 and 1925) and *Schürmann* and *MacMahon* (1933) that there is a form of malignant nephrosclerosis in which renal vascular disease precedes hypertension. *Schürmann* and *MacMahon* called this form of malignant nephrosclerosis "exogenous or toxic malignant nephrosclerosis" in order to distinguish it from "genuine or endogenous malignant nephrosclerosis."

We prefer the term "primary malignant nephrosclerosis" (*Bohle* et al., 1973) to "exogenous" or "toxic exogenous," because we do not know the cause of the disease. Moreover, by using this term we would like to emphasize the fact that during the development of this form of malignant nephrosclerosis, hypertension is not the underlying pathogenic mechanism but rather the consequence of renal vascular disease. On the other hand, we call malignant nephrosclerosis occurring in long-standing accelerated arterial hypertension "secondary malignant nephrosclerosis" (*Bohle* et al., 1973), presuming hypertension to be the cause of the renal vascular disease, as has been shown in animal experiments (*Wilson* and *Byrom*, 1939 and 1941; *Giese*, 1966; *Helmchen* and *Kneissler*, 1976).

In recent years various terms (see Introduction) have been used to define the disease which had been called "exogenous malignant nephrosclerosis" by *Schürmann* and *MacMahon* (1933). The terms "microangiopathic hemolytic anemia" (MHA) or "microangiopathie thrombotique renale" are the ones that have been most frequently applied. *Symmers* (1952a, b and 1956) was the first to use the term "microangiopathy" or "thrombotic microangiopathy." This microangiopathy was characterized by lesions in the distal parts of arterioles, in capillaries and, probably, also in venules of various organs. In these vascular regions vessels were partly or completely occluded by thrombotic material. *Symmers* did not associate the term malignant nephrosclerosis with these vascular lesions.

Since 1962 (*Brain* et al., 1962) *Symmers*' terms "thrombotic microangiopathy" or "thrombotic microangiopathic hemolytic anemia" were changed into "microangiopathic hemolytic anemia" (*Linton* et al., 1969; *Egli* et al., 1969; *Brain*, 1970; *Gavras* et al., 1971 and 1975; *Cohan* et al., 1972). According to *Brain* (1970) MHA is a disease characterized by abnormalities of red blood cells, thrombocytopenia, and moderate or severe renal failure. Thus, MHA has been defined mainly in clinical, and not in morphologic terms (*Gavras* et al., 1975). The morphological changes associated with MHA are very variable. They have been described as a fibrinoid necrosis of the vessel wall, as necrotizing arteritis, as a vascular disease with intraluminal hyaline thrombi in arterioles and capillaries, or, finally, as a vascular disease following tumor cell embolization. Thus, the term MHA covers a large group of different diseases, including the clinical pictures of Moschcowitz syndrome, malignant hypertension, periarteritis nodosa, lupus erythematosus etc.

Fig. 24a and b. Primary malignant nephrosclerosis in sisters: (a) 76/3/701, 21 years, female. Detail from renal cortex (autopsy material). Stenosing intimal edema in the process of organization (interlobular artery). Fibrinoid necrosis of an afferent arteriole, extending into the hilus of the corresponding glomerulus. Wide open tubules and interstitial edema, as in acute renal failure. (b) 74/11/817, 22 years, female. Sister of patient in Figure 24a, biopsy material. Fibrinoid necrosis of an afferent arteriole (above) and hemorrhage into the vessel wall (below). Collapse of glomerular capillaries. (Goldner trichrome, 90:1; reduced to 75%)

Therefore, the term "microangiopathy" used in this very general manner is not acceptable for the disease we call PMN.

We also prefer the term PMN to the term "microangiopathie thrombotique rénale" (*Habib* et al., 1967 and 1969; *Beaufils*, 1972; *Gaubert*, 1973; *Richet*, 1974 and 1975), because the latter is not always a microangiopathy and, moreover, thrombosis is not the essential feature of this disease.

Certainly, one could object to the term PMN as it does not completely outline the nature of the disease because early lesions (stenosing intimal edema, fibrinoid necrosis with thrombosis) do not have the character of a sclerosis. There is no doubt, however, that the early vascular lesions do undergo sclerosing changes leading to the typical picture of malignant nephrosclerosis within a few weeks.

The same objections could also be applied to SMN, which develops from early lesions very similar to those found in PMN. In SMN, however, the development of sclerosis from early lesions becomes more apparent because acute and chronic changes frequently appear in the same biopsy.

Apparently, there is a relationship between PMN and *Gasser*'s "haemolytic uremic syndrome" (*Gasser* et al., 1955; *Gasser*, 1967). More often than any other renal vascular disease PMN takes a course clinically corresponding to that of hemolytic uremic syndrome.

After having had the opportunity of studying the biopsy material of four out of the five original cases with hemolytic uremic syndrome published by *Gasser* et al. (1955), we have to conclude that there is no difference between the vascular and glomerular lesions in these four cases and the lesions observed in the early stages of PMN, including its abortive type.*

In summary, it seems very likely that the special form of "malignant nephrosclerosis" that *Fahr* described in 1924, the "exogenous malignant nephrosclerosis" of *Schürmann* and *MacMahon* (1933), the renal vascular disease in the "haemolytic uremic syndrome" of *Gasser* et al. (1955), at least some cases of the "microangiopathic hemolytic anemia" of *Brain* et al. (1962), and the "microangiopathie thrombotique rénale" of *Habib* et al. (1967 and 1969), may all be the same disease that we called "primary malignant nephrosclerosis" (*Bohle* et al., 1973).

2. Different Morphological Stages

The term "malignant nephrosclerosis" comprises a variety of renal vascular lesions including stenosing intimal edema, fibrinoid necroses and hemorrhage in the intima and media, occluding thrombosis, intimal cell proliferation, and obliterating fibrosis of the vessel lumina and walls. These changes generally may occur in both PMN and SMN, which become morphologically progressively more difficult to distinguish as the vascular lesions progress.

In patients with PMN, however, biopsies are usually performed early because of the sudden and dramatic onset of the disease. Therefore, acute vascular lesions predominate in these patients. In this early stage PMN may be diagnosed without any knowledge of clinical data, by morphological findings only, consisting of widespread acute arterial, arteriolar and glomerular lesions accompanied by tubular changes typical of acute renal failure.

---

* For the histological slides we would like to thank Prof. Dr. R.E. Siebenmann, Zürich, Switzerland.

S.A. 41 years ♀		infusion Catapresan							Lasix	haemo-dialysis	nephrec-tomy
1968 raised B.P.	Hb g %	9.8	9.8	8.8	8.8	8.3	9.8	7.5			
noticed for the	Retic. ‰					52					
first time.	LDH	434		324	394	462					
February 1969	Platelets					133,000		155,000	162,000		
headache,	Bilirubin mg%	1.0	0.5	0.4	0.5	0.7	0.4	0.8			
retching.	Creatinine mg%	3.3	6.3	8.0	8.5	9.6	9.7	13.8	20.2		
B.P. 170/90	BUN mg%	88	65	124	136	151	92	145	234		
7. October	B.P.	290/130	160/110	180/100	220/125	250/130	200/110	210/110	205/110		
headache,	Urine output	2500 ml	1000 ml	1900 ml	1900 ml	2500 ml	1400 ml	600 ml	800 ml		
blurred vision,	Proteinuira	++				+					
nocturia,											
thirst,											
B.P. 290/150											
Creatinine											
1.6 mg%											
		27.10.70	17.11.70	28.12.70	7.1.71	19.1.71	15.2.71	15.3.71	4.4.71	15.4.71	20.10.71

Fig. 25. Clinical data of a patient with SMN. For details see p. 101

In contrast, patchy chronic lesions predominate in SMN because this renal vascular disease develops gradually (Fig. 25), and morphological examination is seldom, if ever, carried out either in later stages or at autopsy.

The progression from early to late lesions can easily be followed by investigating the same case of PMN at an early stage and at a more advanced stage (Fig. 26a and b). We have had the opportunity of examining second biopsies in 14 patients after an interval of up to 10 months. Only the lesions in the second biopsy correspond to those that are generally considered to be typical of MN. They, however, developed from the characteristic early lesions of PMN, i.e., from lesions generally judged to be characteristic of "microangiopathic hemolytic anemia" or "microangiopathie thrombotique rénale." The conversion of early lesions typical of both PMN and SMN into late lesions is probably brought about by the migration of nucleated blood cells into the intima. We presume that these cells are monocytes, because they can be transformed to macrophages or fibroblasts and smooth-muscle cells. Early stages of obliterating endarteritis can be detected by the persisting intimal edema at the intima border. Fibrinoid vessel wall necroses with and without thromboses, such as are characteristic of early lesions of both PMN and SMN, may be digested enzymatically or eliminated by phagocytosis (Fig. 27a and b). Pericellular halos can be observed around macrophages that had migrated into the fibrinoid areas.

The mural thrombi observed in the arteries, arterioles or glomeruli in the early stages develop into an organizing process resulting in a cushion-like intimal fibrosis, vascular occlusions or glomerular scars. Focal glomerular fibrinoid necroses

a 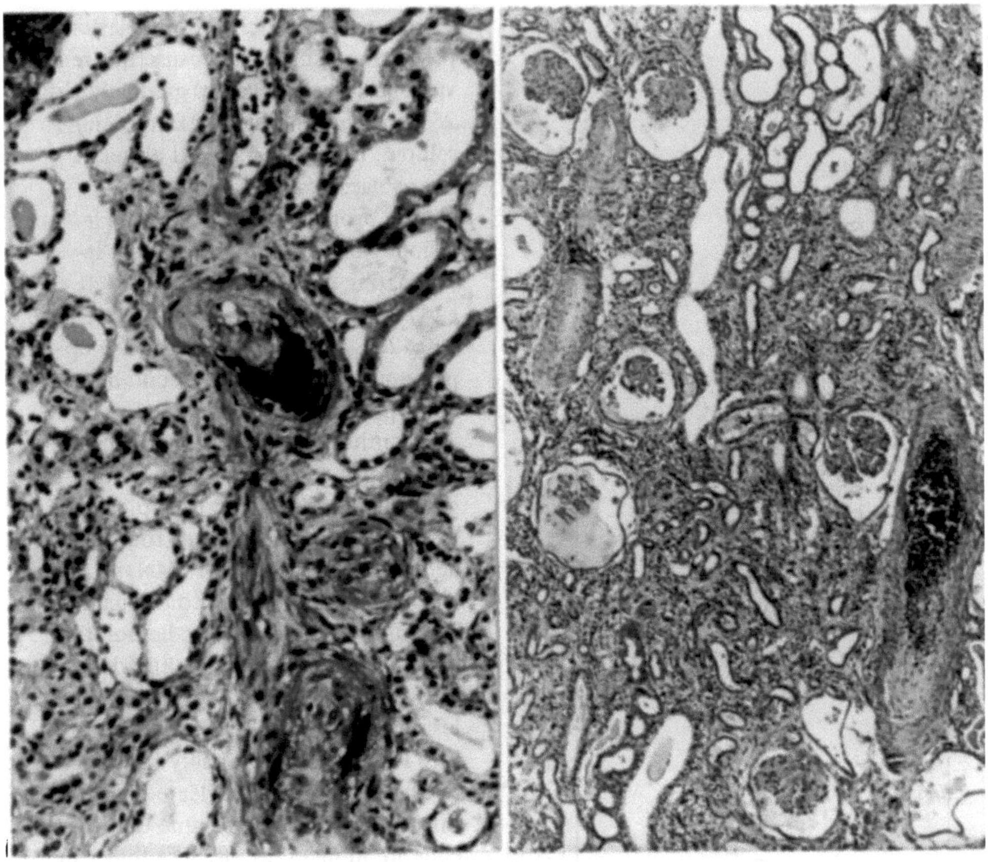 b

Fig. 26a and b. (a) 70/12/1466, 20 years, female. Primary malignant nephrosclerosis. Early stage with fibrinoid necrosis of a branch of an interlobular artery. (Goldner trichrome 210:1). (b) 71/4/338. Same kidney, 4 months later. Fibrous obliteration of vessels, obliterating endarteritis, hemorrhage into the vessel wall. Collapse of glomerular capillaries, atrophy of tubules, interstitial fibrosis. (Goldner trichrome 65:1)

also turn into segmental scars. The swelling of endothelial cells observed in the acute stage disappears again. The splitting of the basement membrane, however, may persist for several months, as has already been described by *Kincaid-Smith* (1975) (Fig. 10).

In kidneys of patients who have suffered from PMN for a longer time tubular atrophy and interstitial fibrosis are observed frequently, as is the case in SMN.

The chronic obliterating vascular processes in the region of the interlobular arteries and the *vasa afferentia* result on average in statistically significant hyperplasia of the juxtaglomerular apparatus (Fig. 28, Table 3).

Thus, the renin-angiotensin system may also be involved in the development of arterial hypertension that frequently occurs in the later stages of PMN.

In a group of patients (predominantly children) suffering from hemolytic uremic syndrome, except for tubular lesions, renal morphological changes are confined to the glomeruli. The glomerular lesions exactly equal those observed in PMN. Infrequently, distal parts of the *vasa afferentia* are also involved.

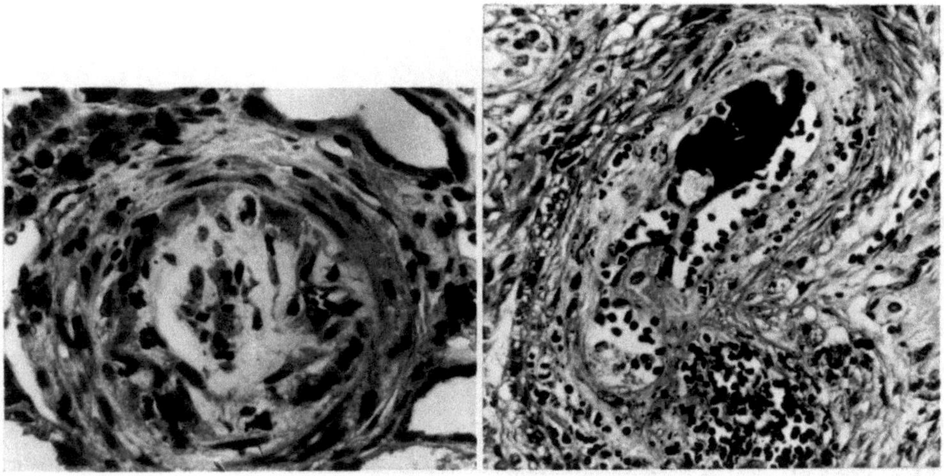

a b

Fig. 27a and b. (a) 73/10/989, 5 years, female. Primary malignant nephrosclerosis. Branch of an interlobular artery with stenosing intimal edema and fibrinoid necrosis of the intima. Nucleated blood cells migrate into the intima forming halos (above). (Goldner trichrome 440:1; reduced to 75%). (b) 68/12/586, 29 years, male. Secondary malignant nephrosclerosis. Intimal edema in the process of organization with fragmentocytes. Mural thrombus, consisting of fibrin (dark), surrounded by macrophages. (Goldner trichrome, 360:1; reduced to 75%)

Table 3. Size of the juxtaglomerular apparatus in primary and secondary malignant nephrosclerosis compared to normals

	Normal controls n = 10	Malignant nephrosclerosis Primary (n = 15)	Secondary (n = 15)
Mean cut area of the JGC-complex ($\overline{x} \pm s$)	689 ± 41 μm^2	929 ± 128 μm^2	841 ± 164 μm^2
Difference		2 p 0.001	2 p 0.001
Calculated mean single volume of a JCG-complex	26 300 μm^3	47 700 μm^3	39 200 μm^3
Volume increase		+ 81%	+ 49%

In our opinion, in these patients, who were clinically almost indistinguishable from those with PMN (Table 2), the development of renal vascular lesions was arrested at this glomerular location, and did not, exceptionally, proceed to the typical picture of malignant nephrosclerosis. It seems to be appropriate, therefore, to call this special morphological pattern an "abortive type of PMN."

Due to the absence of preglomerular lesions, the incidence of secondary hypertension was much lower than in patients with PMN (Table 2). In patients who survived the abortive type of PMN for a long time, the glomeruli in rare instances showed signs of a slight mesangioproliferative glomerulonephritis (Fig. 29), as recently described by *Churg* and *Grishman* (1976).

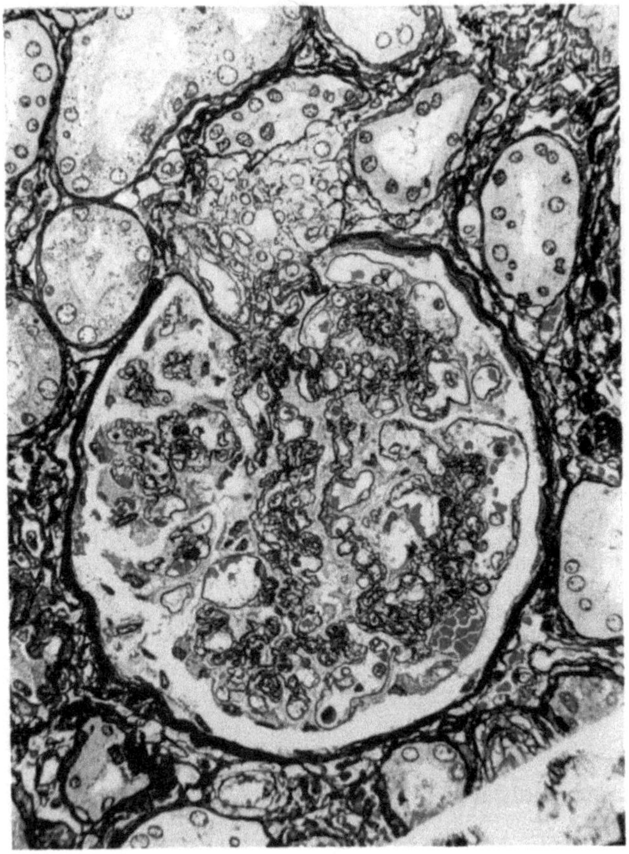

Fig. 28. 70/3/834, 25 years, female. Primary malignant nephrosclerosis, chronic stage. Segmental wrinkling of glomerular capillaries with partial splitting of the basement membrane, hyperplasia of the juxtaglomerular apparatus. (Semi-thin section, MOVAT silver impregnation, 380:1)

Morphologically, it should be possible to distinguish PMN from renal vascular lesions occurring in thrombocytopenic purpura (*Moschcowitz*, 1925) (Fig. 30a-d), or in thrombotic microangiopathy (*Symmers*, 1952a, b), respectively, in generalized Shwartzman-phenomenon, and in chronic transplant rejections.

In agreement with *Churg* and *Grishman* (1976), we presume that the abortive type of PMN, which corresponds to the hemolytic uremic syndrome of these authors (see also *Vitsky* et al., 1969), has many clinical features in common with thrombotic thrombocytopenic purpura of Moschcowitz. In typical cases, Moschcowitz-Symmers disease is usually a generalized vascular disease. Patients suffering from Moschcowitz disease do not all die of uremia, because, here in contrast to PMN, the renal vascular lesions do not predominate [observations made by *Moschcowitz* (1925), *Symmers* (1952a and b) and ourselves]. Furthermore, the PMN and its abortive type can be distinguished from the Moschcowitz syndrome by its severe glomerular lesions, the so-called splitting of the basement membrane,

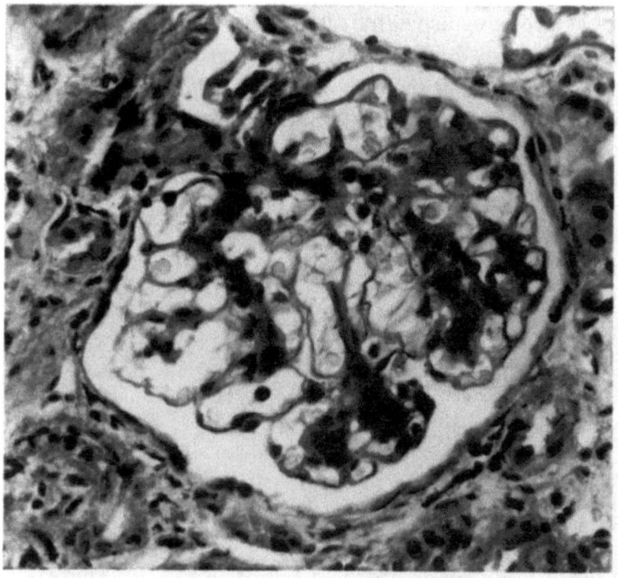

Fig. 29. 73/10/229, 7 years, female. Mild mesangioproliferative glomerulonephritis as a consequence of hemolytic-uremic syndrome. (PAS-reaction, 360:1)

endothelial cell swelling, fatty degeneration of endothelial cells, and the subendothelial edema. In Moschcowitz' syndrome, the basement membranes of the glomerular capillaries usually appear to be normal when examined by light microscopy. Even in the few cases of PMN where extrarenal vascular lesions are also present, these lesions can be distinguished from those of the Moschcowitz syndrome by their heterogeneity.

In PMN we observed extrarenal vascular lesions corresponding to the renal lesions (fibrinoid necroses, stenosing intima edema, vessel wall hemorrhage with fragmentocytes) in 3 out of 14 postmortem examinations. In contrast, only fibrin-rich thrombi in the arterioles, capillaries and venules of the different organs can be observed in the Moschcowitz syndrome. The thrombi can either be disorganized in the vascular lumen or be covered by endothelial cells and thus be incorporated in the vascular wall (Fig. 30c and d).

The generalized Shwartzman phenomenon is characterized by thrombi, rich in thin fibrin fibers located primarily in glomerular capillaries (*Bohle* and *Krecke*, 1959; *Bohle* et al., 1959; *Krecke*, 1964; *Harms* et al., 1973). In 1959 we observed by means of electron-microscopic investigation that the fibrin showed periodicity (*Bohle* et al., 1959). The thrombi usually fill all glomerular capillaries, but subendothelial edema does not develop. In PMN, on the other hand, immune fluorescence investigations have shown that despite occasional positive fibrin reactions, fibrin fibers only rarely reveal periodicity. Furthermore, the preglomerular vessels are rarely involved in the generalized Shwartzman phenomenon. According to our light-microscopy investigations, it is characteristic of the generalized Shwartzman phenomenon that fibrin precipitates appear in the capillaries of the different organs without involving the vessel walls. This does not apply to PMN, which is mainly a renal vascular disease, as already mentioned above.

In typical cases, it is also possible to distinguish early vascular lesions of PMN from corresponding lesions observed in transplants during chronic rejection (*Petersen* et al., 1975; *Magalhaes* et al., 1975) [compare different opinion of *Kincaid-Smith* (1975)]. In chronic transplant rejections one can also observe renal vascular lesions of the intima similar to those of the early stages of PMN. Both types of lesions are characterized by a narrowing of the vascular lumen and by migration of nucleated blood cells into the intima

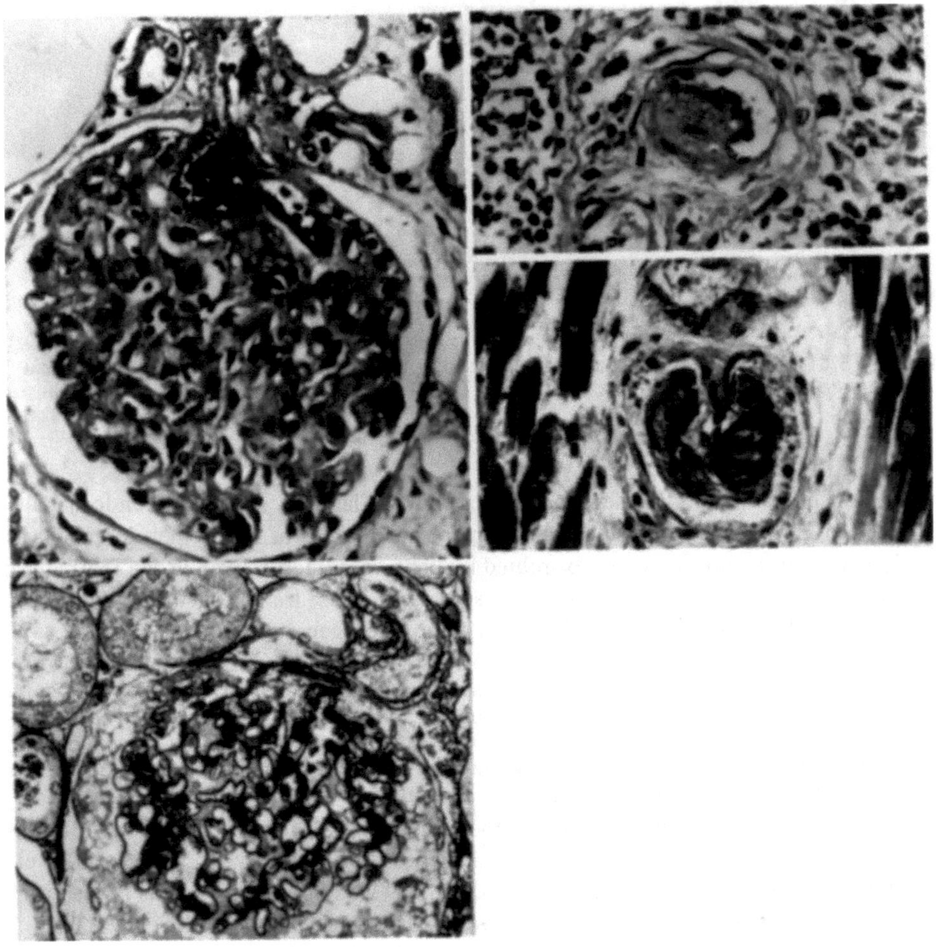

a b c d

Fig. 30a-d. 229/71, 50 years, female. Thrombotic thrombocytopenic purpura (Moschcowitz): (a) Glomerulus with a thrombus in the sinus region, 360:1. (b) Glomerulus showing thin basement membranes. No wrinkling, no splitting. MOVAT silver impregnation, 360:1. (c) Arteriole of the spleen with incorporated fibrin-thrombus in the wall. Goldner trichrome, 440:1. (d) Myocardium, dilated arteriole filled with a fragmented thrombus of fibrin without connection to the vessel wall. Goldner trichrome 360:1. (a-d reduced to 75%)

(*Bohle*, 1972). In contrast, a stenosing edema of the intima with red blood cells and fragmentocytes is usual in chronic transplant rejection. On the other hand, foam cells at the intima-media border can seldom be observed in PMN. Moreover, glomerular lesions such as are typical of PMN can rarely be observed in chronic transplant rejection. Finally, a distinction between transplant rejection and PMN may be made possible by a comparison of the interstitial infiltration: whereas in addition to small and large lymphocytes, a large number of mature and immature plasma cells can be observed in chronic transplant rejection (*Schlüter* et al., 1975), only small and large lymphocytes predominate in PMN (*Mackensen*, unpubl.).

Table 4. Secondary Malignant Nephrosclerose. Clinical data (n = 45)

Sex distribution ♂ : ♀	1.6 : 1
Age (years)	35 ± 10
Hypertension (6 months prior to admission)	72%
Oral contraceptive drugs	26%
Pregnancy or abortion (women aged 15 to 45)	7%
Hemoglobin	
< 8 g/100 ml at onset	15%
< 8 g/100 ml during illness	15%
Signs of severe hemolysis	2%
Platelets < 100 000)mm^3	6%
Proteinuria < 3 g/d	19%
Macrohematuria	23%
Oligoanuria	23%

3. Clinico-Pathological Correlations and Pathogenic Aspects

Except for the acute stage of PMN that can be diagnosed by morphological changes only (acute vascular lesions plus tubular changes as observed in acute renal failure) clinical data including the patient's history may become important for distinguishing later stages of PMN from SMN.

As can be seen by comparing Tables 2 and 4, PMN and SMN differ in several clinical characteristics. PMN often appears after trivial infections. Onset without any prodromal signs and accompanied by severe hemolysis and symptoms of uremia is more frequently acute. Patients with PMN usually have more severe anemia and proteinuria than those with SMN. SMN, in contrast, develops gradually (Fig. 25) over several years of hypertension. Only one of 45 patients with SMN developed severe hemolysis.

PMN is considerably more frequent in women, whereas SMN, as already described by *Volhard* (1918) and *Page* (1939), is more often seen in men. Sex differences, however, could be abolished by excluding all the patients who had developed PMN following abortion, delivery, or oral contraception. This would make the frequency of PMN the same in women and men.

Correlation of the clinical symptoms and morphological alterations in PMN reveals that development of the hemolytic uremic syndrome is not dependent upon the severity of morphological lesions. Patients with the so-called abortive type of PMN revealed the same severe clinical symptoms as are characteristic of typical cases (Table 2). Moreover, as demonstrated by the following example, patients can even die of a hemolytic uremic syndrome without showing any vascular lesions at autopsy.

A 16-year-old girl complained of pain in her legs, nausea, and coughing for 3-4 weeks preceding hospitalization. On admission she was icteric, severely anemic, anuric, uremic, and normotensive. She died 4 days after admission, still normotensive. Neither intravascular thrombi nor lesions of the vessel walls could be detected microscopically* (Fig. 31).

R.B. 16 years ♀				hemo- dialysis	
For 3-4 weeks	Hb g%	4.0		7.6	
feeling	Retic. ‰				
unwell,	LDH		1170		
calf pain	Platelets	166,000		76000	
24.9.73 cough	Bilirubin mg%	25.2			
cold, repeated	Creatinine mg%	6.6		5.8	
vomiting, dark	BUN mg%	116		193	
urine	BP	120/50			
27.9.73	Urine output	anuria	anuria		
icterus	Proteinuria ‰				
	rbc in urine				
	Coagulation factors	consumptive coagulopathy			
		28.9.73	29.9.73	30.9.73	1.10.73 †

Fig. 31. Clinical data of a patient with hemolytic uremic syndrome without any vascular lesions. For details see p. 108

Therefore, as suggested earlier (*Bohle* and *Helmchen*, 1975), PMN, including its abortive type, does not seem to be the cause, but rather a possible complication of a hemolytic uremic syndrome. This hypothesis does not contradict the view that vascular thrombotic diseases, including hypertensive lesions, may cause hemolysis mechanically (*Monroe* and *Strauss*, 1953; *Brain* et al., 1962; *Gavras* et al., 1971 and 1975; *Ferrario* et al., 1976). According to our observations, however, hemolysis in human SMN is usually mild and does not lead to uremia.

Occasionally, PMN may occur repeatedly in the same patient (*Wehinger* et al., 1968; *MacDonald* et al., 1972; *Drukker* et al., 1975).

* For the autopsy material we would like to thank Prof. Dr. W. Remmele, Wiesbaden.

We observed a recurring hemolytic uremic syndrome in 3 patients. The patients were followed up after clinical recovery. Repeated episodes of severe hemolysis and acute renal failure were observed. Seemingly, in one of these patients symptoms first occurred during a relapse of the disease. The patient was a 21-year-old man who first complained of visual disturbances 6 weeks before his death. About 2 1/2 weeks after the onset of the illness he developed severe anemia and uremia and had to be hospitalized. An open renal biopsy was performed 1 1/2 weeks after admission. Macroscopically the surface of the kidney appeared granular. Light microscopic examination revealed hyalinization of 90% of the glomeruli. A splitting of the basement membrane was easily recognized in those glomeruli which were not hyalinized. There was marked tubular atrophy, whereas the vessels showed lesions typical of the chronic stage of PMN or SMN.

The sequence of events leading to PMN, thereby complicating a hemolytic uremic syndrome, has still to be clarified. The main purpose of any hypothesis proposed at present or in the future will have to be to explain the alteration in vascular permeability, i.e. the cause of the so-called "dysorie" of *Schürmann* and *MacMahon* (1933), and the preference for the kidney as target organ. The factor(s) possibly responsible for initiating the process resulting in PMN might be of viral, bacterial, hormonal, immunological, or genetic nature.

The appearance of PMN after infectious diseases, already emphasized by *Fahr* (1944), might indicate a role of viral or bacterial infections. As reported by *Poschmann* and *Fischer* (1974) and *Poschmann* et al. (1976), viral and bacterial neuraminidase can induce severe hemolysis by liberating T-antigens in red blood cells and in endothelial cells of glomerular capillaries. Accordingly, the coagulation cascade might become activated, and, in the presence of glomerular endothelial lesions, PMN might result from hemolysis, hypercoagulability, and altered vascular permeability.

Among patients with PMN, the frequency of pregnancy, delivery, or oral contraception is striking. It might reflect a role of a hormonal shift possibly favoring the development of both the hemolytic uremic syndrome and intrarenal vascular lesions (*Clarkson* et al., 1969 and 1970; *Zacherle* et al., 1972; *Bock* and *Bohle*, 1973; *Brown* et al., 1973; *Ponticelli* et al., 1972; *Girndt* et al., 1976; *Stamler*, 1977). Apparently, the formation of thrombi in the kidney and in different organs can be facilitated by oral contraceptives (*Poltera*, 1972).

On the other hand, it is far from being clear whether thrombosis is a cause or a consequence of acute vascular lesions including fibrinoid necroses in PMN.

Concerning immunological mechanisms possibly involved in the pathogenesis of PMN, in accordance with the results of *McCoy* et al. (1974) IgM and C3 were the most frequent precipitates in the vessel walls of kidneys with positive immunofluorescent results. It is not possible to decide at present whether this positive immunofluorescence does reflect causal immunological mechanisms. On the other hand, negative immunofluorescent results were also obtained in PMN. For several reasons, however, negative immunofluorescence does not necessarily contradict the possibility of an immunological pathogenic mechanism.

The coincidence of PMN in two sisters is really no reason to discuss the possibility of a genetic predisposition. However, *Kaplan* et al. (1975) reported the familial occurrence of hemolytic uremic syndrome, accompanied by renal vascular lesions in some cases, in 83 siblings of 41 families. The authors suggest that an environmental agent may have caused the syndrome in 27 families, and that genetic factors may have been important in the remaining 14 families. Thus, due to this study it is difficult to reject genetic factors generally.

V. Conclusion

Primary malignant nephrosclerosis (PMN), including its abortive type, develops frequently but not necessarily as a complication of the hemolytic uremic syndrome in mostly normotensive patients. In its early stage PMN may be diagnosed by the acute renal vascular lesions and by tubular changes such as are typical for acute renal failure. In later stages it may become impossible to distinguish PMN morphologically from secondary malignant nephrosclerosis (SMN) occurring during long-standing arterial hypertension.

There is no precise information on the cause and pathogenesis of PMN. The possible role of viral and bacterial infections, hormonal and coagulation disorders, and immunological and genetic factors has been discussed.

References

Beaufils, Ph.: Syndrome hémolytique et urémique de l'adulte.(Faculté de Médicine St. Antoine, Paris). Paris: Thèse 1972.

Beller, F.K., Intorp, H.W., Losse, H., Loew, H., Mönninghoff, W., Schmidt, E.H., Grundmann, E.: Malignant nephrosclerosis during pregnancy and in the post partum period (the uremic hemolytic syndrome). Amer. J. Obstet. Gynecol. 125, 633-639 (1976).

Bock, K.D., Bohle, A.: Perakut verlaufende primäre maligne Nephrosklerose mit irreversiblem Nierenversagen und maligner Hypertonie nach Ovulationshemmern. Dtsch. med. Wschr. 98, 757-761 (1973).

Bohle, A.: Pathologische Anatomie des akuten Nierenversagens. Verh. Dtsch. Ges. Path. 49, 54-66 (1965).

Bohle, A.: Neue Ergebnisse der Nierenforschung aus pathologisch-anatomischer Sicht. (Versuch einer Korrelation von Struktur und Funktion beim akuten Nierenversagen). Monatskurse für die ärztl.Fortbildung 17, 528-534 (1967).

Bohle, A.: Die Pathomorphologie der transplantierten Niere. Klin. Wschr. 50, 636-647 (1972).

Bohle, A., Grund, K.E., Helmchen, U., Meyer, D.: Primary malignant nephrosclerosis. Clinical Sci. and Molecular Medicine 51, 23-25 (1976).

Bohle, A., Helmchen, U.: Intrarenale Gerinnung, Anämie und Niereninsuffizienz. VI. Symposion der 4. Med. Klinik Nürnberg über Gerinnungsstörungen und Anämie bei Nierenkrankheiten, 1973. In: Nephrologie in Klinik und Praxis. (W. Schulz, U. Gessler, eds.). Munich: Dustri 1975, Vol. 3, pp. 25-33.

Bohle, A., Helmchen, U., Meyer, D., Bock, K.D., Brünning, L., Edel, H.H., Heimsoth, V., Scheler, F.: Über die primäre und sekundäre maligne Nephrosklerose. Klin. Wschr. 51, 841-857 (1973).

Bohle, A., Helmchen, U., Meyer, D., Christensen, J., Bulla, M., Strauch, M.: Maligne Hypertonie, Hämolyse und maligne Nephrosklerose. In: Hypertension, Current Problems. Symposium, Mainz, 1973. Stuttgart: Thieme 1974.

Bohle, A., Helmchen, U., Meyer, D., Frotscher, U., Mönninghoff, W., Quellhorst, E.: Über verschiedene Formen der malignen Nephrosklerose. In: Aktuelle Probleme der Dialyseverfahren und der Niereninsuffizienz. 5th Symposium, Innsbruck, March 7-9, 1974. Dittrich, P.v., Skrabal, F., Stühlinger, W.D. (eds.). Friedberg/Hessen: Carl Bindernagel 1975.

Bohle, A., Jahnecke, J., Meyer, D., Schubert, G.E.: Morphology of acute renal failure: Comparative data from biopsy and autopsy. Kidney International 10, S9-S16 (1976a).

Bohle, A., Jahnecke, J., Rauscher, A.: Vergleichende histometrische Untersuchungen an bioptisch und autoptisch gewonnenem Nierengewebe mit normaler Funktion und bei akutem Nierenversagen. Klin. Wschr. 42, 1-12 (1964).

Bohle, A., Krecke, H.J.: Über das Sanarelli-Shwartzman-Phänomen (sog. generalisiertes Shwartzman-Phänomen) des Menschen. Klin. Wschr. 37, 803-814 (1959).

Bohle, A., Krecke, H.J., Miller, R., Sitte, H.: Über die Natur des sog. Fibrinoids bei der generalisierten Shwartzman'schen Reaktion. Elektronenmikroskopische Untersuchun-

gen an Kaninchennieren. In: Immunopathologie, I. Internat. Symposium, Basel-Seelisberg, 1959. Basel: Schwabe 1959, pp. 339-350.
Brain, M.C.: Microangiopathic hemolytic anemia. Ann. Rev. Med. 21, 133-144 (1970).
Brain, M.C., Dacie, J.V., Hourihane, D.O.B.: Microangiopathic hemolytic anemia: the possible role of vascular lesions in pathogenesis. Brit. J. Haemat. 8, 358 (1962).
Brain, C.B., Clarkson, A.R., Robson, J.S., Cameron, J.S., Thomson, D., Ogg, C.S.: Haemolytic uraemic syndrome in women taking oral contraceptives. Lancet **1973** I, 1479-1481.
Churg, J., Grishman, E.: Electron microscopy of glomerulonephritis. Current Topics in Pathology 61, 107-153 (1976).
Clarkson, A.R., Meadows, R., Lawrence, J.R.: Post partum renal failure. The generalized Shwartzman-reaction. Aust. Ann. Med. 18, 209-216 (1969).
Clarkson, A.R., Lawrence, J.R., Meadows, R., Seymoor, A.E.: The haemolytic uraemic syndrome in adults. Quart. J. Med. 39, 227-239 (1970).
Cohan, M., Pittman, G., Hoffman, C.: Hemolytic anemia, tumor cell emboli and intravascular coagulation. Arch. Path. (Chicago) 93, 305-307 (1972).
Drukker, A., Winterborn, M., Bennett, B., Churg, J., Spiter, A., Greifer, I.: Recurrent hemolytic uremic syndrome: a case report. Clinical Nephrology 4, 68-72 (1975).
Egli, F., Stalder, G., Gloor, F., Duckert, F., Koller, F., Hottinger, A.: Heparintherapie des hämolytisch-urämischen Syndromes. Helv. paediat. Acta 24, 13-37 (1969).
Fahr, T.: Über atypische Befunde aus den Kapiteln des Morbus Brightii nebst anhangsweisen Bemerkungen zur Hypertoniefrage. Virchows Archiv 248, 323-336 (1924).
Fahr, T.: Pathologische Anatomie des Morbus Brightii. Nephrosklerose. In: Handbuch der speziellen pathologischen Anatomie und Histologie. Berlin: Springer, 1925, pp. 368 ff.
Fahr, T.: Die Nephrosklerose. In: Nierenkrankheiten (Becher, E., ed.). Jena: Fischer 1944, Vol. 1, pp. 638-650.
Ferrario, C.M., Helmchen, U.M., McCubbin, J.W.: On the differences and similarities between the benign and malignant phases or renal hypertension. In: Recent Advances in Hypertension (Milliez, P., Safar, M., eds.). Ingelheim: Boehringer 1976, pp. 159-169.
Gasser, C.: Haemolytisch-urämisches Syndrom. In: Handbuch der Kinderheilkunde (Opitz, H., Schmid, F., eds.). Berlin-Heidelberg-New York: Springer 1967, Vol. VI, pp. 951-963.
Gasser, C., Gautier, E., Steck, A., Siebenmann, H.E., Oechslin, R.: Hämolytisch urämische Syndrome. Bilaterale Nierenrindennekrosen bei akuten erworbenen hämolytischen Anämien. Schweiz. med. Wschr. 85, 905-909 (1955).
Gaubert, D.: Angiographie dans les nephropathies vasculaires. Thèse Med. Paris 1973.
Gavras, H., Brown, W.C.B., Brown, J.J., Lever, A.F., Linton, A.L., MacAdam, R.F., George, M.B., McNicol, P., Robertson, J.I.S., Wardrop, Ch.: Microangiopathic hemolytic anemia and the development of the malignant phase of hypertension. Suppl. II to Circulat. Res. 28 and 29, 127-141 (1971).
Gavras, H., Oliver, N., Aitchinson, J., Begg, C., Briggs, J.D., Brown, J.J., Horton, P.W., Lee, F., Lever, A.F., Prentice, C., Robertson, J.I.S.: Abnormalities of coagulation and the development of malignant phase hypertension. Kidney International 8, 252-261 (1975).
Giese, J.: The pathogenesis of hypertensive vascular disease. Copenhagen: Munksgaard 1966.
Girndt, J., Kramer, P., Quellhorst, E., Held, K., Bohle, A., Scheler, F.: Ovulationshemmer, Hypertonie und Nephrosklerose. Dtsch. med. Wschr. **101**, 1246-1251 (1976).
Habib, R., Courtecuisse, V., Leclerc, F., Mathieu, H., Royer, P.: Etude anatomo-pathologique de 35 observations de syndrome hémolytique et urémique de l'enfant. Arch. franç. Péd. 26, 391-416 (1969).
Habib, R., Mathieu, H., Royer, P.: Le Syndrome hémolytique et urémique de l'enfant. Nephron 4, 139-172 (1967).
Hammond, D.D., Liebermann, E.: The hemolytic uremic syndrome. Renal cortical thrombotic microangiopathy. Arch. intern. Med. 126, 816-822 (1970).
Harms, D., Pape, G.R., Bohle, A.: Pathologische Anatomie des Waterhouse-Fridrichsen-Syndroms unter besonderer Berücksichtigung der disseminierten intravaskulären Koagulation. Dtsch. med. Wschr. 98, 542-547 (1973).
Helmchen, U., Kneissler, U.: Role of the renin-angiotensin system in renal hypertension. An experimental approach. Current Topics in Pathology 61, 203-238 (1976).
Kaplan, B.S., Chesney, R.W.: Hemolytic uremic syndrome in families. New Engl. J. Med. 282, 1090-1093 (1975).

Kincaid-Smith, P.: Participation of intravascular coagulation in the pathogenesis of glomerular and vascular lesions. Kidney International 7, 242-253 (1975).
Krecke, H.J.: Zum generalisierten Shwartzman-Phänomen. Suttgart: Fischer 1964.
Linton, A.L., Gavras, H., Gledale, R.I., Hutchinson, H.E., Lawson, D.H., Lever, A.F., MacAdam, R.F., McNicol, G.P., Robertson, J.I.: Microangiopathic haemolytic anaemia and the pathogenesis of malignant hypertension. Lancet **1969 II**, 1277-1282.
Luke, R.G., Talbert, W., Siegel, R.R., Holland, N.: Heparin treatment for post-partum renal failure with microangiopathic haemolytic anaemia. Lancet **1970 II**, 750-752.
MacDonald, M.K., Clarkson, A.R., Davison, A.M.: The role of coagulation in renal disease. In: Glomerulonephritis. Proc. Internat. Symposium, Melbourne, 1972. (Kincaid-Smith, P., Mathew, T.H., Becker, E.L., eds.). New York-London-Sydney-Toronto: Wiley 1972, pp. 809 ff.
Magalhaes, R.L., Braun, W.E., Straffon, R.A., Hoffman, G.C., Shainoff, J.R., Osborne, G., Deddhar, S.D.: Microangiopathic hemolytic anemia in renal allotransplantation. Amer. J. Med. **58**, 862-868 (1975).
Mattern, W.D., Sommers, S.C., Kassirer, J.P.: Oliguric acute renal failure in malignant hypertension. Amer. J. Med. **52**, 187-197 (1972).
McCoy, R.C., Abramowsky, C.R., Krueger, R.: The hemolytic uremic syndrome with positive immunofluorescence studies. J. Pediatrics **85**, 170-174 (1974).
Meadows, R., Lawrence, J.R.: Postpartum renal failure and the hemolytic uremic syndrome. In: Glomerulonephritis. Proc. Internat. Symposium, Melbourne, 1972 (Kincaid-Smith, P., Mathew, T.H., Becker, E.L., eds.). New York-London-Sydney-Toronto: Wiley 1972
Meyer, D., Helmchen, U., Bohle, A.: Hypertensive glomeruläre Schäden. Verh. Dtsch. Ges. Path. **57**,392 (1973).
Monroe, W.M., Struass, A.F.: Intravascular hemolysis. A morphologic study of schizocytes in thrombotic purpura and other diseases. Southern Med. J. **46**, 837-842 (1953).
Moschcowitz, E.: An acute febrile pleiochronic anemia with hyaline thrombosis of the terminal arterioles and capillaries. Arch. intern. Med. **36**, 89-93 (1925).
Movat, H.U.: Silver impregnation methods for electron microscopy. Amer. J. clin. Path. **35**, 528-537 (1961).
Page, I.H.: A clinical study in malignant hypertension. Ann. intern. Med. **12**, 978 (1939).
Petersen, V.P., Olsen, T.S., Kissmeyer-Nielsen, F., Bohmann, S.O., Hansen, H.E., Hansen, E.S., Skov, P.E., Sølling, K.: Late failure of human renal transplants. Medicine **54**, 45-71 (1975).
Poltera, A.A.: The pathology of intracranial venous thrombosis in oral contraception. J. Path. **106**, 209-220 (1972).
Ponticelli, C., Imbasciati, E., Tarantino, G., Graziani, G., Repaelli, B.: Post partum renal failure with microangiopathic haemolytic anaemia. Long-term survival after anticoagulant therapy. Nephron **9**, 27-41 (1972).
Poschmann, A., Fischer, K.: Hämolytisch-urämisches Syndrom. Überblick und neue pathogenetische Aspekte. Med. Klinik **69**, 1821-1834 (1974).
Poschmann, A., Fischer, K., Grundmann, A., Gjirad, A. von: Neuraminidase-induzierte Hämolyse. Mschr. Kinderheilk. **124**, 15-24 (1976).
Richet, G.: Insuffisances rénales aigues d'origine vasculaire. Rev. Med. de Liège **29**, 1-6 (1974).
Richet, G.: Hämolytisch urämisches Syndrom bei Erwachsenen. In: Gerinnungsstörungen und Anämie bei Nierenerkrankungen (W. Schulz, V. Gessler, eds.). Munich: Dustri 1975, pp. 13-24.
Robson, J.G., Martin, A.M., Ruckley, V.A., MacDonald, M.K.: Irreversible post-partum renal failure. Quart. J. Med. 37, 423-435 (1968).
Scheer, R.L., Jones, D.B.: Malignant nephrosclerosis in women post partum. J. Amer. med. Ass. **201**, 600-604 (1967).
Schlüter, E., Lennert, K., Bohle, A.: The immunological significance of cellular infiltrates in chronic rejection of human kidney transplants. Virchows Archiv Abt. A **368**, 191-204 (1975).
Schürmann, P., MacMahon, H.E.: Die maligne Nephrosklerose, zugleich ein Beitrag zur Frage der Bedeutung der Blutgewebsschranke. Virchows Archiv Abt. A **291**, 47-218 (1933).
Sraer, J.D., Beaufils, P., Morel-Maroger, L., Richet, G.: Vascular nephropathies with acute renal failure. In: Glomerulonephritis. Morphology, Natural History and Treatment (Kincaid-Smith, P., Mathew, T.H., Becker, E.L., eds.). New York-London-Sydney-Toronto: Wiley 1974, pp. 1035-1046.

Stamler, F.W.: Disseminated intravascular coagulation induced by progesteron in the pregnant rat. Am J. Path. **86**, 603-622 (1977).
Sun, N.C.J., Johnson, W.J., Sung, D.T.W., Woods, J.E.: Idiopathic postpartum renal failure. Mayo Clinic Proc. **50**, 395-401 (1975).
Symmers, W.St.C.: Thrombotic microangiopathic haemolytic anemia (thrombotic microangiopathy. Brit. med. J. **1952 a II**, 897-903.
Symmers, W.St.C.: Über die thrombotische Mikroangiopathie und ihre Beziehungen zu den sog. Kollagenkrankheiten. Verh. Dtsch. Ges.Path. **36**, 224-233 (1952b).
Symmers, W.ST.C.: Thrombotic microangiopathy. Histological diagnosis during life. Lancet **1956 I**, 592-596.
Vitsky, B.H., Suzuki, Y., Strauss, L., Churg, J.: The hemolytic uremic syndrome. Amer. J. Path. **57**, 627-639 (1969).
Volhard, F.: Die doppelseitigen hämatogenen Nierenerkrankungen. Berlin: Springer 1918.
Wagoner, R.D., Holley, K.E., Johnson, W.J.: Accelerated nephrosclerosis and postpartum acute renal failure in normotensive patients. Ann. intern. Med. **69**, 231-248 (1968).
Wehinger, H., Zollinger, H.U., Schenk, W., Künzer, W.: Hämolytisch-urämisches Syndrom (Gasser). Bericht über zwei Kinder mit ungewöhnlichem Verlauf. Klin. Wschr. **46**, 874-881 (1968).
Wilson, C., Byrom, F.B.: Renal changes in malignant hypertension. Experimental evidence. Lancet **1939 I**, 130-139.
Wilson, C., Byrom, F.B.: The vicious circle in chronic BRIGHT's disease. Experimental evidence from the hypertensive rat. Quart. J. Med. **10**, 65-93 (1941).
Zacherle, B.J., Richardson, J.A.: Irreversible renal failure secondary to hypertension induced by oral contraceptives. Ann. intern. Med. **77**, 83-85 (1972).

Liver Carcinogenesis in Rats After Aflatoxin B_1 Administration

A Light- and Electron-Microscopic Study

Anna M. NOVI

Abstract

The sequential development of light- and electron-microscopic changes in rat liver was monitored during the induction of hepatocellular carcinomas by an 8-weeks aflatoxin B_1 dosage regimen that produces minimal toxic effects. By 16 weeks only an increased number of megalocytes was detected by light microscopy. Electron microscopy revealed profound changes of the liver parenchyma. Depending on their location within the liver lobule, the hepatocytes underwent two main patterns of modification. While periportal hepatocytes rapidly degenerated, more peripherally located parenchymal cells first showed a high proliferation of ER, of the type observed in hepatocytes actively engaged in drug metabolism, and then peripheral hepatocytes underwent degenerative changes of a pattern similar to that observed in periportal hepatocytes. ER appeared to be affected first, then depletion of glycogen and alteration of the Golgi zones occurred, followed by damage to mitochondria and cell membrane. Between 17 and 37 weeks, light-microscopic observations showed: a) the appearance of small periportal foci of newly born hepatocytes that successively degenerated, b) a progressive disappearance of megalocytes. Electron microscopy revealed sublobular changes resembling the ones reported in the previous period. Only glycogen-storing hepatocytes became more frequent in the centrilobular zone. From 42 weeks onward, light microscopic observations showed a diffuse proliferation of periportal hepatocytes resulting in the appearance of islands of neoplastic cells by histological standard. Degenerative changes of the newly born hepatocytes consisted either in addensation of their basophilic cytoplasm toward the periphery of the cell, which assumed a ground-glass appearance in paranuclear location, or in vacuolation of their cytoplasm. Ultrastructural equivalents of all these cellular changes were reported.

On the basis of the present observations it was concluded that: 1) the lag time preceding the appearance of recognizable cancer by morphological criteria is characterized by a constant spectrum of ultramicroscopic changes that are dependent on the location of the hepatocytes within the liver lobule. Since liver parenchymal cells disclosed identical phenotypical changes after AFB_1 was discontinued, it postulates an endogenous mechanism of storage and release of the carcinogen. Ultramicroscopic features supporting this mechanism have been described. 2) Basophilic periportal hepatocytes represent the cellular type responding to AFB_1 by proliferation. 3) The cellular proliferative response to AFB_1 is diffuse in nature. 4) Newly born hepatocytes correspond to neoplastic cells by histological standards.

I. Introduction

Among the *in-vivo* models of experimental carcinogenesis, the aflatoxin one is of special interest, since these toxins are at present strongly suspected of being carcinogenic in man. The aflatoxins are a group of metabolites elaborated by some strains of the mold *Aspergillus flavus*, which grows readily on peanuts and other crops, such as maize, when these are stored in warm weather and humid conditions (*Lancaster* et al., 1961; *Wogan* 1966, 1973). These fungal metabolites exert pronounced hepatotoxic effects in a wide variety of laboratory and farm animals (*Newberne* and *Butler*, 1969). Aflatoxin B_1, the most potent of these toxins, produces hepatocellular carcinomas in rats, mice, ferrets, tree shrews, rhesus monkeys, rainbow trout, and guppies (*Carnaghan*, 1965; *Halver*, 1969; *Newberne* and *Wogan*, 1968; *Newberne* and *Butler*, 1969; *Sato* et al., 1973; *Adamson* et al., 1976; *Reddy* et al., 1976). In addition, the available epidemiological data from various developing countries of the world reveal a definite correlation between the risk to man of developing acute or chronic liver disease, including the occurrence of primary hepatocellular carcinoma, and the degree to which food products are contaminated with aflatoxins (*Shank* et al., 1972; *Van Rensburg* et al., 1975; *Peers* et al., 1976). Furthermore, aflatoxin B_1 was recently identified in a sample of liver tissue obtained at biopsy from a US patient suffering from liver carcinoma (*Phillips* et al., 1976).

The availability of chemically pure AFB_1 and well-defined technics for inducing liver tumors in rats provide a model that allows investigation of the sequences of essential cellular events that are unfolded during carcinogenesis. One approach to investigation of how the biological properties of cells are altered during cancerous growth is to monitor the morphological changes of target cells after carcinogen treatment. Although considerable research has been undertaken on the chemical nature and biological effects of the aflatoxins and their metabolism (for a review, cf. *Goldblatt*, 1969; *Wogan*, 1973; *Campbell* and *Hayes*, 1976), the sequential morphological changes in rat liver during carcinogenesis induced by aflatoxin B_1 have been the subject of few reports of studies based on either light or electron microscopy (*Newberne* and *Wogan*, 1968; *Kalengayi* and *Desmet*, 1975; *Newberne*, 1976; *Svoboda* et al., 1966; *Svoboda* and *Higginson*, 1968).

Therefore, in an attempt to complete the morphological investigations on aflatoxins, a correlated light and electron microscopic study was undertaken of the sequential morphological changes induced in rat liver by aflatoxin B_1 under conditions that minimize toxic effect.

II. Materials and Methods

1. Animals and Toxin

The animals used were Wistar II female rats from the Zentralinstitut für Versuchstierzucht, Hanover, Germany. The rats were obtained as weanlings and maintained in conventional cages with food (Altromin pellets) and water *ad libitum* until they weighed 100 g, at which time the experimental treatment was begun. Throughout the experiment, they were housed in screen-bottomed cages, five to a cage, in an air-conditioned room with a 12-hour light-dark cycle. The rats were given water and food (Altromin) *ad libitum*, and weighed monthly and just before sacrifice. They remained healthy up to the end of the experiment. The schedule of sacrifice was as follows: weekly for eight weeks, then 10, 13, 14, 16, 17, 19, 25, 28, 32, 37, 42, 48, 52, 61, and 66 weeks after the beginning of treatment. Experimental animals were randomly killed in groups of 3-4, together with 1 or 2 controls. Sacrifice always took place between 10 and 11 a.m., without previous starvation, to avoid diurnal variations of glycogen and endoplasmic reticulum (*Chedid* and *Nair*, 1972). Detailed autopsies were performed on all animals sacrificed during the course of the experiment or at its termination.

Crystalline aflatoxin B_1 (AFB_1) (Makor chemicals Inc., Jerusalem, Israel) dissolved in spectral grade dimethylformamide (DMF) (Merck, Darmstadt, Germany), was given by stomach tube. The rats were intubated on five consecutive days per week for eight consecutive weeks: each experimental animal received 25 μg AFB_1 in 2.5 μl DMF per day (total dose, 1 mg AFB_1; 0.1 ml DMF); control animals received 2.5 μl DMF only per day. (Preliminary experiments have demonstrated that such an amount of DMF does not influence the incorporation of appropriate precursors into DNA, RNA and protein of rat liver; *Novi* in preparation.) Prior to intubation, the solutions were made up to 1 ml in volume with distilled water.

2. Electron Microscopy

The fixative for all experiments was a mixture of cold 2.5% glutaraldehyde and 0.8% paraformaldehyde in 0.1 M cacodylate buffer, pH 7.4. The final osmolality of the solution was 358 mOsmoles. Animals were anesthetized with ether and the liver fixed by perfusion through the portal vein according to *Fahimi* (1967). Immediately after the completion of perfusion, the liver was removed and cut in blocks with sides about 0.5 mm, which were placed for another 2.5 h in the same fixative at 4°C. The specimens were postfixed in 1% osmium tetroxide (in 0.1 M phosphate buffer, pH 7.3), dehydrated and embedded in Araldite. 1-μm-thick large survey sections of plastic-embedded liver tissue were cut from 24 blocks from each rat and stained with toluidine blue for light microscopy. This allowed us: 1) to locate specific sublobular zones of hepatic lobules in the cut surface of the tissue blocks, and 2) to make an exact comparison of changes seen by light and by electron microscopy. Small areas were then selected and trimmed, and ultrathin sections were cut with a glass or diamond knife on a Reichert ultratome and routinely stained with uranyl acetate and lead citrate. For identification of glycogen particles, ultrathin sections were stained with 1% phosphotungstic acid (PTA). The sections were examined with a Siemens 101 electron microscope at 60 kV, with double condensor illumination.

3. Light Microscopy

Tissue was removed from the liver while the animals were under ether anesthesia, and fixed in 10% neutral formalin. Paraffin sections were stained with hematoxylin and eosin, periodic acid-Schiff, Van Gieson, and cresyl-fast violet. Frozen sections were stained with oil red 0.

4. Mitotic Index

The mitotic index of the liver parenchymal cells was determined by examination of a minimum of 40 adjacent microscopic fields (an average of 5000 nuclei) in each of the liver lobes, and expressed as the number of mitoses per 1000 nuclei. Only parenchymal cells in metaphase and anaphase were scored as mitoses.

The terms periportal zone, midzone and centrilobular zone, when referred to changes observed in this experiment, correspond to *Rappaport*'s concept of liver acinus, 1st, 2nd, and 3rd zone, respectively (1976).

III. Results

The livers of control rats sacrificed at the same time as the AFB_1-treated animals showed no morphological changes. Throughout the experiment, the lesions were totally confined to parenchymal cells. Bile ductus and oval cell proliferation were absent. No cirrhosis or fibrosis was observed.

IV. Morphological Changes During AFB_1 Administration (0-8 Weeks)

1. Light-Microscopic Findings

The livers of AFB_1-treated animals sacrificed within the first four weeks showed no histological changes. By five weeks occasional large liver cells (megalocytes) began to appear in the midzone of the lobule. By eight weeks, the megalocytes had become more evident.

2. Electron-Microscopic Findings (1-2 Weeks)

The ultrastructural changes in the parenchymal cells were more profound than light microscopic studies had suggested. The modified cells showed a typical lobular distribution, being mainly located in the periportal zone and the midzone of the lobule. Centrilobular cells appeared to be unaffected.

Periportal cells exhibited alterations of the endoplasmic reticulum (ER). As shown in Figure 1, stacks of rough endoplasmic reticulum (RER) displayed dilatation and cisternal irregularity without evident loss of ribosomes attached to the membrane surface. The most prominent changes occurred in the cisternal membranes, which showed focal loss of continuous visualization with membranous profiles like blebs protruding into the cisternal space. Here and there, degenerating tubular structures bridged the dilated cisternae. The dilatation of the cisternae was mainly segmental in type, and in several sections repeating segmental dilatations could be found. The membranes limiting the dilated portions were usually ill-defined but retained a normal complement of ribosomes at least at one side. A very constant feature was the presence of filamentous, rodlike structures in the cisternal lumen. In some areas of the cytoplasm there was a decrease in the number of elongated profiles and a preponderance of circular and elliptical images partially or totally devoid of ribosomes. This may in part have resulted from vesiculation and fragmentation of the RER cisternae. The ribosomes observed in close proximity to disrupted vesicles appeared as randomly dispersed particles within the cytoplasmic ground substance.

The other cytoplasmic organelles and nuclei in these cells usually exhibited a normal appearance. More rarely, besides the changes described above the cells showed a segmental dilatation of the nuclear envelope, and swelling of the mitochondria that appeared to be transformed into empty vacuoles outlined by membrane.

On the basis of their ultrastructural changes, the parenchymal cells within the midzone of the lobule formed a heterogeneous population composed of different cell types. The latter may represent intermediate steps in the same functional process. One type of cells (ER-hyperplastic cells) (Fig. 2) exhibited the ultrastructural features that are a characteristic aspect of liver cells after the administration of phenobarbital (*Chiesara* et al., 1967; *Smuckler* and *Arcasoy*, 1969). Large areas of cytoplasm were filled with tightly packed vesicles and tubules of the smooth endoplasmic reticulum (SER), which mainly showed the same appearance as in untreated animals. An increase in RER profiles also occurred. No significant alterations other than those mentioned above were observed.

The following types of parenchymal cells (transitional basophilic cells) predominated in the midzone of the liver lobule. Large areas of cytoplasm were occupied by agglomerates

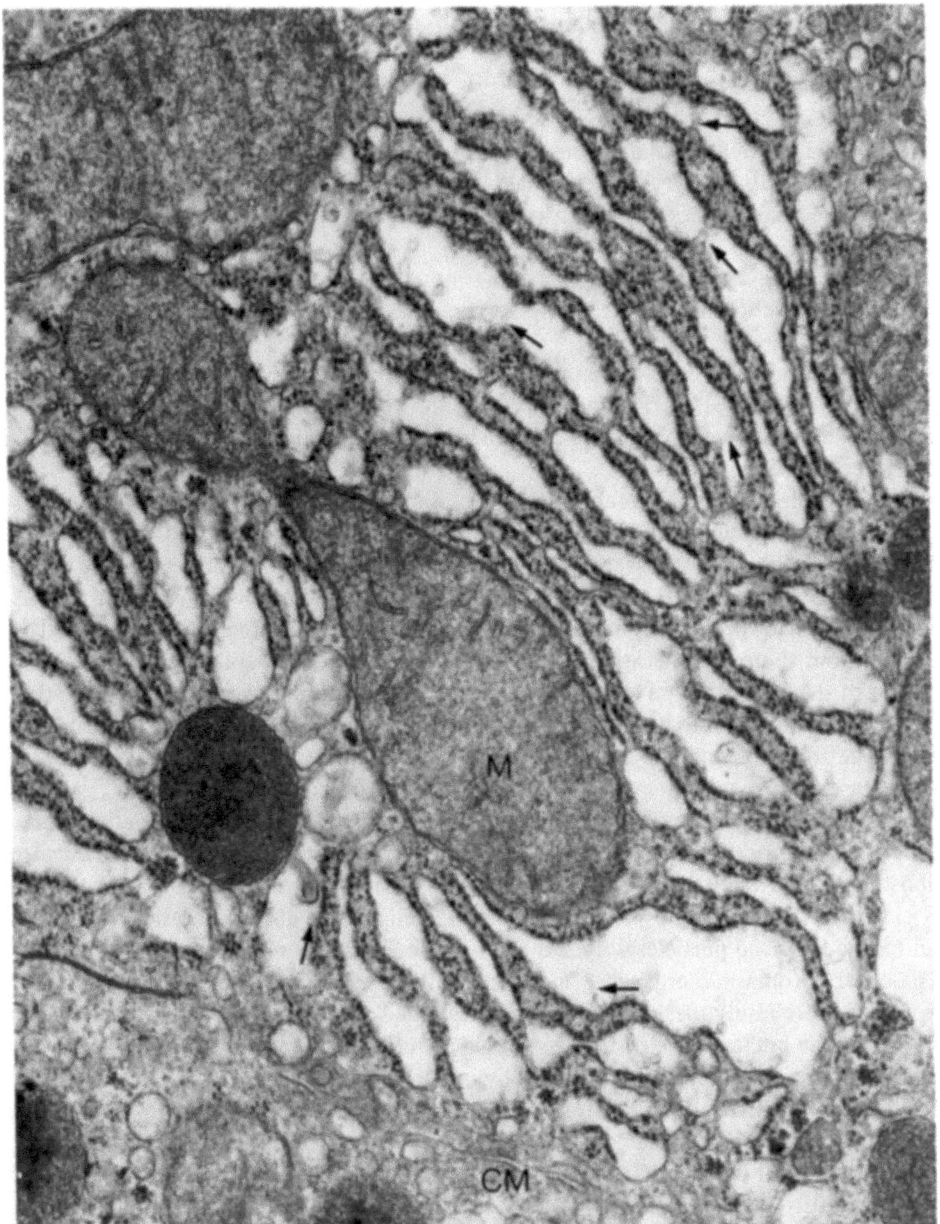

Fig. 1. Cytoplasmic portion of a periportal hepatocyte after 1 week on AFB_1. Irregular dilatation of RER cisternae without evident loss of ribosomes from membranes. Arrows indicate degenerating membranous profiles bridging or protruding into dilated cisternae. *M* = mitochondria; *CM* = cell membrane. X 30 800

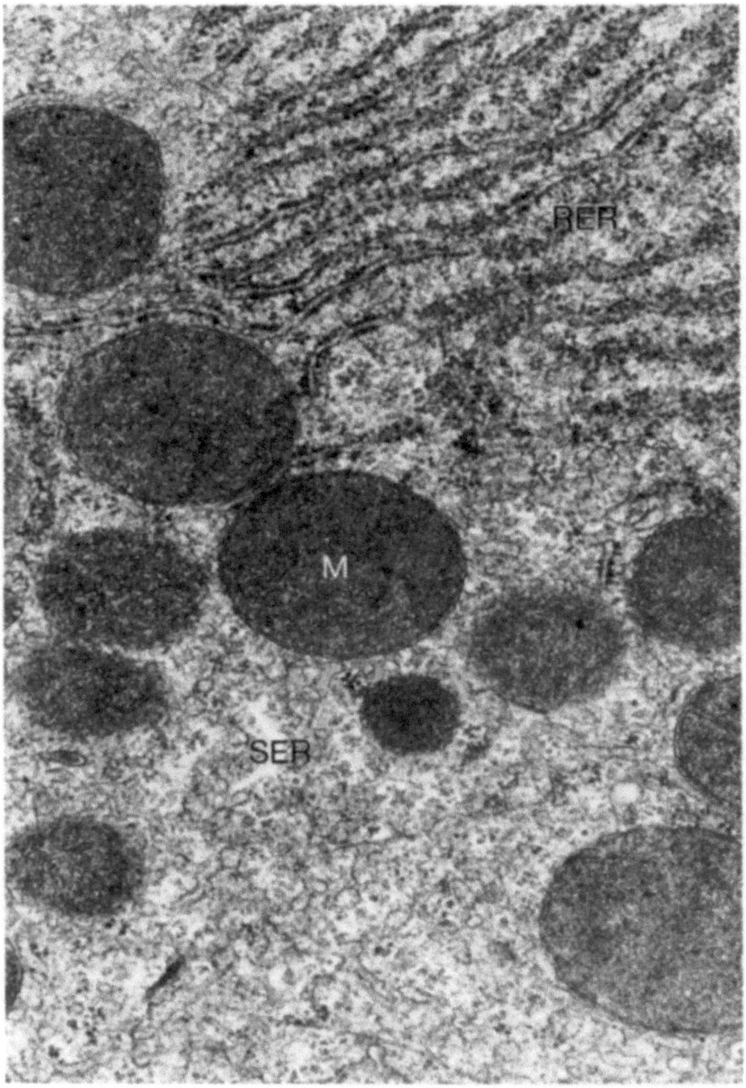

Fig. 2. Cytoplasmic part of a midzonal "ER-hyperplastic" hepatocyte after 1 week on AFB_1. *SER* = smooth endoplasmic reticulum; *RER* = rough endoplasmic reticulum; *M* = mitochondria. X 33 700

of rough-surfaced tubular profiles arranged in parallel arrays (Fig. 3). The RER conglomerates were characterized by an increased concentration of ribosome particles within the intercisternal spaces (asterisks in Fig. 3), which did not show any special pattern of arrangement and appeared to be distributed in a random fashion. The SER was also increased (Fig. 4). Slightly dilated smooth-surfaced tubules and vesicles intermingled with glycogen particles occupied some areas of the cytoplasm. The expansion of the SER occurred mainly in glyco-

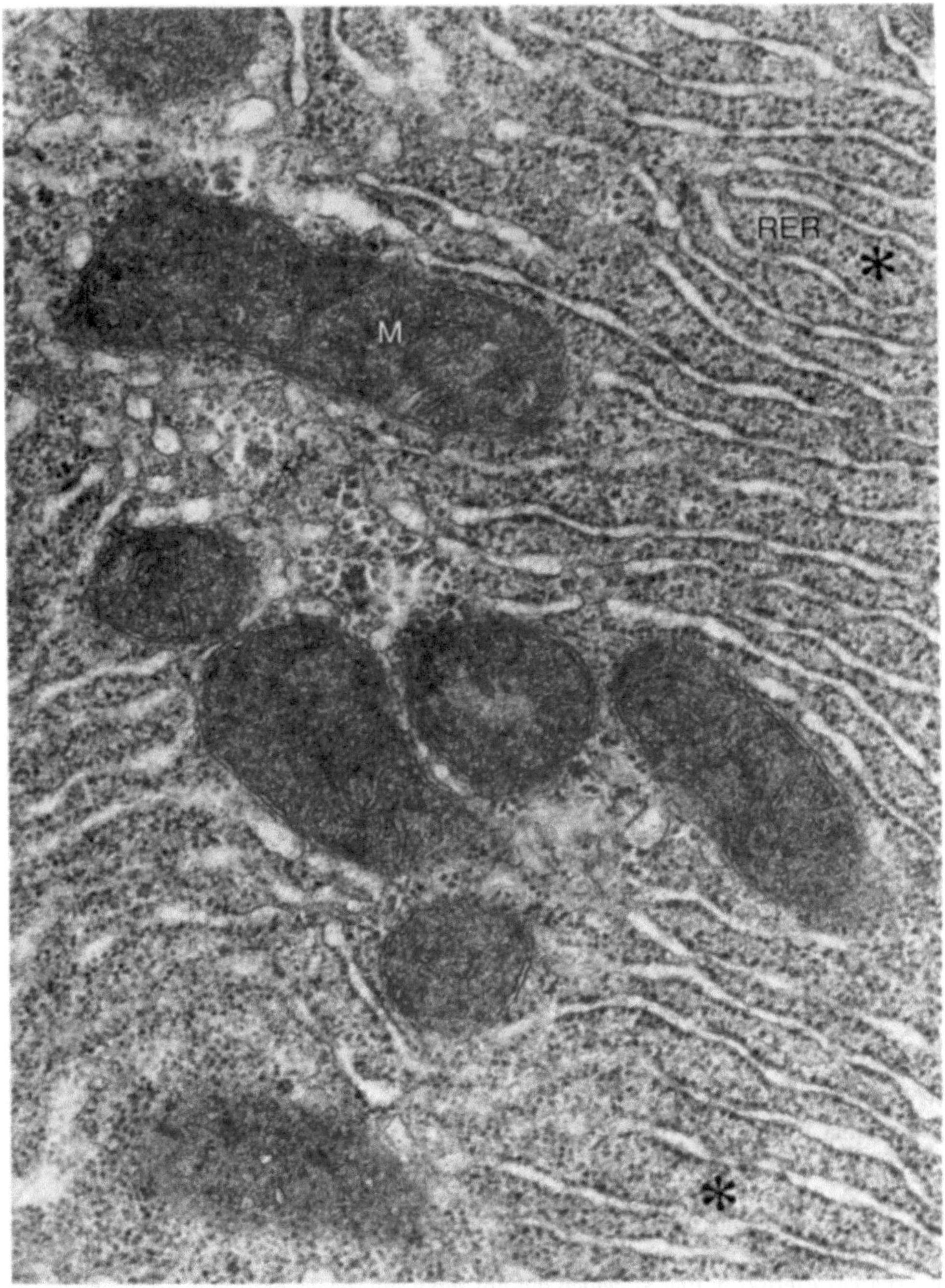

Fig. 3. Cytoplasmic portion of a midzonal "transitional basophilic" hepatocyte after 1 week on AFB_1. Note increase of free ribosomes in the intercisternal spaces (asterisks). *RER* = rough endoplasmic reticulum; *M* = mitochondria. X 38 500

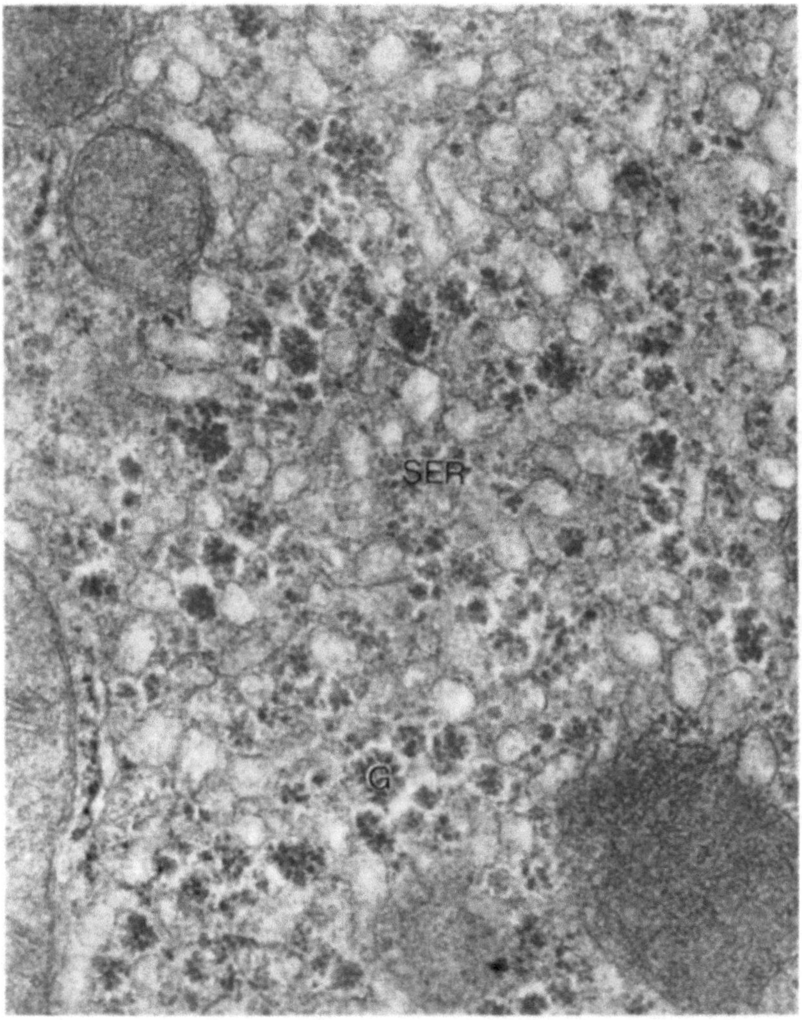

Fig. 4. Cytoplasmic portion of a midzonal, "transitional basophilic" hepatocyte after 1 week on AFB_1. Slightly dilated smooth endoplasmic reticulum profiles *(SER)* are intermingled with glycogen *(G)*. X 34 200

gen areas, which were progressively permeated by the agranular profiles. These contained finely granular material of low electron density and small aggregates of osmiophilic substance.

Microbodies showing a regular lattice-like structure in their center were increased in number. Golgi zones were abundant and rather conspicuous. The tubuli and secretory vesicles were slightly dilated and filled with a material of moderate density. More electron-dense material was observed in the peripheral portions of the secretory cisternae and in secretory vacuoles localized in the vicinity of the Golgi complex. Some changes in the cell membrane were observed, consisting in moderate enlargement of the microvilli along the bile canaliculi and along the sinusoids. Dilatation of these structures into blebs was also occasionally encountered. Pynocytotic vesicles were frequently seen at the cell membrane along the sinusoids. Here and there, the spaces of Disse were filled up with coarsely granular material. The other cellular constituents, including mitochondria, nuclei, and nucleoli, were unaffected by any detectable change.

After one week of treatment, occasional transitional basophilic cells showed ultrastructural evidence of involution (variant no. 1 of degenerating transitional basophilic cells). The membranes of the ER and the Golgi complex were widely affected. The common alteration was a loss of continuous visualization. The profiles of the SER became attenuated and partially disrupted, and progressively disappeared. The RER cisternae arranged in parallel arrays seemed to be better preserved. However, vesiculation of the RER cisternae, especially at their margins, was frequently found. Aggregates of images resembling the Golgi zone were recognizable in some areas. The glycogen was also affected. Glycogen particles were usually ill-defined, smaller in size, and of lower electron density. Although intermediate aspects easily allowed morphological identification of these granula as glycogen particles, their identity was confirmed by specific staining. The glycogen areas appeared enlarged, probably as a consequence of loss of SER profiles. However, the distribution of modified glycogen particles in the glycogen areas was rather uneven, and foci of glycogen depletion were often encountered. Mitochondria showed a slightly denser matrix; otherwise they appeared well preserved. The nuclear outline was slightly indented; the nucleoplasm showed an increase in electron density.

After two weeks of treatment there was an increase in number of this variant of degenerating transitional basophilic cells. In several of them (variant no. 2 of transitional basophilic cells), the lesions had progressed to a complete depletion of glycogen and deterioration of all membranous structures, including the mitochondrial ones, into a smudgy-looking material.

3-8 Weeks

After 3 weeks most periportal cells exhibited a high degree of disorganization of the RER, reflected by a decrease in the number and length of the parallel cisternae. Wrapping of RER cisternae around mitochondria was usually found. In some areas no parallel profiles were observed and RER occurred only in the form of isolated profiles, which appeared to be irregularly distributed in the cytoplasm. The RER cisternae were mostly dilated with disrupted membranes and filamentous rodlike structures in their lumen. However, no obvious degranulation of the membranes was apparent. Foci of cytoplasmic degradation occupied the spaces among the disorganized RER and the mitochondria. They consisted of degenerating vesicles flanked by smudgy material. Glycogen particles had disappeared. Golgi zones and SER could no longer be identified. Mitochondria exhibited a rather dense matrix, with loss of visualization of the cristae. Microbodies and lysosomes were decreased in number. Centrioles were occasionally encountered. Nuclei were mostly round in shape, although slight indentations were sometimes observed. No evident modifications of the nucleoli were detected. The nuclear envelope was slightly distended. Significant alterations of the cell membrane were not noticed. The capillary lumen contained coarsely granular material.

The hepatocytes showing the ultrastructural details reported above were mainly situated close to the terminal afferent vessels. As the distance from the supplying vessels increased,

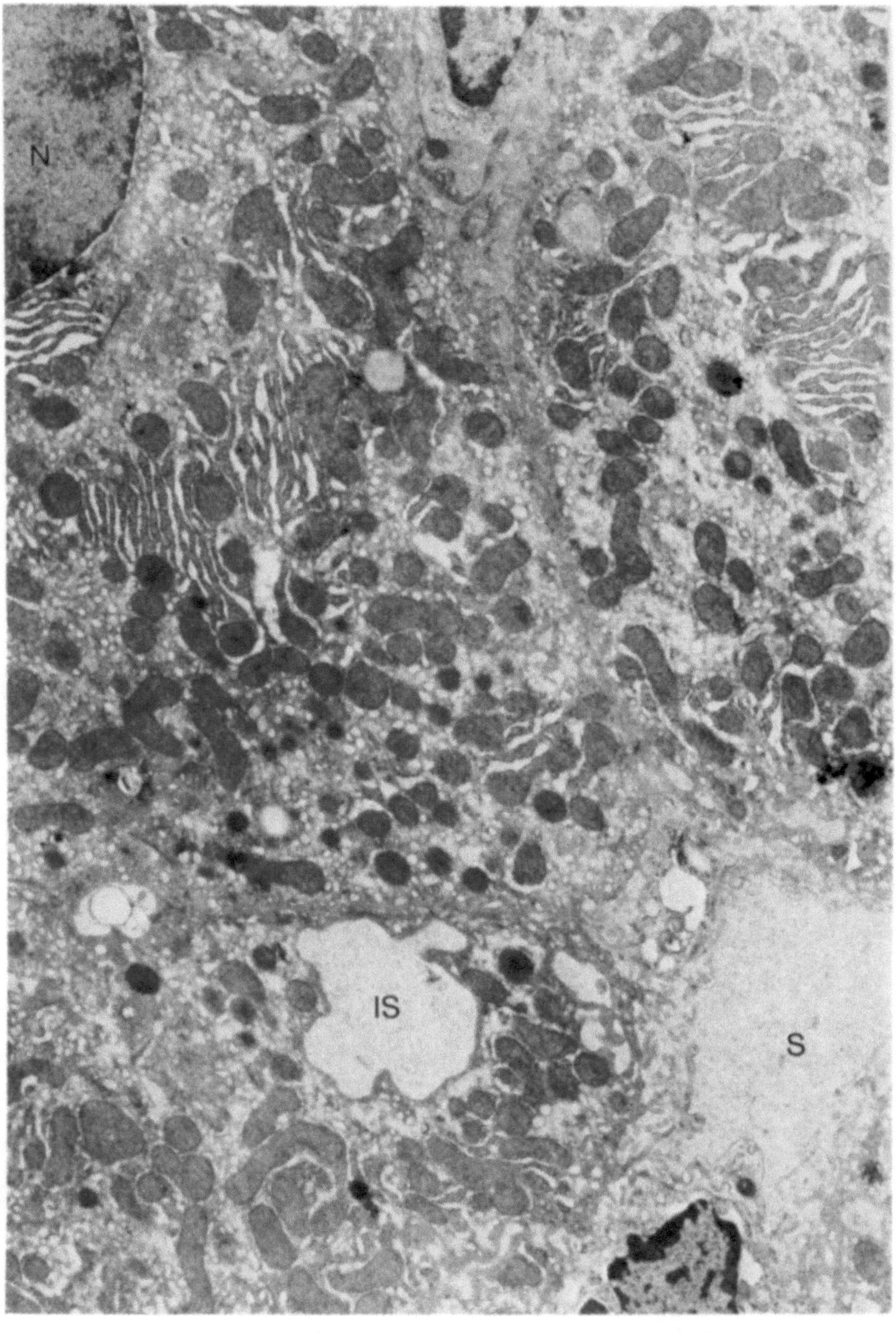

Fig. 5. Periportal hepatocytes after 3 weeks on AFB_1. Note disorganization of RER and prominence of vesicular profiles. *IS* = intracytoplasmic space. A portion of a nucleus *(N)* appears in the upper left and a sinusoid *(S)* at the lower right. X 9600

the vesicular profiles of the ER and mitochondrial structures appeared better preserved. A conspicuous abnormality in these cells was the presence through the cytoplasm of irregular spaces (Fig. 5), even in paranuclear locations. They appeared to arise from dilated tortuosity of the cell membrane and usually contained granular material, as did the slightly dilated intercellular spaces.

After 4 weeks there was clear evidence that the cytoplasm of periportal hepatocytes had deteriorated further. In a considerable number of cells, it exhibited large empty spaces among disorganized ergastoplasm, denser mitochondria, and patchy agglomerations of membranous debris. In comparison with the cytoplasmic alterations, the nuclei were better maintained and appeared similar to those found in periportal hepatocytes at the end of the third week. Zonal disintegration of the cell membrane along the spaces of Disse was occasionally found. Cytoplasmic components of the liver cells were easily identified in the space of Disse and capillary lumen.

The midzone of the lobule mainly consisted of transitional basophilic cells and their degenerative variants.

Centrilobular hepatocytes showed ultramicroscopic changes similar to those observed in ER-hyperplastic cells. However, degeneration of cytoplasmic structures occurred with increased frequency from the 4th to the 8th week. The membranes of the SER underwent degenerative changes resulting in irregular electron-dense annuli or small whorls of filamentous material scattered in the rarefied ground substance. In these areas glycogen became rare. Focal interruptions in the continuity of the limiting membrane of the RER cisternae were also observed. The ribosomes occurred as small clusters of randomly dispersed particles located in close proximity to the degenerating RER cisternae, or as patchy aggregates mirrowing stacks of RER. The Golgi complex was often difficult to identify. When this was possible, however, its components appeared dilated and partially filled with electron-dense material. Cytoplasmic vacuoles partially limited by a single membrane and containing either whorls of filamentous material or electron-dense flecks were a consistent feature. Fat droplets were usually found free in the cytoplasm at the cell periphery. Nuclear structures showed no apparent modification. Slight changes of the cell membrane were often observed. They consisted of shortening and rarefaction of the microvilli. At the sinusoidal border, focal ruptures of the cell membrane were often seen.

V. Morphological Changes After Withdrawal of AFB_1 (9-66 Weeks)

1. Light-Microscopic Findings (9-16 Weeks)

The only histological change observed was an increase in the number of megalocytes, which showed a progressive vacuolation of the cytoplasm.

2. Electron-Microscopic Findings (9-16 Weeks)

At this point the ultramicroscopic changes within the hepatocytes were, in general, comparable to those observed during AFB_1 administration (0-8 weeks). However, advanced cytoplasmic lesions were now more common.

The majority of periportal cells showed ultramicroscopic features similar to those observed at the end of the third week in the most peripheral areas of the periportal zone (cf. Fig. 5). As reduction and vesiculation of the RER had progressed, these cells were characterized by the presence of large areas of cytoplasm filled up with ill-defined, circular profiles partially denuded of ribosomes. Small aggregates of granular material were scattered within the ground substance among the vesicles. Although morphological identification of this material was rather difficult, specific staining demonstrated that most of it was made up of ribosomes. The mitochondria were lightly stained and had gathered among the residual RER. Lysosomes were rarely seen and, when present, they were located close to mitochondria. Nuclei showed reduced electron density of the nucleoplasm and smaller nucleoli with increased electron opacity. Focal membrane degeneration and rupture of the hepatocytes were often observed. Membranous debris, and especially mitochondria, were found inside the capillary lumen. As a consequence of the paucity in specialized cytoplasmic organelles and the decreased electron density of the cytoplasmic background, these cells appeared "clear" under the electron microscope.

Hepatocytes showing ultramicroscopic changes, which up to now had only been found in the periportal area (cf. Fig. 5), had extended to the midzone of the lobule. Besides a marked alteration of the ER, these cells exhibited mitochondrial lesions consisting in segmental membrane alterations with focal deficit in the subjacent mitochondrial matrix.

In addition to the degenerating hepatocytes mentioned above, the midzone of the lobule contained a heterogeneous cell population mainly consisting of ER-hyperplastic and transitional basophilic cells with their degenerative variants. ER-hyperplastic hepatocytes were now a very common finding. However, most of them displayed some cytoplasmic modifications. The most striking was the presence of large clusters of ribosome particles, some of which were arranged in polysomal patterns. They were usually observed close to RER stacks, the cisternae of which exhibited ill-defined limiting membranes. The RER cisternae did not show apparent dilatation, and they were frequently arranged in a ruffled pattern. The Golgi apparatus consisted mainly of dilated vesicles containing finely fibrillar material of low electron density.

Hepatocytes showing a high vacuolated cytoplasm were often encountered (Fig. 6). These cells retained the major ultrastructural characteristic of transitional basophilic cells, i.e. conglomerates of RER tubular profiles with packed ribosome particles in the interspaces (Fig. 7), but otherwise their cytoplasm consisted of smudgy dense outlines delimiting empty areas, and dark mitochondria. The mitochondria were characterized by a very electron-dense matrix and increased numbers of irregularly oriented cristae. All the mitochondrial membranes showed a loss of ultrastructural definition. Lysosomes and microbodies were either rare or absent. Other cytoplasmic structures, including SER, glycogen, and Golgi apparatus, could not be identified. Partial interruptions of the plasma membrane were observed. Despite the high level of cytoplasmic alterations, the nuclei maintained an almost normal appearance.

Intermediate aspects of damage in hepatocytes located side by side with the highly vacuolated cells allowed us to reconstruct the degeneration process. The first structures to show signs of alteration in typical transitional basophilic cells were the SER profiles. They appeared to be fragmented, with some ill-defined and some more electron-dense, limiting membranes, whereas the glycogen particles located among them showed aggregation and loss of ultramicroscopic definition. A progressive loss of these structures occurred, which

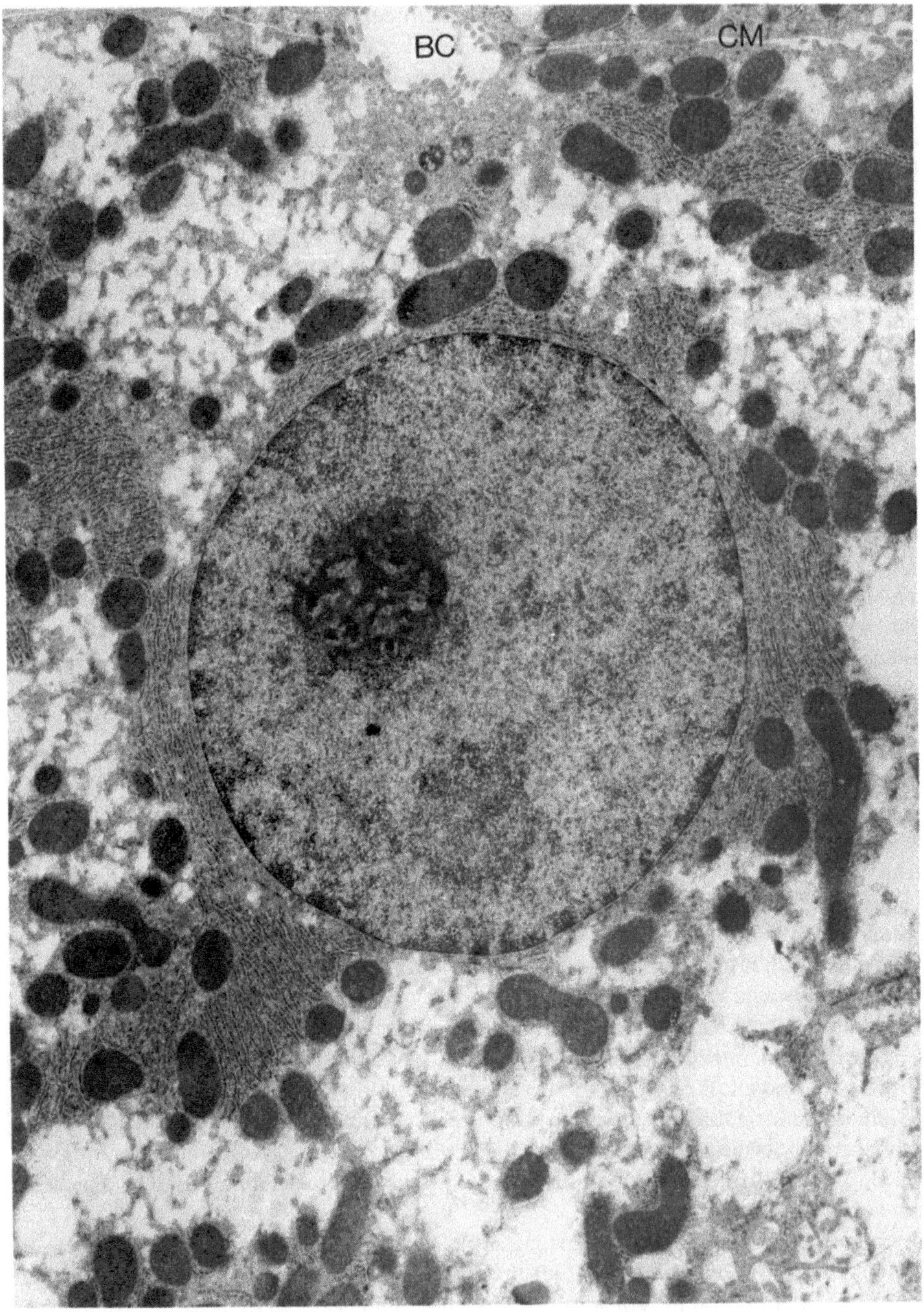

Fig. 6. Electron micrograph of a midzonal, "transitional basophilic" hepatocyte in advanced stage of degeneration, 8 weeks after AFB_1 withdrawal. In spite of the remarkably altered cytoplasm, nuclear structures are well preserved. *CM* = cell membrane; *BC* = bile canaliculus. X 11 400

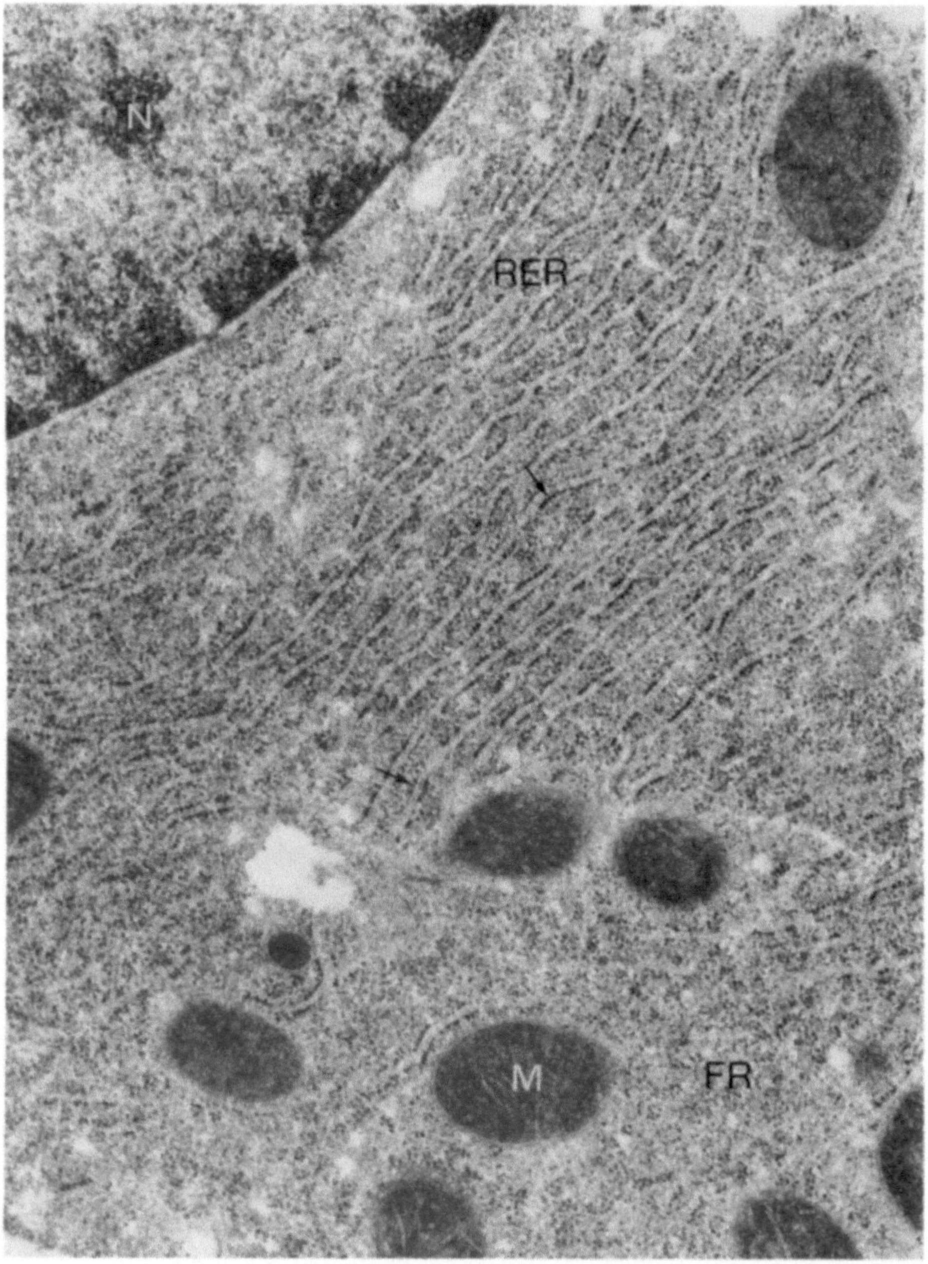

Fig. 7. Portion of a midzonal, "transitional basophilic" hepatocyte in intermediate stage of degeneration 8 weeks after AFB_1 withdrawal. Agglomerates of rough endoplasmic reticulum *(RER)* and free ribosomes *(FR)* widely extended throughout the cytoplasm. As shown at arrows, wall of RER cisternae appears as a transparent layer. Note increase of free ribosomes in the intercisternal spaces. *M* = mitochondria; *N* = nucleus. X 32 400 (reduced to 90%)

appeared to be transformed into small flecks of low electron density among small whorls of filamentous material of high electron density. Alteration of the Golgi zone occurred almost in parallel. Damage to the RER was observed first at the periphery of the RER conglomerates and at the isolated tubular profiles in the cytoplasm. The RER cisternae appeared fragmented but no loss of ribosomes or dilatation was observed. On careful examination, the wall of the RER cisternae appeared as a transparent layer (arrows in Fig. 7) delimited outside by ribosomes and inside by granular material of moderate electron opacity. The membranes of the nuclear envelope showed a similar modification. Small fragments of RER profiles displaying the ultramicroscopic features reported above were fre-

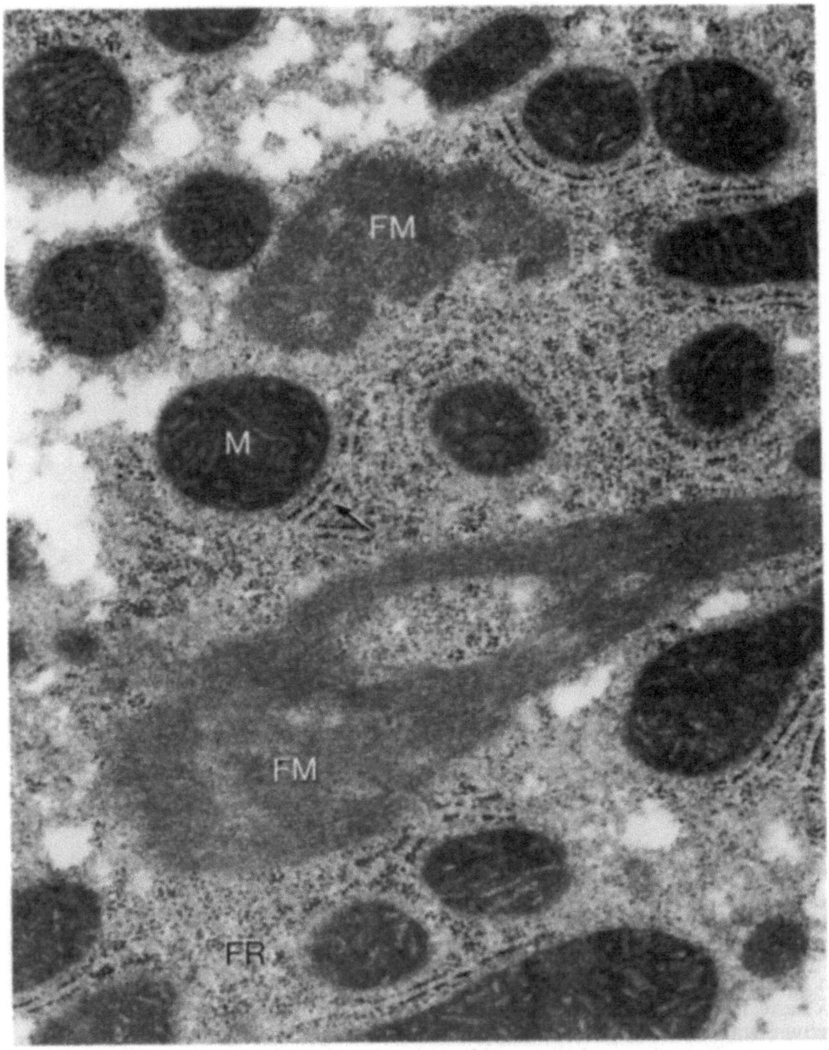

Fig. 8. Cytoplasmic portion of a degenerating "transitional basophilic" hepatocyte 11 weeks after withdrawal of AFB_1. Note aggregates of electron-dense fibrillar material *(FM)* among dark mitochondria *(M)*, fragments of RER cisternae (arrows), and free ribosomes *(FR)*. X 21 000

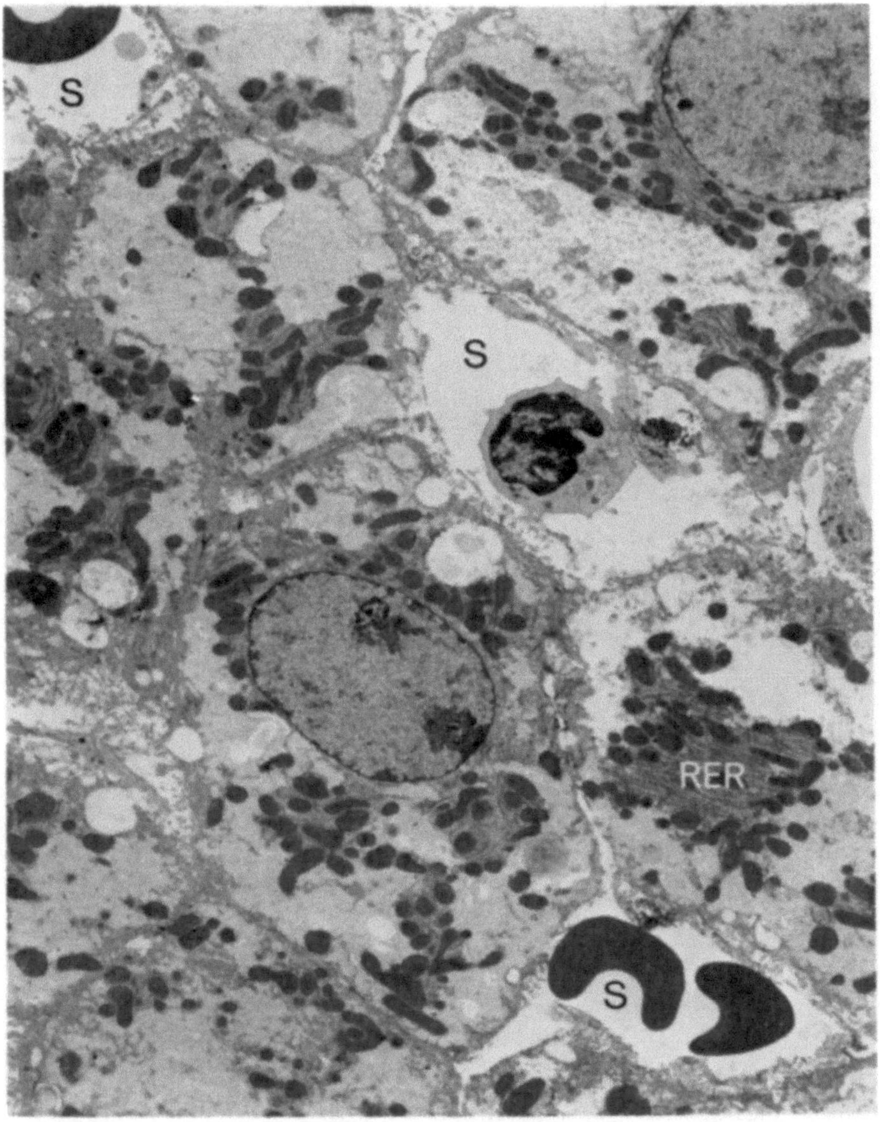

Fig. 9. Centrilobular, glycogen-storing hepatocytes 11 weeks after AFB_1 withdrawal. Note large cytoplasmic areas devoid of organelles but filled with granular material. The rough endoplasmic reticulum *(RER)* is crowded aside and seems to surround mitochondria more prominently. *S* = sinusoid. X 5000 (reduced to 90%)

quently observed among ribosome particles, dark mitochondria, and aggregates of fibrillar material of high electron density (Fig. 8). The fibrillar material closely resembled linear profiles of the degenerating membranous material often encountered in hepatocytes with ER alterations. In parallel with the loss of RER membranes, huge conglomerates of ribosome particles with no special pattern of arrangement were observed in the cytoplasm (cf.

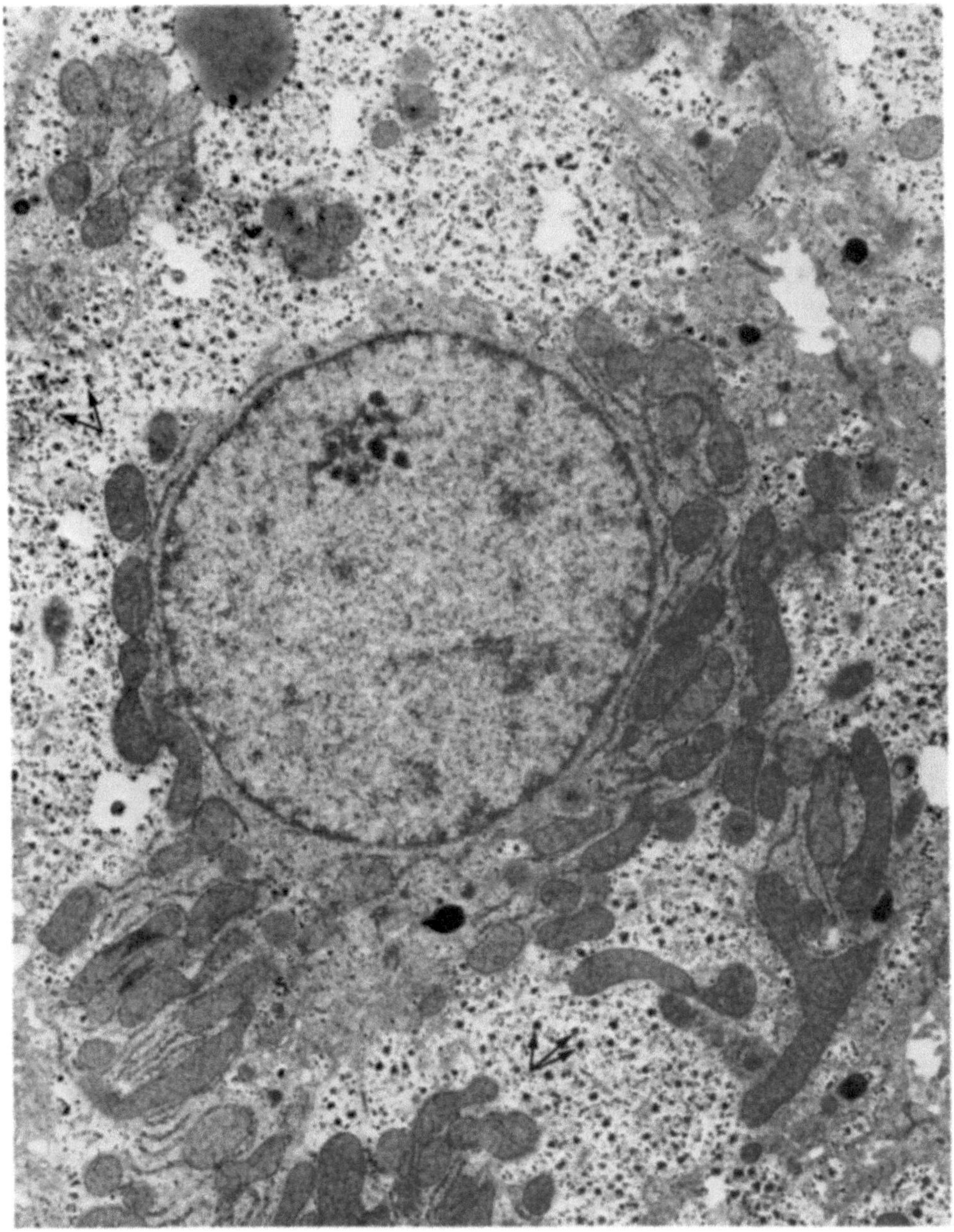

Fig. 10. Electron microscopic demonstration of glycogen in the cytoplasm of a centrilobular hepatocyte 11 weeks after AFB_1 withdrawal. Note selective location of PTA precipitates (arrows) within large cytoplasmic areas devoid of organelles. 1% PTA stain. X 10 300

Fig. 7). Focal empty areas were then observed among the ribosomes, resulting in progressive disappearance of these structures. It is noteworthy that loss of ribosome aggregates was often detected close to lysosomes showing focal interruptions in the continuity of the limiting membrane.

ER-hyperplastic hepatocytes and their variants were the only type of cells observed in the centrilobular zone of the lobule. Variant one showed a reduction of the agranular profiles, which were rather widely separated and formed a loose lattice with glycogen particles inside. Most of the profiles were made of vesicles arranged in a row. Transition of rough and smooth membranes was commonly encountered. Parallel stacks of RER cisternae were usually present; only rarely were they partially disarranged or curved around mitochondria. Dilatation of RER cisternae was not observed. The Golgi zones contained abundant partially dilated vesicles filled up with material of moderate density. More electron-dense material was observed in enlarged secretory vacuoles located close to the Golgi complex. Microbodies and lysosomes were numerous. Degenerating membranous material, in the form of either large aggregates or linear profiles, was scattered in the cytoplasm. Microfoci of cytoplasmic degeneration, consisting in single-membrane-limited areas with structureless material inside, were occasionally observed. Nuclei and other cytoplasmic organelles were normal. The cell membrane showed no apparent modification except for a slight reduction in number of the microvilli.

Variant two was characterized by the presence of limited cytoplasmic areas containing degenerating fragments of SER profiles scattered among ill-defined granular material. The RER profiles were correspondingly reduced, so that isolated RER cisternae of decreased length, showing clear continuity with the SER profiles, were often encountered. Small clusters of ribosomes with no special pattern of arrangement frequently occurred among the degenerating profiles of the RER.

The third variant of ER-hyperplastic cells was characterized by the presence of large areas of cytoplasm devoid of organelles and filled up with ill-defined granular material (Fig. 9). As shown in Figure 10, this material is mainly glycogen. The residual cytoplasmic structures consisted only of partially disarranged RER cisternae, slightly dark mitochondria, and rare lysosomes. As the degenerative process had progressed further, empty zones were observed in the cytoplasm. They were mainly a consequence of zonal loss of glycogen particles. Rupture of cell membrane, especially at the sinusoid borders, was a common finding at this stage. In these cells, the nuclei had a normal configuration except for the nucleoli, which showed a depletion of the granular component while the fibrillar component assumed a clumped reticulated pattern.

3. Light-Microscopic Findings (17-37 Weeks)

Little difference was usually noted between the body weight of control (DMF) and AFB_1-treated rats. At this point the body weight of controls (11 animals) ranged between 195 and 280 g. Most of AFB_1-treated rats (17 out of 24 killed at this time) weighed approximately the same as their controls. The other seven rats weighed about 30-40 g less than control animals within the same experimental group. Livers taken from rats with no differences in weight from their controls contained a few scattered foci of small parenchymal cells with round nuclei and slightly basophilic cytoplasm (Fig. 11a). The microfoci were usually surrounded by a rim of compressed hepatocytes. More frequently, aggregates of small parenchymal cells showing apparent degeneration were found (Fig. 11b). The cells were irregularly arranged, with spaces containing cellular debris among them. The peripheral cytoplasm displayed intense RNA staining, while the central cytoplasm had a ground-glass appearance. The nuclei were mostly pycnotic and peripherally located.

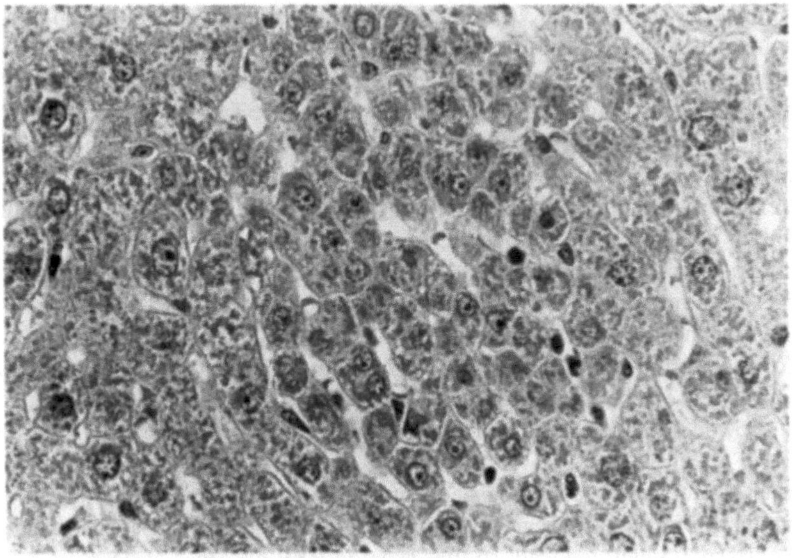

a

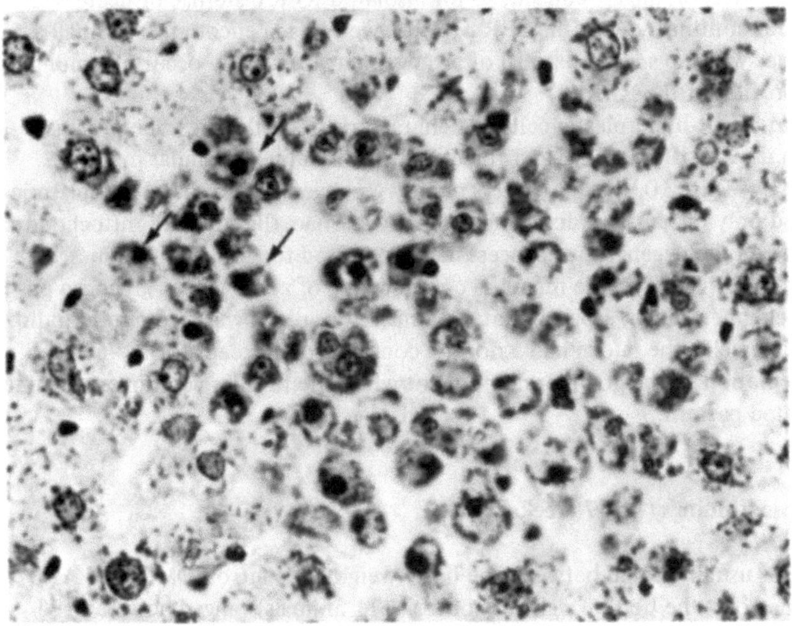

b

Fig. 11a and b. Paraffin sections of livers of rats killed 17 weeks after AFB_1 withdrawal. (a) Early island of small parenchymal cells compressing the surrounding parenchyma. H.E., 250 x. (b) Island of small parenchymal cells undergoing degeneration. Note the irregular addensation of RNA-staining material at the cell periphery. Pycnotic nuclei are indicated by arrows. Fast cresyl violet, 400 x

The small cellular foci were usually found in the periportal zone, though some of them had extended into the midzone of the lobule.

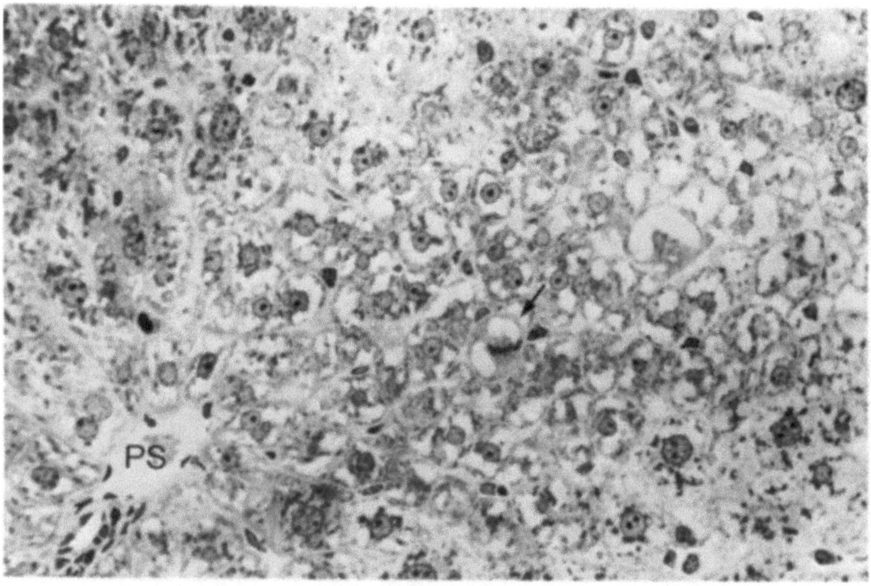

Fig. 12. Thick section of Araldite-embedded liver tissue from a rat killed 20 weeks after AFB_1 withdrawal. Vacuolated periportal hepatocytes in pseudonodular formation extend out into lobule. At arrow, vacuolated hepatocyte in mitosis. *PS* = periportal space. 250 x

Megalocytes were especially in evidence, though they later decreased in number and the residual ones appeared as large vacuolated cells.

Livers taken from rats with lower body weight than controls were characterized by cytoplasmic vacuolation of the hepatocytes. The change was particularly evident in the periportal zone of the lobule. Vacuolated mitotic figures were often seen among the altered hepatocytes. In tangential sections, groups of hepatocytes with a clear vacuolated cytoplasm appeared as nodular formations (Fig. 12). In such a group of cells mitotic figures were often found. However, compression of the surrounding parenchyma was not detected. Megalocytes were not evident.

4. Electron-Microscopic Findings (17-37 Weeks)

a) Liver of Rats with Normal Range of Body Weight

The majority of periportal cells appeared severely damaged. Their cytoplasm consisted of fragments of enlarged RER cisternae still retaining their complement of attached ribosomes, smudgy material, and electron-dense bodies totally devoid of a limiting membrane. The cell membrane was partially disrupted and cellular debris was easily identified in the capillary lumen. In spite of the remarkably altered cytoplasmic structures, the nuclei were rather well preserved. The only alteration observed was a lessening of the density of the nucleoplasm and an increase in electron opacity of the fibrillar component of the nucleolus.

The ultramicroscopic features of the small basophilic hepatocytes observed in the nodular formations by light microscopy (cf. Fig. 11a) are shown in Figure 13. The cytoplasm of these cells consisted mainly of partially fragmented RER cisternae. Clusters of ribosomes arranged as polysomes were often seen. They were usually located in close proximity to or intermin-

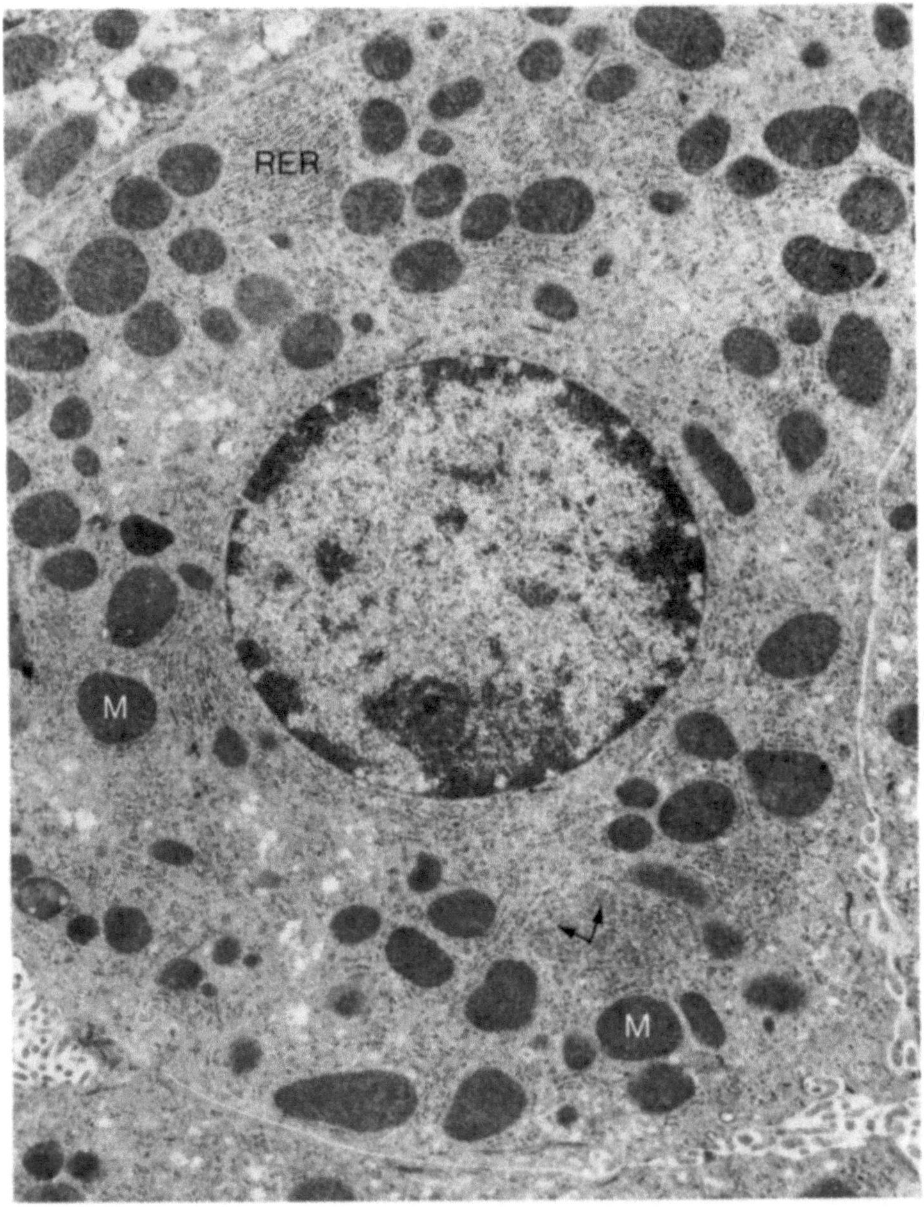

Fig. 13. Electron microscopic equivalent of small basophilic hepatocytes within early islands. Note diffuse fragmentation of rough endoplasmic reticulum *(RER)* cisternae among dark mitochondria *(M)*, and lack of SER, glycogen and Golgi zone. At arrow, a cluster of polysomes. Rat liver 11 weeks after AFB_1 withdrawal. X 14 500

gled with fragments of RER cisternae. Mitochondria showed an electron-dense matrix and ill-defined cristae. Centrioles were often seen. Glycogen, SER, and Golgi apparatus could not be identified. The nuclei showed no sign of alterations. There was, however, an increase in heterochromatin aggregates around the nucleus, which often formed a complete ring. No definable alteration in nucleolar structures was discerned.

Hepatocytes in the mid- and centrilobular zone of the lobule showed similar ultramicroscopic features to those observed in the previous time interval (8-16 weeks). However, at this time, the third variant of ER-hyperplastic hepatocytes predominated in the centrilobular zone of the lobule.

b) Liver of Rats with Lower Body Weight

The ultramicroscopic features of the clear vacuolated hepatocytes observed in the nodular formations by light microscopy (cf. Fig. 12), are shown in Figure 14. In these cells the nucleus was unremarkable except for the presence of prominent nucleoli, whereas the cytoplasm was characterized by the occurrence of empty spaces in which a few degenerating membranous profiles could still be traced. Disorganized ergastoplasm limited the empty spaces peripherally. Mitochondria were usually located in close association with RER cisternae and exhibited rather indistinct internal cristae, apparently in part because of an increase in the density of the intercristal matrix. The remainder of the cytoplasm contained conglomerates of RER cisternae, prominent Golgi zones, and lysosomes, which were usually grouped. Lipid droplets of various sizes and exhibiting a low degree of osmiophilia were found, especially in close proximity to the cell membrane. Evident alterations of the latter were not observed. However, the microvilli at the bile canaliculi appeared to be slightly reduced in number. The intercellular spaces were variably dilated and contained a coarsely granular material, as did the capillary lumen. Lipid droplets like the ones observed in the cytoplasm of vacuolated hepatocytes were either found in the perisinusoidal spaces or filled up the cytoplasm of interstitial cells.

Hepatocytes showing extreme vacuolation of their cytoplasm were frequently observed in the periportal zone. Intermediate aspects of damage in hepatocytes located close to highly vacuolated cells made it possible to reconstruct the degeneration process. The earliest alterations were seen at the endoplasmic reticulum, and these included dilatation and disruption of the RER cisternae, together with dissolution of the adjacent structures. It resulted in spaces containing scattered membranous profiles. Since these areas of cytoplasmic disintegration were at first delimited by cytoplasmic components showing structural integrity, the impression of acute damage was gained.

Corresponding to the light microscopic observations (cf. Fig. 12), mitotic figures were often observed among the vacuolated hepatocytes. Alterations of the chromosomes, which were easily recognized standing out clearly against a background of granular material, were not detected (Fig. 15). In contrast, the periphery of dividing cells, where cytoplasmic organelles are usually located, showed alterations of the RER profiles. These changes were similar to those observed in adjacent vacuolated hepatocytes. Although lipid droplets of the size observed in the cytoplasm of adjacent vacuolated hepatocytes were not detected in mitotic cells, most vesicles of RER were filled up with or contained a core of material that was similar in aspect and electron density. Mitochondria were normal. Lysosomes were rarely encountered. Golgi apparatus, SER, and glycogen could not be detected.

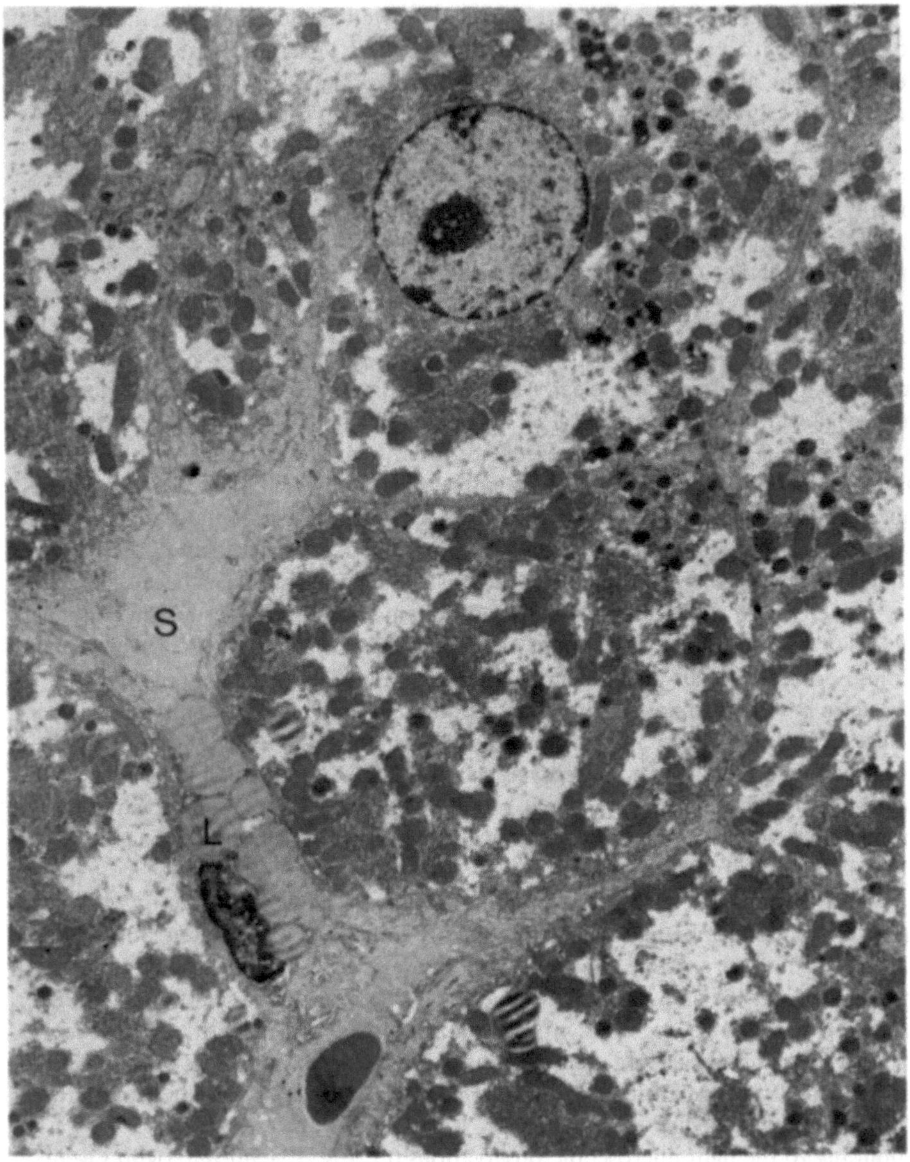

Fig. 14. Low magnification electron micrograph of vacuolated hepatocytes from the nodular formation shown in Figure 12, 20 weeks after AFB_1 withdrawal. Note large areas of cytoplasmic dissolution but integrity of nuclear structures with prominent nucleolus. *S* = sinusoid; *L* = lipid droplet. X 4000 (reduced to 90%)

At this stage a few round hepatocytes were encountered in the periportal zone. They showed similar ultramicroscopic changes to the surrounding vacuolated cells.

The hepatocytes located within the mid- and centrilobular zones of the liver lobule were characterized by the presence of large cytoplasmic areas containing ill-defined granular

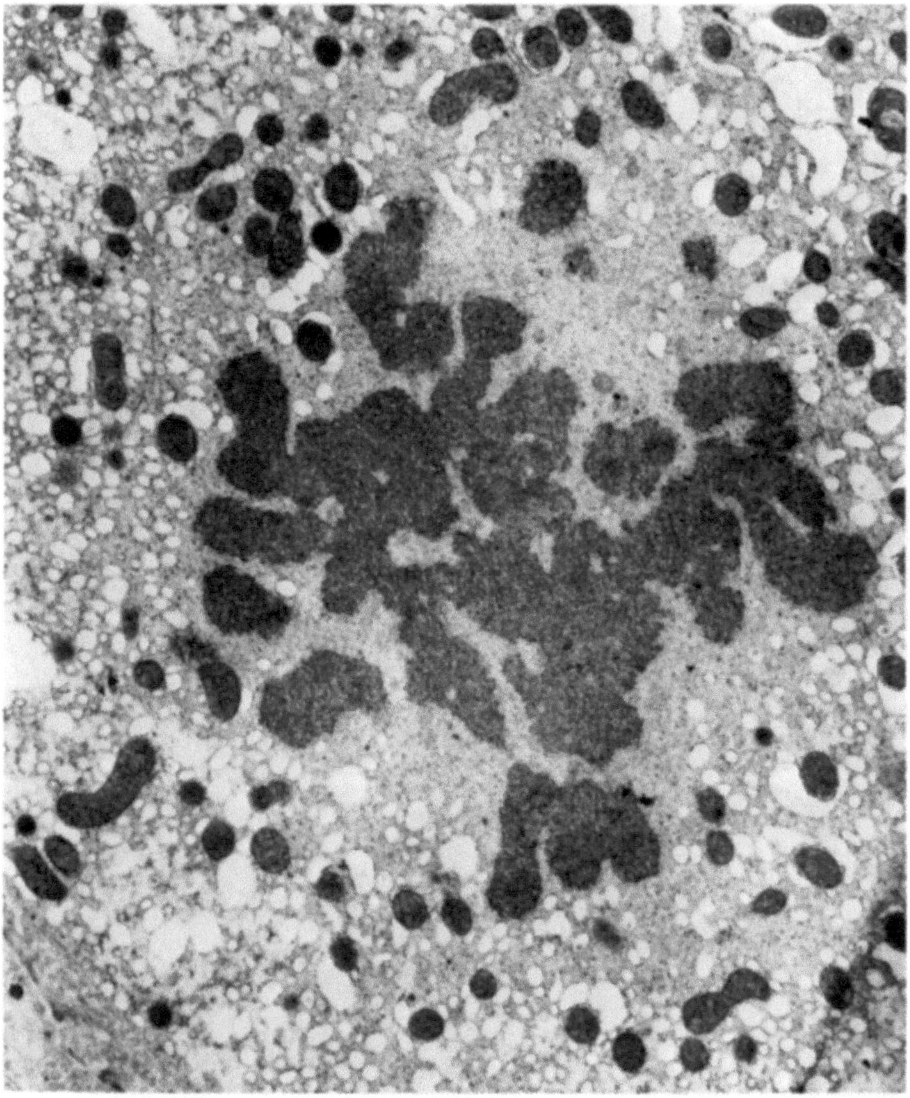

Fig. 15. Electron micrograph of periportal hepatocyte in mitosis 20 weeks after AFB_1 withdrawal. This cell was in pseudonodular formation composed of vacuolated hepatocytes. Note diffuse vesiculation and dilatation of RER cisternae around apparently undamaged chromosomal mass. X 8600 (reduced to 90%)

material. Intermediate aspects of damage showed that such cytoplasmic areas resulted from a progressive loss of ergastoplasmic structures. The pattern of RER disorganization seemed to be a constant one and consisted first of segmental dilatation of the cisternae with disruption of the membrane, while filamentous rodlike material accumulated in the cisternal lumen (cf. Fig. 1). Vesiculation of the RER profiles occurred first at their margins, which appeared to be surrounded by dilated vesicles still retaining a few ribosomal particles. A

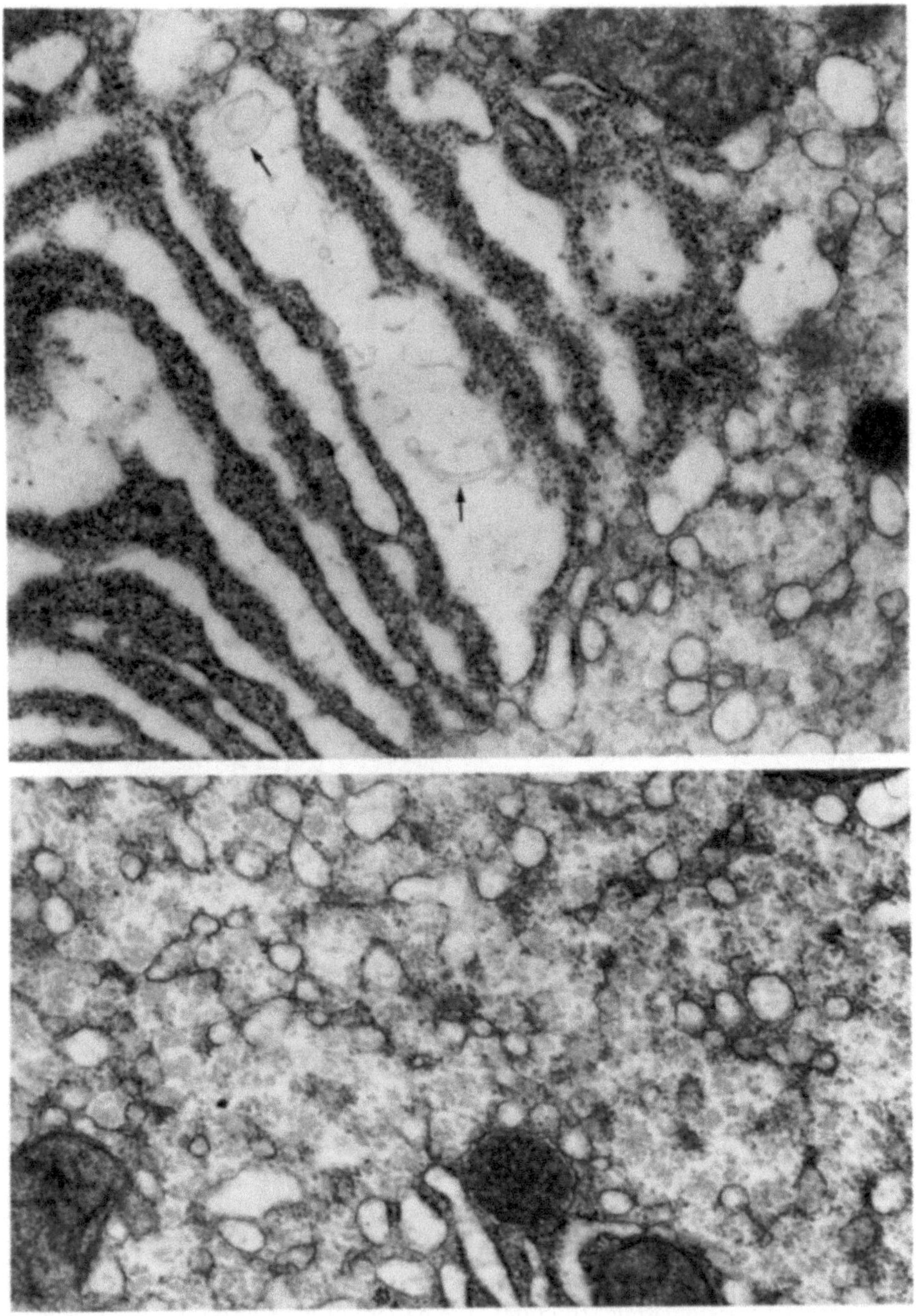

a

b

Fig. 16 a and b. Cytoplasmic portions of midzonal hepatocytes showing more advanced aspects of degeneration of RER, 24 weeks after AFB_1 withdrawal. (a) Stage B of RER disorganization. Note extensive dilatation of the cisternae with degenerating membranous profiles in lumen (arrows). X 33,300. (b) Stage C of RER disorganization. Note residual profiles of ER within a granular background of low electron density. X 40 8000 (reduced to 85%)

granular background surrounded the vesicular profiles. Specific staining demonstrated a lack of glycogen in these areas. Extensive dilatation of the cisternae then occurred (Fig. 16a), while ribosome particles among the vesicular profiles became less defined. As the damage had progressed further, the RER stacks were reduced to small groups of RER profiles, usually located around isolated mitochondria and lysosomes, and surrounded by large cytoplasmic areas consisting of scattered degenerating profiles partially or totally devoid of ribosomes, within a granular matrix of low electron density (Fig. 16b). A low magnifica-

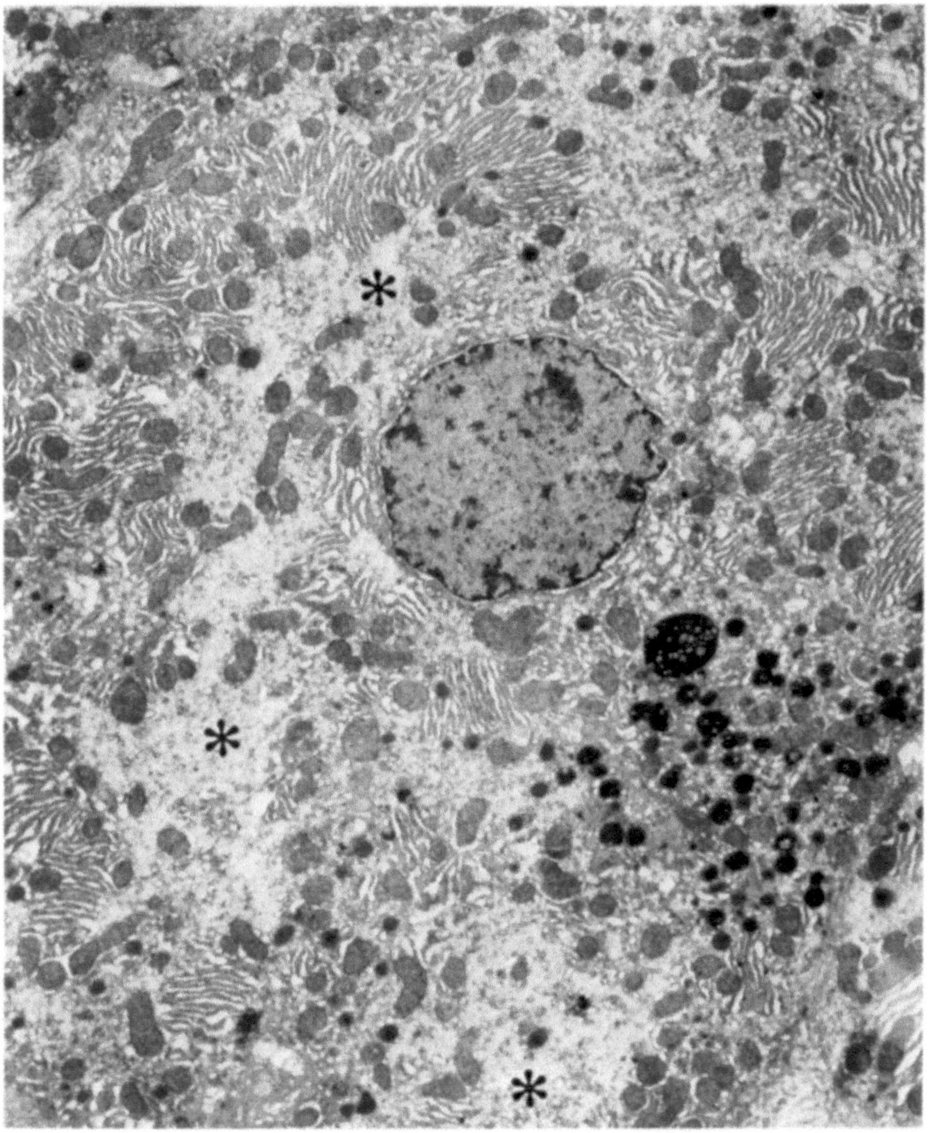

Fig. 17. Low-magnification electron micrograph of a midzonal hepatocyte, showing zonal loss of ergastoplasmic structures. Asterisks indicate stage C of RER disorganization. Liver from rat killed 24 weeks after AFB_1 withdrawal. X 4400

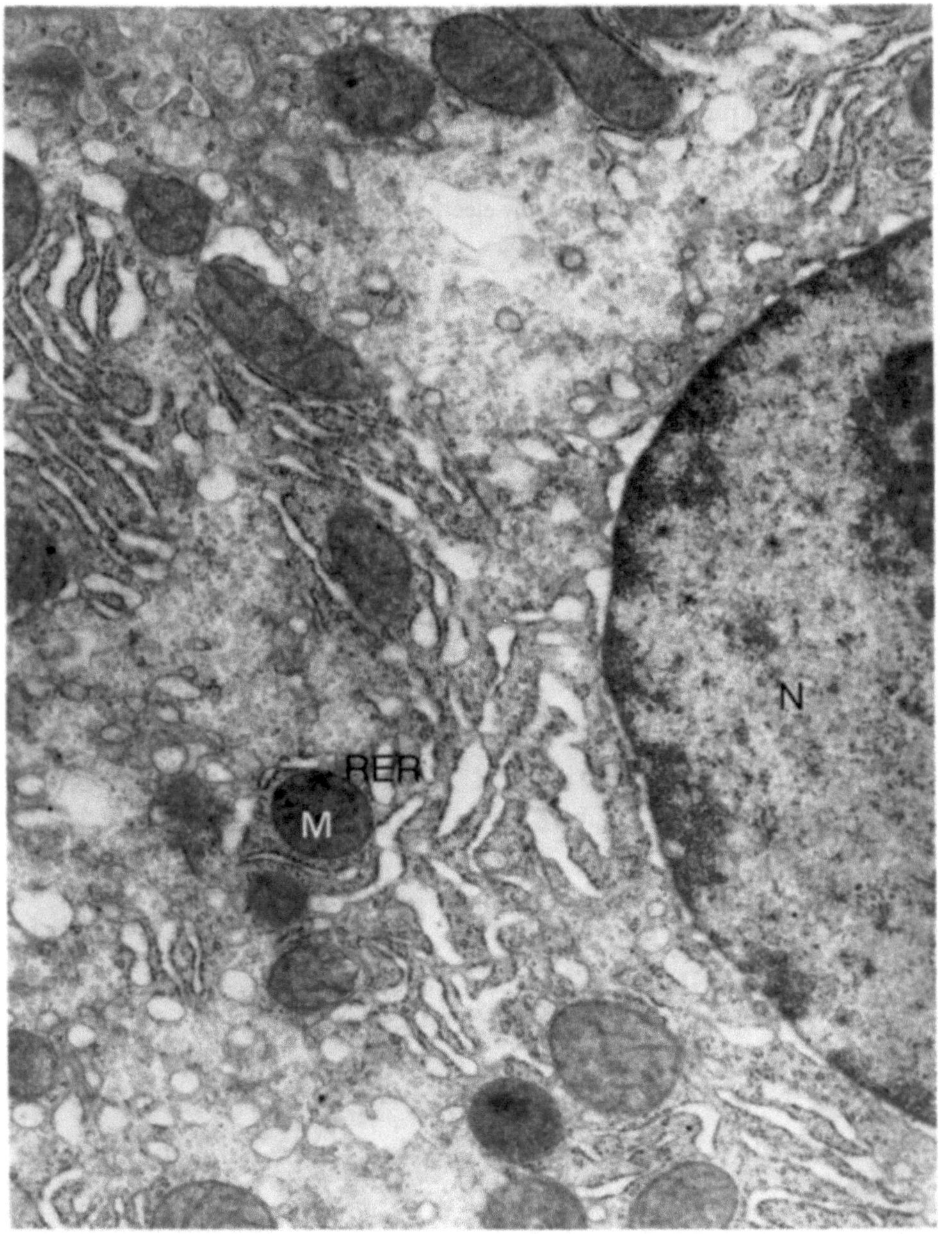

Fig. 18. Portion of midzonal hepatocyte, illustrating a late stage of chronic cytoplasmic degeneration, 24 weeks after AFB_1 withdrawal. Note sparse cytoplasmic organelles. *RER* = rough endoplasmic reticulum cisternae; *M* = mitochondria; *N* = nucleus. X 19 000 (reduced to 90%)

Fig. 19a and b. (a) Low magnification of strikingly injured midzonal hepatocytes *(A, B)* 28 weeks after AFB_1 withdrawal. Note focal loss of cell membranes (arrows). Nuclear structures *(N)* appear better preserved. X 6700. (b) Portion of cytoplasm in hepatocyte B (cf. Fig. 19a) at higher magnification. Note maintenance of ribosome-membrane relation- (Continuation see p. 143)

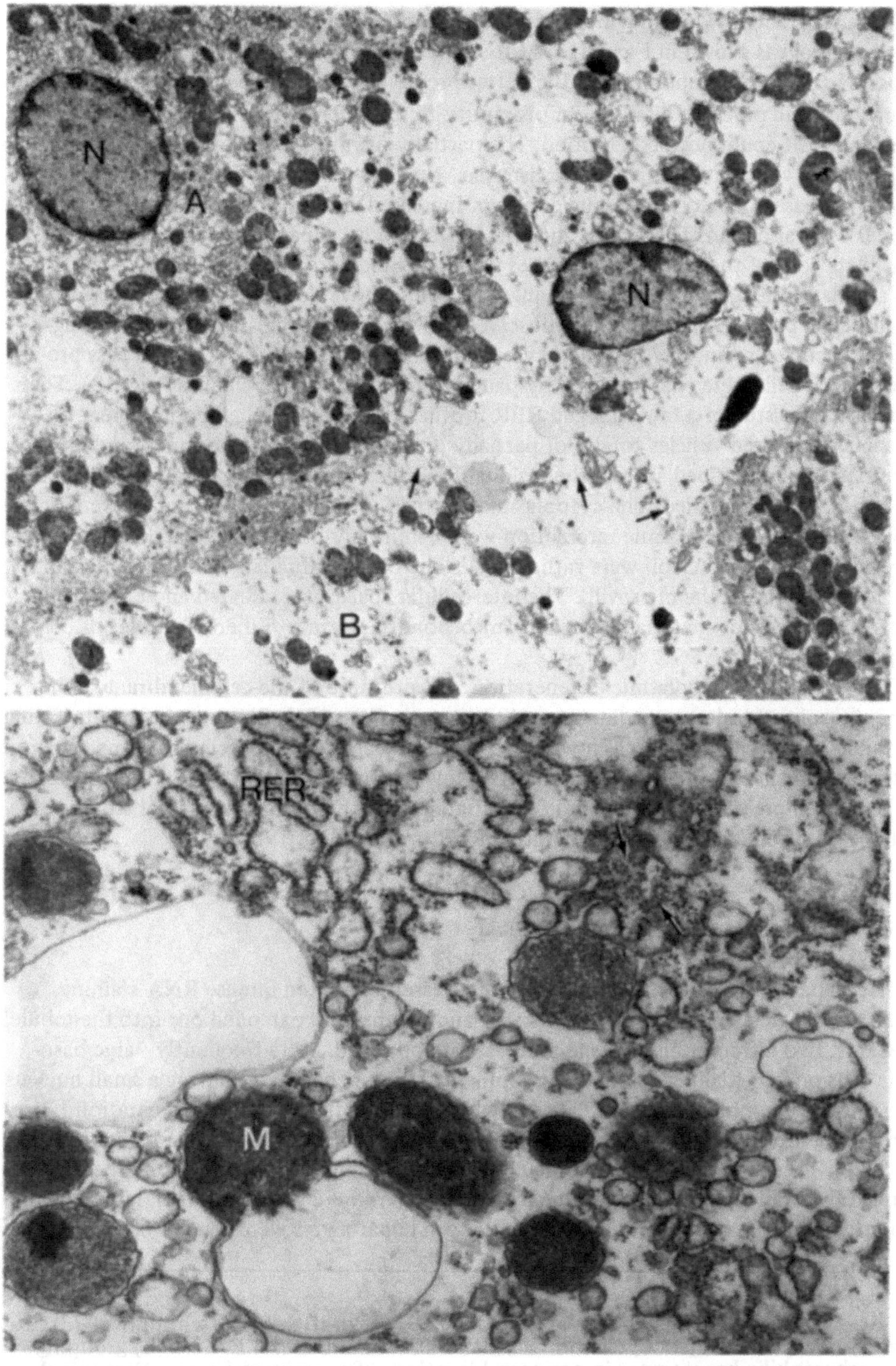

a

b

Fig. 19a and b

ship at the enlarged rough ER cisternae *(RER)*. Arrows indicate well-preserved polysomal structures among disintegrating RER profiles. *M* = mitochondrium with segmental alteration of the limiting membranes. X 32 600 (reduced to 85%)

tion of a hepatocyte exhibiting intermediate and more advanced aspects of the alterations described above is shown in Figure 17. Mitochondria displayed no evident modifications. Lysosomes were rather abundant in the better-preserved areas of the cytoplasm, while they became rare and partially dissolved in proximity to the disorganized ER. Golgi zones, glycogen and SER could not be identified. The partially disrupted vesicles devoid of ribosomes resulted from vesiculation of the RER cisternae. Nuclei were mainly irregular in shape and showed increased density of the nucleoplasm. Increased amounts of heterochromatin aggregates were also seen. The plasma membrane showed no apparent modifications. However, dilatations of the intercellular spaces were detected here and there.

Variants of the ultramicroscopic changes reported above occurred in some hepatocytes. For instance, parenchymal cells were observed in which the progressive loss of RER aggregates occurred mainly by peripheral vesiculation of the cisternae. As the process progressed, such cells were characterized by paucity in cytoplasmic organelles (Fig. 18). Their cytoplasm consisted of a few enlarged RER profiles still retaining their complement of ribosomes, scattered vesicles totally or partially devoid of attached ribosomes, and mitochondria, usually grouped around the residual RER cisternae. Golgi apparatus and glycogen could not be identified. The cytoplasmic matrix was finely granular, but unevenly distributed. Zones of cytoplasmic rarefaction were commonly observed. Nuclei did not show any evident change. Nucleoli were rather small. The cell membrane exhibited reduction and slight swelling of the microvilli. The intercellular spaces were dilated and contained debris of cytoplasmic material, especially mitochondria. Here and there, bundles of collagen were found.

The next step in cytoplasmic degeneration was a rupture of the cell membrane, either at the sinusoidal borders or at the intercellular spaces (Fig. 19a). Close to the disintegrating membranes the residual cytoplasm was represented by clusters of degenerating membranous profiles within an extremely rarefied matrix. However, nuclei and mitochondria appeared still to be well preserved. It is worth noting that apparently normal polysomal structures could be observed among the disintegrating RER profiles (Fig. 19b).

5. Light Microscopic Findings (42-66 Weeks)

At first, hepatocytes adjacent to the supplying vessels exhibited intense RNA staining. Then they progressively increased in number and volume and extended out into the lobule. After this, two different histological aspects were observed. More frequently, large basophilic cells only partially surrounded groupings of small hepatocytes having a small nucleus and similarly basophilic cytoplasm. The newly born cells (hepatocytes of generation II) appeared to be irregularly arranged in columns or plates, or showed gland-like formations (Fig. 20a). These cell groupings extended out into the lobule, where they could be surrounded by a rim of compressed parenchyma. Later (from 52 weeks onward), large islands composed of trabecular formations of newly born hepatocytes were usually observed. They

---

Fig. 20a-c. Paraffin sections of liver of rats killed 53 weeks after AFB_1 withdrawal. (a) Late island of newly born hepatocytes showing gland-like formations. H.E. 63x; (b) grouping of hyperbasophilic hepatocytes in periportal location. *PS* = periportal space. Fast cresyl violet. 160x; (c) large island of hyperbasophilic hepatocytes partially compressing the surrounding parenchyma (arrow). H.E. 37x

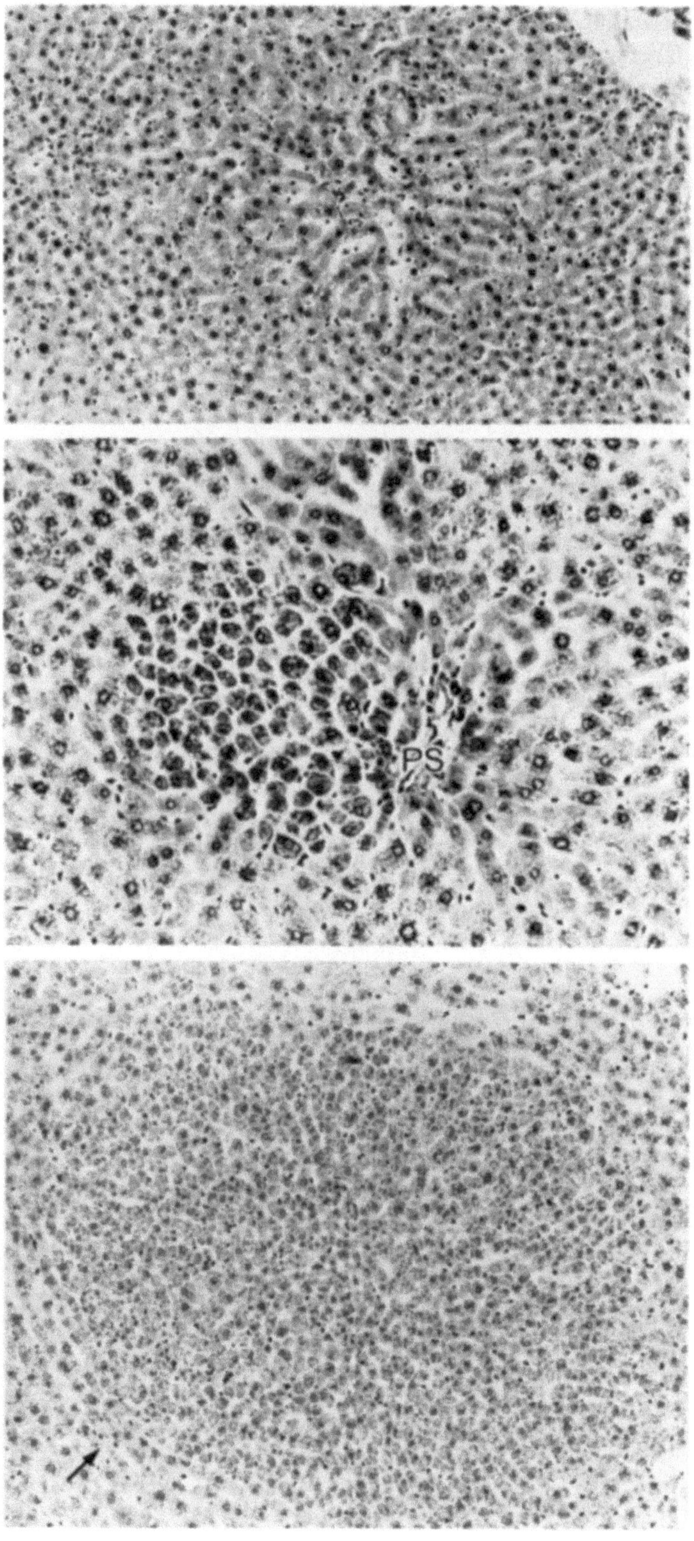

a

b

c

Fig. 20a-c (Legend see p. 144)

were classified as well-differentiated liver cell carcinomas on the basis of their microscopic appearance. Less frequently, large basophilic cells appeared to be irregularly intermingled with newly born hepatocytes. Small foci of necrosis partially replaced by inflammatory infiltrates were scattered among the large basophilic cells, some of them showing either a further increase in RNA staining or vacuolation of their cytoplasm. Transitional aspects between large basophilic cells and frankly abnormal hepatocytes were frequently encountered. The latter were characterized by an altered nuclear-cytoplasmic ratio and prominent nucleoli (Fig. 21a), or by the presence of three nuclei (Fig. 21b). The cytoplasm around the nucleus or nuclei usually appeared rarefied.

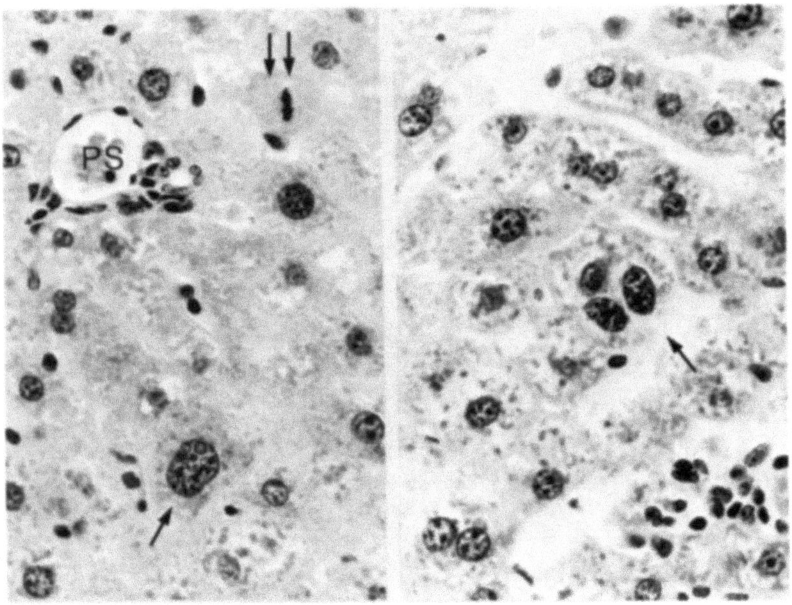

a b

Fig. 21a and b. Paraffin sections of livers of rats killed 48 weeks after AFB_1 withdrawal. H.E. 250x. (a) Arrow indicates frankly abnormal hepatocyte. Note a parenchymal cell in mitosis (double arrow) in close proximity to a periportal space *(PS)*; (b) at arrow, abnormal hepatocyte with three nuclei

Table 1. Mitotic index in liver parenchyma during AFB_1 carcinogenesis

Time after beginning of experiment (weeks)	Mean mitotic index [a]	
	DMF	AFB_1
0- 8	0 (4)	0.10 (8)
10-16	0 (3)	0.03 (6)
17-37	0 (4)	0.23 (6)
42-66	0 (4)	1.0 (11)

[a] Number of mitoses/1000 parenchymal nuclei. Figures in parantheses give the number of animals

Mitotic cells were a frequent finding, as confirmed by the sharp increase in mitotic activity shown in Table 1. They were diffusely distributed within the periportal areas and were about the same size as large basophilic cells. When newly born hepatocytes occurred in groups, the mitotic figures were located at their periphery.

Newly born hepatocytes exhibited two main routes of degeneration. The cells lost their spatial arrangement and progressively separated. Parallel to this, tightly packed hyperbasophilic material irregularly accumulated at the periphery of the cell, which in its central portion exhibited a ground-glass appearance. Nuclei became peripherally located. As shown in Figure 20b and c, groupings of hyperbasophilic hepatocytes could appear as periportal nodular formations or occupy larger areas of the liver parenchyma. The other main mode of degeneration of newly born hepatocytes consisted of vacuolation of their cytoplasm. Afterwards they showed nuclear pycnosis and underwent necrosis, as did hyperbasophilic hepatocytes. More rarely, hepatocytes of generation II were characterized by a progressive enlargement of their cytoplasm, which either showed a loose structure with a progressive decrease in RNA staining (large pale-staining hepatocytes), or stained intensely with eosin while failing to show any change with RNA or glycogen staining (large eosinophilic hepatocytes). Subsequently, both types of large degenerating hepatocytes underwent vacuolation of their cytoplasm, nuclear pycnosis, and necrosis.

Very large islands of degenerating hepatocytes were only rarely observed in our experimental conditions. They occurred in five animals out of 27 killed during this time interval (42-66 weeks), and only seldom bulged from the surface of the liver to be visible on gross examination (0.2-0.5 mm in diameter). At histological examination, these islands consisted of either large, pale-staining or eosinophilic hepatocytes.

An additional change observed on gross examination consisted of areas of hemorrhagic necrosis, especially on the liver surface. Histologically, these areas were made up of blood-filled spaces irregularly lined with hepatocytes.

6. Electron-Microscopic Findings (42-66 Weeks)

Between 42 and 52 weeks most hepatocytes within the liver lobule showed ultramicroscopic features closely resembling those observed in transitional basophilic cells. However, agglomerates of rough-surfaced profiles occupied larger areas within their cytoplasm (basophilic hepatocytes) (Fig. 22).

Two main variants of degenerating basophilic cells were observed. Variant one was characterized by loss of SER profiles, glycogen and Golgi zones, while agglomerates of RER cisternae appeared to be progressively substituted by large clusters of polysome particles. Mitochondria showed an increase in density of their matrix. Except for highly degenerating cells, evident alterations of nuclear structures and cell membrane were not noticed. Such cells were especially evident at the periphery of the liver lobule.

Variant two was observed from 52 weeks onward. These cells exhibited diffuse fragmentation and vesiculation of the RER cisternae. As a consequence of this process, the cytoplasm appeared to be filled with vesicles devoid of content and delimited by ill-defined membrane. The vesicular images then progressively disappeared, followed by dissolution of the adjacent cytoplasmic structures. This process was especially evident in the paranuclear area (Fig. 23). Golgi areas were difficult to identify. When this was possible, they

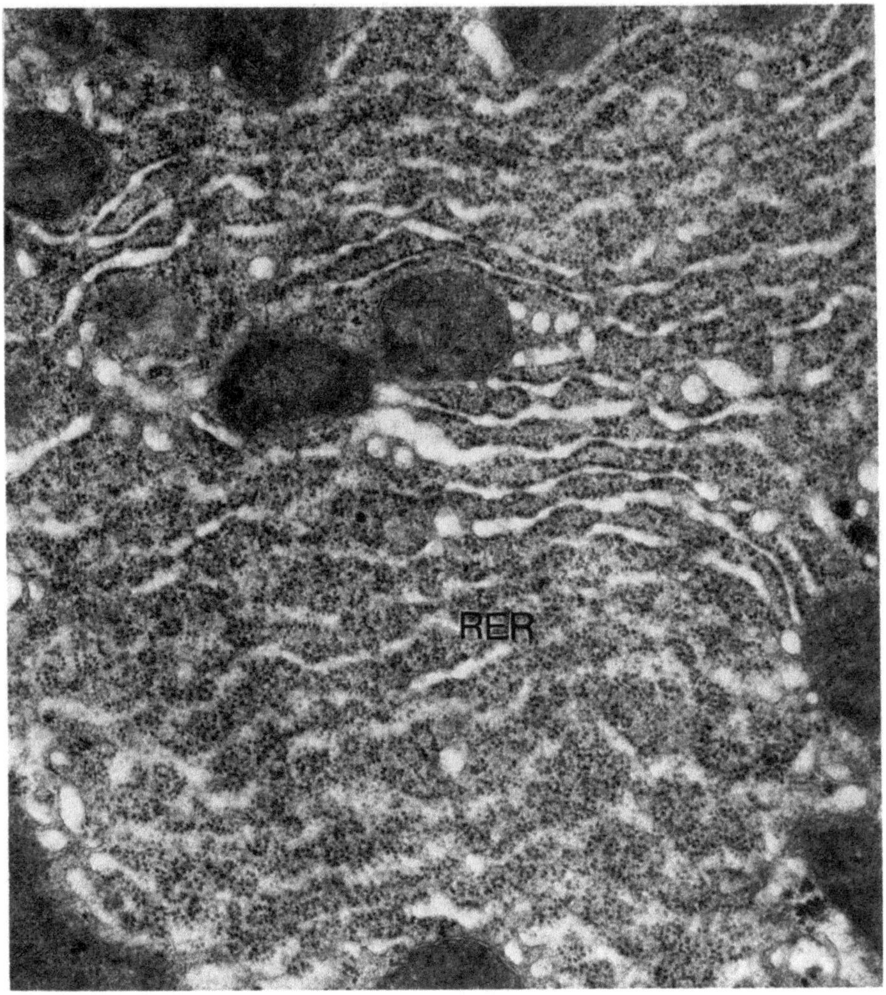

Fig. 22. Cytoplasmic portion of periportal, "basophilic" hepatocyte 44 weeks after AFB_1 withdrawal. Marked increase of rough endoplasmic reticulum *(RER)* is apparent. X 28 000 (reduced to 90%)

consisted of a few enlarged vesicles partially filled with electron-dense material. Here and there, a few glycogen particles could be detected. Nuclei were usually enlarged, irregular in outline with a scalloped pattern of the nuclear envelope. Large clumps of chromosomal material appeared to be irregularly distributed in the nucleoplasm. When present, nucleoli did not show evident modifications. Frequently, the ultramicroscopic aspect of nuclei resembled that in mitotic prophase. These changes were especially evident in hepatocytes identified as transitional or frankly neoplastic cells by light microscopy in thick sections.

Newly born hepatocytes were mainly round in shape and did not show any special ultramicroscopic details except for an increased tendency for individual RER cisternae to surround single mitochondria. The mitochondria exhibited a slight increase in the electron

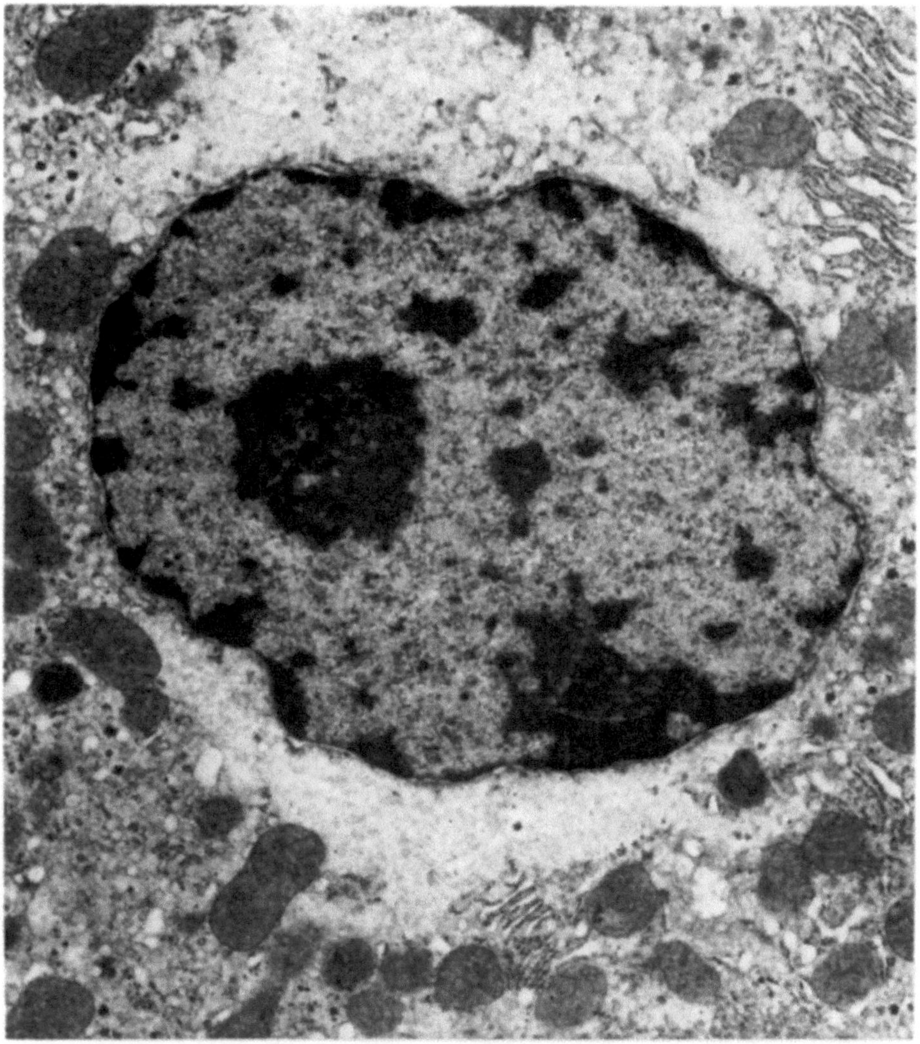

Fig. 23. Electron microscopic equivalent of frankly abnormal hepatocytes by light microscopy. Note dissolution of cytoplasmic structures in paranuclear location and addensation of chromatin within nucleus. X 15 000 (reduced to 90%)

density of the intercristal matrix. Parallel arrays of RER cisternae were less frequent. Lipid droplets free in the ground substance were observed. Nuclei were either round or slightly indented. Evident changes of the nuclear structures were not detected. The cell membrane appeared intact. When the cells began to disjoin, the intercellular spaces were continuous with sinusoidal recesses at one extremity and closely approximated biliary canaliculi at the other. Near their confluence with sinusoidal recesses, some of these intercellular spaces contained bundles of collagen.

Newly born hepatocytes evolved to show ultramicroscopic features resembling those of their mother cells. Their development was characterized by a constant pattern of changes.

It consisted of an initial increase of RER cisternae (step I), which subsequently regressed while SER and glycogen increased in extent (step II) (Fig. 24). Degenerative changes were observed at either step of the evolution pattern mentioned above. In early degenerating cells (step-I degenerating hepatocytes), RER cisternae showing segmental dilatation and disruption of the limiting membrane occupied most of the cytoplasm. Lysosomes and fat droplets accumulated in a paranuclear location close to the Golgi zone. Glycogen and SER, initially present in very small amounts, progressively disappeared, while clusters of ribo-

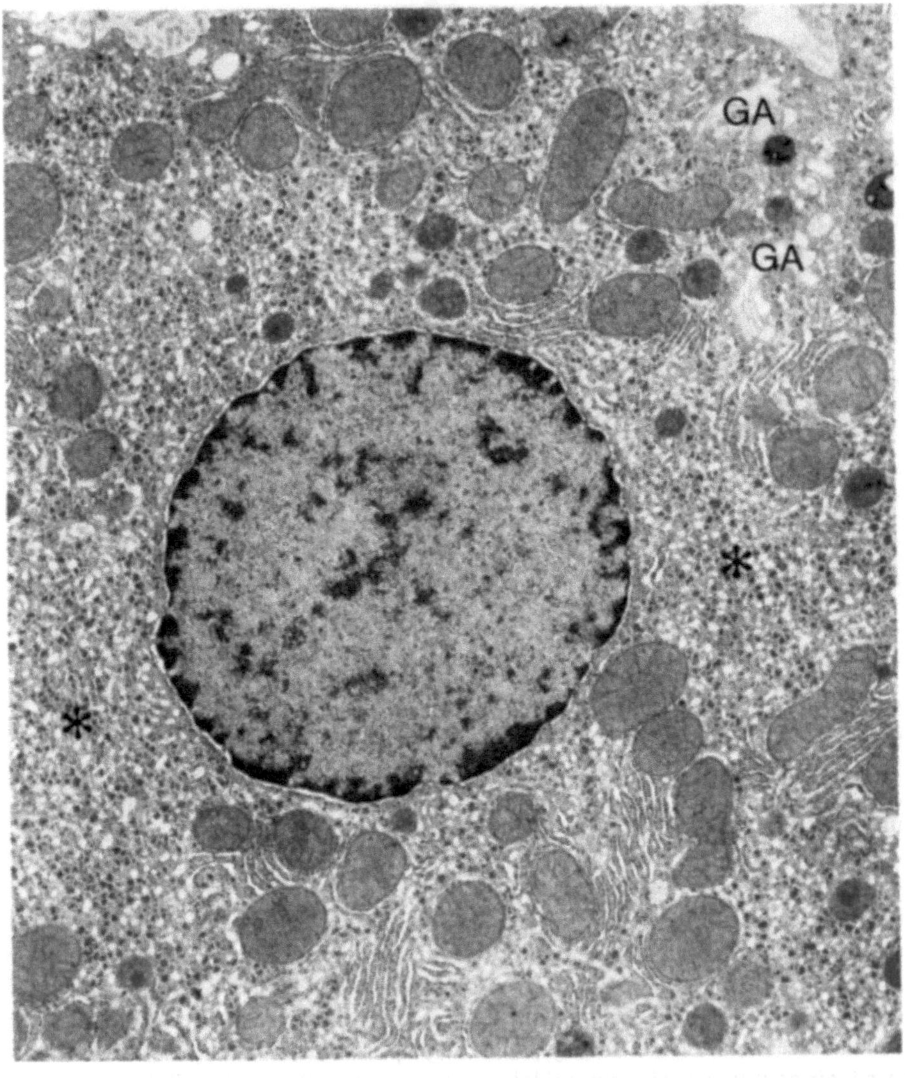

Fig. 24. Electron micrograph of a newly born hepatocyte at step II of its evolution pattern, 53 weeks after AFB_1 withdrawal. Note increase in SER profiles interspersed among glycogen particles (asterisks). Nuclear outline slightly indented. *GA* = Golgi area. X 11 000 (reduced to 90%)

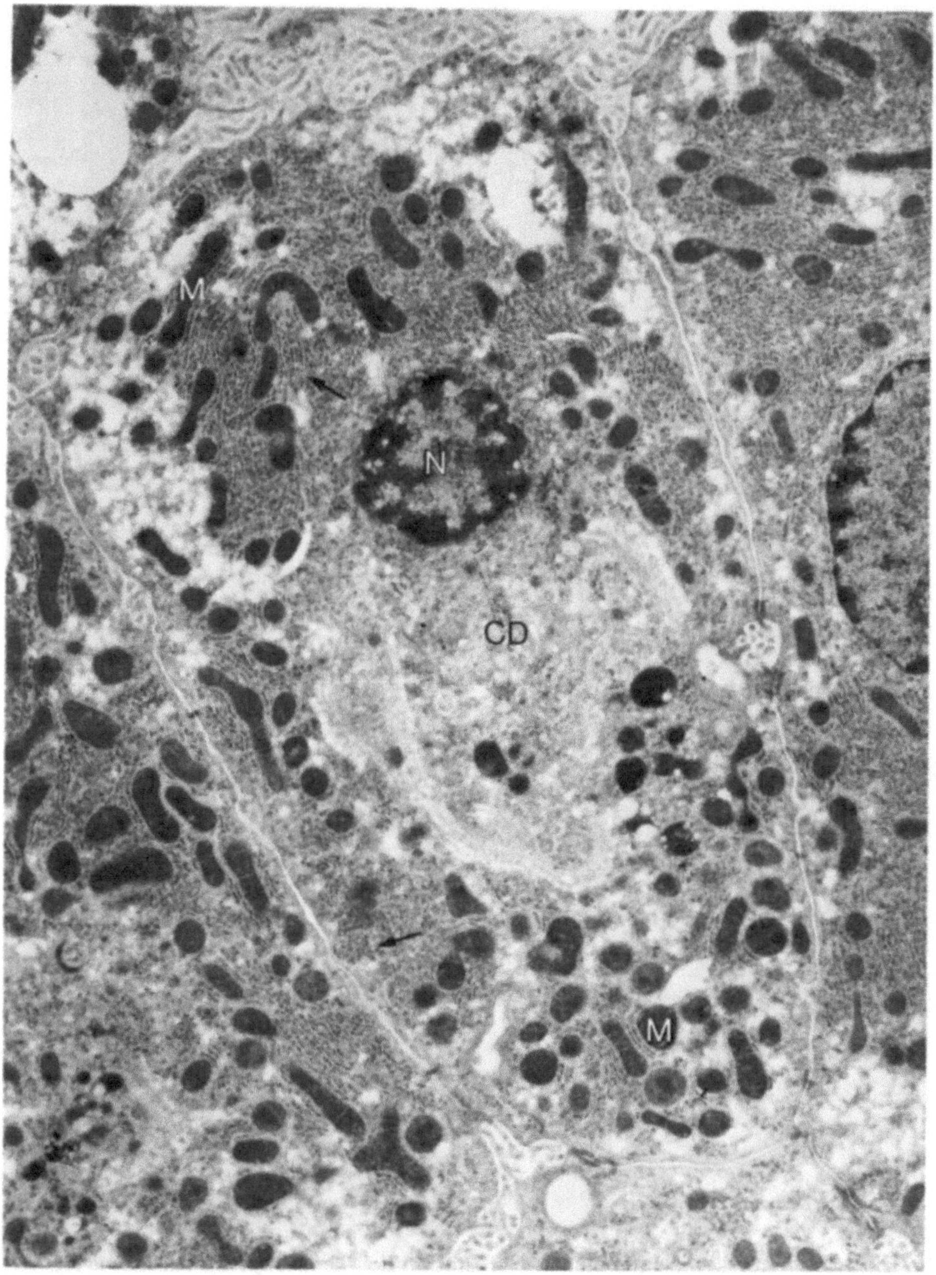

Fig. 25. Electron micrograph of "hyperbasophilic" hepatocyte 44 weeks after AFB_1 withdrawal. Note central area of cytoplasmic degradation *(CD)* surrounded by clusters of degenerating ergastoplasmic structures (arrow) and dark mitochondria *(M)*. Nucleus tangentially cut, peripherally located. X 7400

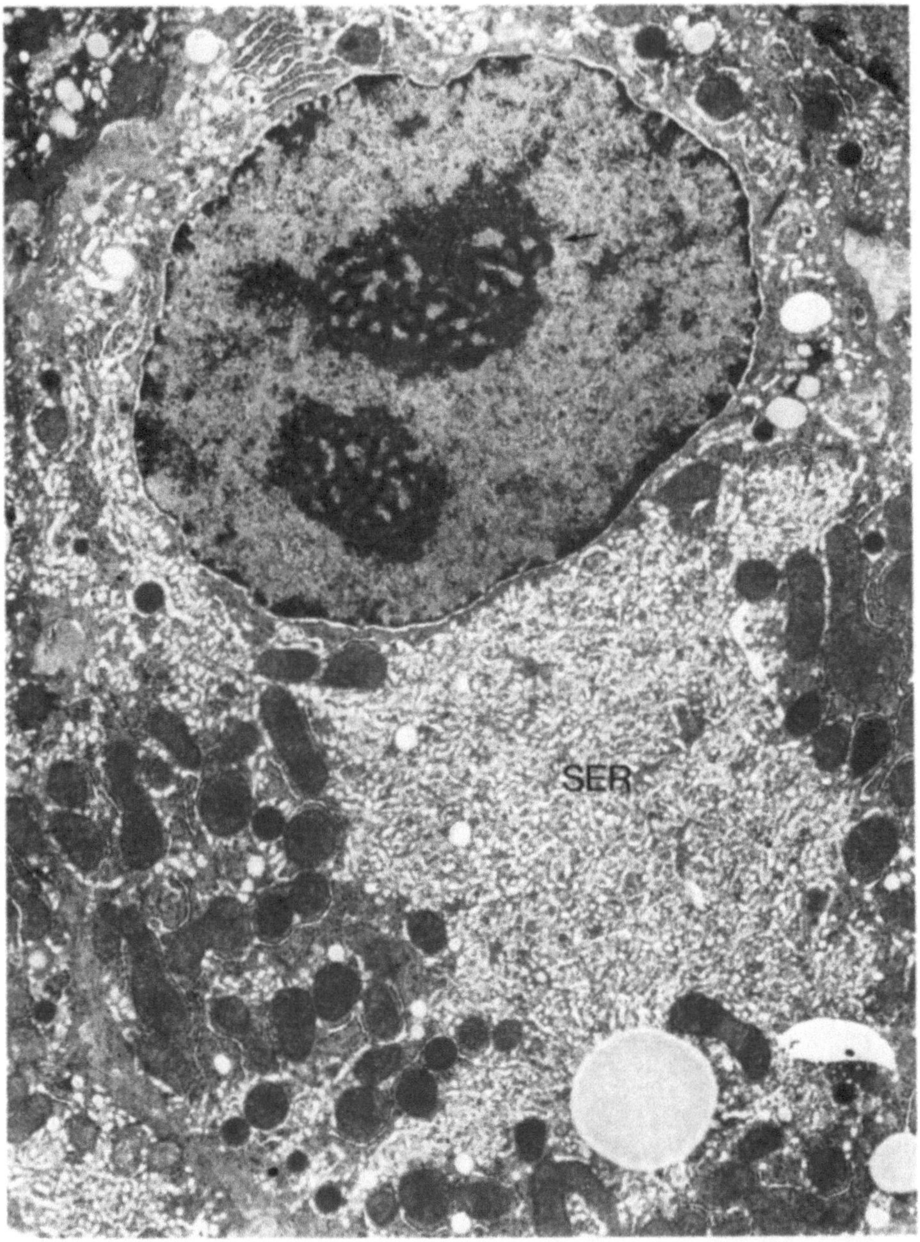

Fig. 26. Electron microscopic equivalent of "eosinophilic" hepatocytes 58 weeks after AFB_1 withdrawal. Partially degenerating smooth ER profiles *(SER)* occupy most of cytoplasm. Arrow indicates microsegregation of nucleolar structures. X 11 000 (reduced to 85%)

somes, mainly arranged as polysomes, became evident. Mitochondria showed ill-defined cristae and limiting membranes. These cells were found especially at the periphery of hyperbasophilic islands (cf. Fig. 20b, c). Deeper in these islands the hepatocytes showed marked aspects of degeneration. As shown in Figure 25, the cytoplasm of these cells consisted of clusters of partially degenerating ribosomes among fragments of RER cisternae, lysosomes and dark mitochondria, the whole surrounding a central area of cytoplasmic degeneration. The nuclei were usually pycnotic and occupied the periphery of the cells.

A special variant of hepatocytes of generation II was often encountered from 62 weeks onward. Such cells were characterized by the presence of large cytoplasmic areas containing partially disrupted SER profiles intermingled with scarcely defined glycogen particles (Fig. 26). Lamellary formations of SER, consisting of multiple layers of concentrically disposed membranes encircling a core of ill-defined cytoplasmic material, were often found. The residual cytoplasmic structures were confined to the periphery of the cell and consisted of scattered RER cisternae, slightly dark mitochondria, and lipid droplets free in the ground substance. The nucleoli showed microsegregation. These cells displayed a progressive disappearance of SER profiles and glycogen particles, resulting in vacuolation of the cytoplasm. These ultramicroscopic changes were found in parenchymal cells identified as eosinophilic hepatocytes by light microscopy.

VI. Discussion

1. Sequential Histopathological Changes During AFB_1-Induced Carcinogenesis

Our long-term experiment has been designed in such a way as to minimize the early toxic effect of AFB_1. This has involved: 1) a dosage regimen that has previously been shown to produce minimal toxic effects while yielding a 100 percent incidence of hepatocellular carcinomas after one year (*Wogan*, 1973; *Busby* et al., 1976), 2) the use of female rats, which have been found to be less sensitive than males to the acute toxic effects of AFB_1 (*Wogan* and *Newberne*, 1967; *Newberne* and *Butler*, 1969; *Purchase* et al., 1973). The absence of biliary proliferation, fibrosis, and cirrhosis throughout the experiment indicates that our experimental premises have been fulfilled.

Our histological findings clearly indicate that the precancerous lesions are characterized by a very slow rate of progression. Up to 16 weeks (8 weeks after AFB_1 was discontinued), the only change observed was an increase in the number of megalocytes. During the next interval (from 17 to 37 weeks), a few periportal islands of small hepatocytes were seen. However, they did not show any further enlargement and successively disappeared. These histological modifications were paralleled by a decrease in the number of megalocytes. After 42 weeks a sequence of cellular events became apparent. First periportal hepatocytes started to undergo mitosis. Islands of newly born hepatocytes appeared, which could be limited to one side of, or lay concentrically around, the periportal space. Identification of such islands was only made possible by the small size of their cellular components or by the occurrence of pathological cell arrangements, such as in plates more than one cell thick or gland-like formations.

Histological modifications due to AFB_1 became especially evident as degenerative changes took place. The most typical of them was the occurrence of hyperbasophilic hepatocytes. Transitional aspects showed that hepatocytes of generation II progressively lost their intercellular connections, while their basophilic cytoplasm gathered irregularly at the periphery of the cell. Like vacuolated or large hepatocytes, hyperbasophilic cells underwent nuclear pycnosis and necrosis.

Mitoses were found among degenerating cells. They either exhibited pathological changes resembling those in the cells they were intermingled with, or lay at the periphery of the cell islands where degenerative and proliferative changes were closely mixed. Evidence indicated that altered mitotic cells did not evolve any further and underwent necrosis, as did adjacent degenerating hepatocytes. After 52 weeks, most of the liver parenchyma consisted of large islands of newly born hepatocytes undergoing degeneration.

Considering that apart from the appearance of megalocytes all the changes reported above occurred several months after AFB_1 was discontinued, it clearly indicates that such changes reflect the carcinogenic effect of AFB_1. Furthermore, two findings are of special interest: 1) basophilic periportal hepatocytes represent the cellular type responding to AFB_1 by proliferation. 2) Newly born hepatocytes correspond to "neoplastic cells" by histological standards.

2. Ultramicroscopic Analysis of Intracellular Changes

It is evident from the results of this study that productive and degenerative changes of intracellular structures are related to development of liver carcinogenesis. Indeed, both types of change not only persist after the withdrawal of AFB_1, but progressively increase in extent during neoplastic transformation.

a) Productive Changes

Productive changes consist mainly of an increase in the quantity of smooth and rough endoplasmic reticulum. Such intracellular modifications mirror the ones observed in parenchymal liver cells involved in drug metabolism. It is now widely accepted that agents such as phenobarbital, which are capable of inducing a rapid increase of drug-metabolizing enzymes, as determined chemically in the microsomal fraction, produce a large increase of smooth- and rough-surfaced ER (*Orrenius* et al., 1965; *Smuckler* and *Arcasoy*, 1969; *Chedid* and *Nair*, 1972). Furthermore, the morphological similarity is supported by biochemical analyses that have clearly indicated that AFB_1 requires metabolic activation for its carcinogenic and toxic effect (for review, see *Campbell* and *Hayes*, 1976), and is capable of inducing a net synthesis of microsomal enzymes connected with its metabolism (*Schabort* and *Steyn*, 1972).

b) Degenerative Changes

Depending on the zonal location of the hepatocytes within the liver lobule, degenerative changes can occur first in otherwise unmodified cells or overlap productive modifications. In both cases, degenerative changes can affect all the cellular structures, the involvement of which appears to follow a well-defined sequential pattern. Endoplasmic reticulum appears to be affected first, and alterations of glycogen and Golgi areas then occur, which are followed by damage to mitochondria and cell membrane. Changes of nuclear structures, such as irregularity in the shape of the nucleus and increased electron density of the nucleoplasm, only occur in hepatocytes with intensely damaged cytoplasm. These findings do not support a role of primary importance for the nucleus in carcinogenesis.

Degenerative changes of ER seem to suggest that the membranes, *per se*, are the major target of AFB_1 injury. Indeed, the first change observed in otherwise intact hepatocytes was in the membranes of the ER. Ruptured membranes are characterized by increased contrast, which suggests a localized degradation of the lipoprotein composition of the reticulum membranes, resulting in the release of osmiophilic unsaturated lipid. Similar alterations of ER membranes have been reported after irradiation (*Ghidoni*, 1967; *Hendee* and *Alders*, 1968).

The relation of SER to glycogen stores is of particular interest. In the experiments reported in the present paper, hypertrophy of smooth ER occurs in the presence of intact and abundant glycogen stores. This finding militates against the concept that SER hypertrophy necessarily accompanies or is the consequence of glycogenolysis (*Porter*, 1961; *Rosen* et al., 1966). However, the observation that glycogen breakdown constantly accompanies alterations of SER suggests that SER membranes are in some way related to glycogen metabolism.

RER disorganization seems to follow three main patterns, which probably reflect different degrees of lesion. Pattern 1 consists of cisternal dilatation with parallel dissolution of membranes and ribosomal particles, and clearing of the adjacent cytoplasm. The lack of intermediate aspects of damage, and the observation that these changes are firstly delimited by cytoplasmic components showing structural integrity, suggest a high-grade acute lesion. Release of toxic substances from altered RER cisternae into the adjoining cytoplasm is suggested by the lack of cytoplasmic material around the ruptured RER cisternae. Pattern 2 includes a generalized vesiculation of RER cisternae, which appear to be transformed into empty round images still retaining their complement of ribosomes. Such changes have been observed in hepatocytes closely located to necrotic ones. The clearing of the cytoplasmic matrix at one side and the partial reduction in cytoplasmic organelles at the other suggest a subacute degree of injury. Pattern 3 has been subdivided into sequential steps (cf. Fig. 16a, b). It consists of segmental disruption of the limiting membranes and marginal vesiculation of the cisternae, which at first retain their complement of ribosomes (Stage A of RER disorganization). Extensive dilatation of the affected cisternae follows, while ribosomes, mainly arranged in spirals and rosettes, are released into the contiguous cytoplasm (Stage B). As the dissolution of membranous profiles takes place faster than that of ribosome particles, areas devoid of organelles but still containing granular material appear in the cytoplasm (Stage C). The occurrence of multiple areas of cytoplasmic degradation at different evolution stages within the cytoplasm of individual hepatocytes suggests a low-grade, recurrent cell injury.

Ribosome changes seem to be secondary to membrane alterations. This is suggested by the observation that detachment of ribosomes usually follows alterations of cisternal membranes. Biochemical evidence supports a minor effect of AFB_1 on ribosomes, since purified polysomes isolated from AFB_1-treated rats synthesize proteins *in vitro* to the same extent as those from controls (*Sarasin* and *Moulé*, 1975), and monosomes produced by AFB_1 resemble runoff ribosomes (*Hayes* et al., 1975).

A special feature is the presence of agglomerates of polysomes situated close to disintegrating RER cisternae. Unless concomitant functional analyses are performed, it is not possible to determine whether they result from new synthesis of polysomes or from transformation of preexisting agglomerates of RER, which undergo progressive loss of cisternal membranes while ribosomes are released as mRNA-bound particles. However, the observation that these ultramicroscopic aspects are only observed in hepatocytes showing degenerative changes seems to support the latter mechanism. Furthermore, the presence in these cells of nuclei characterized by small nucleoli and increased heterochromatin aggregates hardly suggests an active transcription of messenger and ribosomal RNA.

It has been demonstrated that in normal liver parenchymal cells, protein synthetic mechanisms are associated with RER (*Palade* and *Siekevitz*, 1956). Biochemical studies have shown that AFB_1 has a direct inhibitory action on protein synthesis (*Harley* et al., 1969; *Williams* and *Rabin*, 1971; *Sarasin* and *Moulé*, 1973). In the present study, the morphological evidence support a similar correlation; that is, the disorganization of RER is consistent with the reported decrease in protein synthesis in AFB_1 administration.

Changes in Golgi apparatus, mitochondria, lysosomes, and cell membrane may not necessarily reflect the primary effect of AFB_1 at the cellular level. They could very probably result from altered intracellular metabolism following inhibition of protein synthesis. For instance, lipid depositions has been attributed to decreased protein available for triglyceride transport from the liver (*Robinson* and *Seakins*, 1962; *Hamilton* et al., 1967). In the present study the morphological evidence supports a similar correlation, since disruption of RER has been found associated with lipid accumulation. Since the Golgi apparatus is the site of addition of carbohydrates to glycosphingolipids and plays a role in the origin of specific receptor molecules of the cell surface (*Richardson* et al., 1975), alteration of the cell membrane may be secondary to damage of this organelle.

Mitochondria with special features occur in hepatocytes with degeneration of cytoplasmic structures. They show a high increase in the density of the matrix with irregularly arranged, "clear"-staining cristae (cf. Fig. 8). Other abnormal forms of mitochondria, including enlargement, focal rupture of the limiting membranes, and bizarre shapes with abnormal number and sitribution of the cristae, are confined to a very small number of cells and therefore considered nonspecific to aflatoxin administration.

At no stage of our study were virus-like particles observed.

3. Analysis of Ultramicroscopic Cell Types

The cellular heterogeneity that follows AFB_1 administration is due to the simultaneous presence within the liver lobule of hepatocytes showing productive or degenerative changes only, or an overlap of both ultramicroscopic modifications.

a) "Productive" Hepatocytes

The main variants of hepatocytes with productive changes only are summarized in Table 2. ER-hyperplastic hepatocytes probably represent the first adaptation of liver parenchymal cells to AFB_1 metabolism. The increased amount of RER structures, which is a hallmark of transitional basophilic and basophilic cells, probably reflects an increased demand for newly synthesized enzyme molecules.

Transitional basophilic cells may be the ultramicroscopic equivalent of megalocytes observed by light microscopy. This assumption is based on their similarity in lobular location and mode of degeneration. Furthermore, transitional basophilic cells and megalocytes si-

Table 2. Summary of ultramicroscopic features of "productive" hepatocytes

Features observed	ER-hyperplastics	Transitional basophilics	Basophilics
Nucleolus	N	N	Prominent
Nucleoplasm	N	N	N
RER	increased +	increased ++ intercisternal free ribosomes ++	increased +++ intercisternal free ribosomes ±
SER	increased ++	increased ++	increased +
Golgi	N	conspicuous	conspicuous
Mitochondria	N	N	N
Microbodies	N	increased ++	N
Cell membrane	N	slight enlargement of microvilli	N

± = slightly increased; + = increased; ++ = markedly increased; +++ = much increased; N = normal

multaneously disappear from the liver parenchyma. A major ultrastructural characteristic of transitional basophilic hepatocytes is the presence of packed free ribosomes within the intercisternal spaces of RER agglomerates. The question of the possible significance of these structures to the carcinogenic process is of interest because their release from degenerating transitional basophilic cells is temporally related to the phase of generalized cell proliferation. One suggestion is that ribosomes closely located to RER cisternae, where drugs can be metabolized at the same rate as at the smooth-surfaced membranes (*Conney*, 1967; *Alvares* et al., 1973), may in some way interact with AFB_1 or its metabolites, so that they become unable to attach again to membranes and initiate protein synthesis. As a consequence, free ribosomes accumulate in the intercisternal spaces and may represent carcinogen storage particles. The lack of enlarged nucleoli constantly noted in transitional basophilic hepatocytes seems to support our assumption, that free ribosome accumulation in the intercisternal spaces results from decreased turnover rather than increased synthesis of these structures. Binding of the carcinogen to ribosomes may act to protect them from microsomal hydrolase attack. Morphological findings in this study have shown that agglomerates of packed free ribosomes are the last cytoplasmic component left apparently intact in extremely degenerating transitional basophilic cells. It supports a high resistance of these structures.

In spite of their morphological analogy to basophilic hepatocytes, transitional basophilic cells can be considered true variants in view of their different location (midzonal, while basophilics are periportal), and evolution (degeneration only, while basophilics proliferate as well).

While retaining their phenotypic characteristics of drug-metabolizing cells, basophilic hepatocytes display ultramicroscopic features (cf. Table 2) which have usually been associated with high rates of ribosomal and protein synthesis. This indicates that an increased functional demand is imposed on these cells, which, according to the "increased functional demand hypothesis" (*Novi*, 1976), should progress through the G_1 phase of the cell cycle, synthesize DNA and divide. That this is indeed the case is demonstrated by the finding that shortly after their appearance basophilic hepatocytes undergo mitosis.

b) Degenerating Hepatocytes

From a morphological point of view, hepatocytes showing degenerative changes only can easily be distinguished from productive hepatocytes undergoing degeneration. The latter are referred to as degenerating ER-hyperplastic, degenerating transitional basophilic, and degenerating basophilic hepatocytes.

Hepatocytes showing certain signs of dedifferentiation, as recognized by loss of organized endoplasmic reticulum, glycogen, Golgi apparatus and surface specialization, were frequently encountered. However, transitional aspects clearly point out that such hepatocytes represent degenerative variants.

Variant 2 of degenerating basophilic cells seems to be of special interest, since it has been found to represent the ultramicroscopic equivalent of frankly neoplastic cells by light microscopy. At the ultramicroscopic level, such cells are characterized by: 1) a progressive loss of RER agglomerates; 2) concentration of toxic substances in paranuclear location, as indicated by complete dissolution of cytoplasmic material around the nucleus; 3) progressive increase of chromosomal material in the nucleus, which frequently becomes similar to that observed in mitotic prophase. These results indicate that such cells undergo cytoplasmic degeneration during or after completion of DNA synthesis (S/G_2-degenerating hepatocytes). This finding is not surprising, considering that at this time most basophilic hepatocytes are in mitosis.

The ultramicroscopic features of degenerating basophilic cells summarized above suggest a very tempting functional correlation. There is general agreement in the literature that strongly reactive electrophilic forms of chemical carcinogens are capable of attacking nucleophils (RNA, DNA, and proteins) in the cell with little discrimination and usually without the aid of enzymes (for a review, see *Miller* and *Miller*, 1974). In view of their metabolic situation, S/G_2-degenerating hepatocytes are characterized by an inverted nucleo-cytoplasmic gradient of nucleophilic centers (decrease of RNA in the cytoplasm, increase of DNA in the nucleus), which for electron affinity may direct the reactive electrophilic carcinogens towards the nucleus. This suggestion is supported by the paranuclear dissolution of cytoplasmic material, which only occurs in this type of cell. If this premise is correct, it implies two postulates: 1) DNA-bound carcinogen may represent an alternative pattern of carcinogen storage. 2) Indiscriminate binding of carcinogen to DNA may interfere with or prevent further evolution of the mitotic process, resulting in S/G_2-arrested cells, or atypical cell division. It may explain the morphological heterogeneity of nuclear structures within neoplastic cells, which is one of the hallmarks of cancer seen at histological examination.

4. Distribution of AFB_1-Induced Ultramicroscopic Cell Types Within the Liver Lobule

The distribution of AFB_1-induced ultramicroscopic cell types within the liver lobule during and after AFB_1 administration is summarized in Tables 3 and 4, respectively. From these data some main conclusions can be derived: 1) Ultramicroscopic changes within the hepatocytes are clearly dependent on the cell location in the liver lobule. For instance, periportal hepatocytes are rapidly damaged, while centrilobular parenchymal cells, which are located at the most peripheral part of the hepatic microcirculation (*Rappaport*, 1976), are affected the least. One reason for this is that being periportal hepatocytes situated close to the sup-

Table 3. Distribution of the ultramicroscopic cell types within the liver lobule during AFB$_1$ administration

Time (weeks)	Periportal zone	Midzone	Centrilobular zone
1-2	degenerating only +	ER-hyperplastic + transitional basophilic ++ degenerating transitional basophilic +	–
3-8	degenerating only ++	ER-hyperplastic ± transitional basophilic ++ degenerating transitional basophilic +++	ER-hyperplastic + degenerating ER-hyperplastic ++

– = absent; ± = rare; + = quite frequent; ++ = frequent; +++ = very frequent

Table 4. Distribution of the ultramicroscopic cell types within the liver lobule after AFB$_1$ withdrawal

Time (weeks)	Periportal zone	Midzone	Centrilobular zone
8-16	degenerating only +++	degenerating only ++ ER-hyperplastic +++ degenerating ER-hyperplastic ++ transitional basophilic ++ degenerating transitional basophilic ++	ER-hyperplastic ++ degenerating ER-hyperplastic ++
17-37	degenerating only ++	degenerating only + ER-hyperplastic +++ degenerating ER-hyperplastic ++ transitional basophilic ++ degenerating transitional basophilic +++	ER-hyperplastic ± degenerating ER-hyperplastic +++
42-66	basophilic degenerating basophilic	hepatocytes II generation degenerating hepatocytes II generation	

± = rare; + = quite frequent; ++ = frequent; +++ = very frequent

plying vessels (*Rappaport*, 1976), they are bathed by blood containing the highest concentration of AFB$_1$. Though it may play a substantial role, carcinogen concentration alone does not seem to be the only factor in inducing a differential distribution of cellular changes within the liver lobule. This is highlighted by the observation that similar zonal modifications are still evident months after withdrawal of the carcinogen. It suggests that enzymatic specificity and metabolic heterogeneity of hepatocytes in different lobular zones must be implicated in the cellular response to AFB$_1$. This seems to be the case, for example, after phenobarbital administration. It has been found that after phenobarbital there is a significant increase of SER, mainly confined to the pericentral and midzonal regions but seen to a lesser degree in periportal zones (*Chedid* and *Nair*, 1972). In addition, the existence of a porto-central gradient in various enzyme activities and glycogen content has been reported (*Wachstein*, 1963). In our experimental conditions, glycogen-storing hepatocytes have only been found within the centrilobular zone.

If we admit that hepatocytes in different zones of the lobule have different metabolic potentialities, it may imply that there could be a single biochemical cause for even deviant cellular responses within the lobule. For instance, similar concentrations of AFB_1, which could be easily metabolized by midzonal hepatocytes, resulting in the induction of new drug-metabolizing enzyme molecules, could induce degenerative changes in periportal hepatocytes having a more limited capability for detoxication. Modulation upon two different parameters, such as drug concentration and metabolic capability of zonal hepatocytes, could explain the variation in ultrastructural features observed after AFB_1.

2) Phenotypic ultramicroscopic features of liver parenchymal cells are essentially the same during and after AFB_1 administration. These findings indicate a continuous process with a constant biochemical cause, though AFB_1 has been administered for a short time only. It implies a mechanism of storage of the carcinogen, the progressive release of which results in a constant spectrum of cellular changes.

3) The appearance of productive modifications in periportal hepatocytes seems to represent the "switching mechanism" toward cell proliferation. Indeed, location of hepatocytes within the liver lobule appears to determine their further evolution: this is indicated by the findings that "productive" peripheral hepatocytes degenerate while periportal parenchymal cells showing similar modifications undergo cell division. It suggests that periportal hepatocytes are still in cycle (G_1 or Go cells) while more peripherally located cells have permanently left the cell cycle and are destined to die without dividing again.

The length of the lag period before the appearance of generalized cell proliferation might be dependent on the time needed by the liver parenchyma to "dilute" the toxic effect of the carcinogen on periportal hepatocytes, so that productive changes are allowed to show.

VII. Conclusions

Our findings have demonstrated that:

1. The lag time preceding the appearance of recognizable cancer by morphological criteria is characterized by a constant spectrum of ultramicroscopic changes. When the hepatocytes do not rapidly degenerate, they specifically differentiate toward drug metabolism. These cellular changes cannot be considered as nonspecific reactions to toxicity or a manifestation of enzyme induction unrelated to the initiation of carcinogenesis, since they persist after withdrawal of AFB_1.

2. Basophilic periportal hepatocytes represent the cellular type that responds to AFB_1 by proliferation. Correlated light- and electron-microscopic findings have demonstrated that these cells are phenotypically differentiated toward drug metabolism.

3. The proliferative response to AFB_1 is diffuse in nature, as indicated by the occurrence of synchronous waves of mitoses within the periportal zones. The few small islands of newly born hepatocytes observed earlier result from asynchronous division of groupings of periportal heptaocytes. This is demonstrated by: a) the constant location of early islands in the periportal zone; b) the morphological identity (light and electron microscopy) of cellular components within early and late islands.

4. Newly born hepatocytes evolve to differentiate toward drug metabolism, as did their mother cells.

Our findings seem to suggest that the main action of AFB_1 on liver parenchymal cells is to act as a substrate for drug-metabolizing enzymes. An increased rate of formation of metabolically activated AFB_1 may result in the appearance in the cytoplasm of free radicals (strong electrophilic reagents) that interact by electron affinity with nearby intracellular structures bearing the opposite charge, such as ribosome particles. The binding may protect the ribosomes from nuclease attack, resulting in storage of AFB_1 within the hepatocytes. Increased production of unfavorable metabolites may lead to cell degeneration whereby the carcinogen is released again in the liver parenchyma. This endogenous mechanism of storage and release of carcinogen may be responsible for the persistence of the cellular changes induced by AFB_1 after the exogenous supply of carcinogen is withdrawn.

Acknowledgments. I wish to thank Prof. *H. Meessen* for advice, criticism and encouragement. The skilled technical assistance of Ms. *L. Hensel* (electron microscopy) and Mrs. *H. Schmidt* (light microscopy), and the photographic work of Ms. *R. Bentele* are gratefully acknowledged. I am also indebted to Prof. *V. Marinozzi* for advice on histochemical procedures. The experiments were generously supported by Research Grant IIB8-FA4404 from the Ministerium für Wissenschaft und Forschung des Landes Nordrhein-Westfalen.

References

Adamson, R.H., Correa, P., Sieber, S.M., McIntire, K.R., Dalgard, D.W.: Carcinogenicity of aflatoxin B_1 in rhesus monkeys: two additional cases of primary liver cancer. J. natl. Cancer Inst. 57, 67-78 (1976).

Alvares, A.P., Parli, C.J., Mannering, G.J.: Induction of drug metabolism. VI. Effects of phenobarbital and 3-methylcholanthrene administration on N-demethylating enzyme systems of rough and smooth hepatic microsomes. Biochem. Pharmacol. 22, 1037-1045 (1973).

Busby, W.F., Jr., Paglialunga, S., Newberne, P.M., Wogan, G.N.: Transfer RNA methylase activity and capacity during aflatoxin B_1-induced hepatocellular carcinogenesis. Cancer Res. 36, 2013-2018 (1976).

Campbell, T.C., Hayes, J.R.: The role of aflatoxin metabolism in its toxic lesion. Toxicol appl. Pharmacol. 35, 199-222 (1976).

Carnaghan, R.B.A.: Hepatic tumors in ducks fed a low level of toxic groundnut meal. Nature (Lond.) 208, 308 (1965).

Chedid, A., Nair, V.: Diurnal rhythm in endoplasmic reticulum of rat liver: electron microscopic study. Science 175, 176-179 (1972).

Chiesara, E., Clementi, F., Conti, F., Meldolesi, J.: The induction of drug-metabolizing enzymes in rat liver during growth and regeneration. A biochemical and ultrastructural study. Lab. Invest. 16, 254-267 (1967).

Conney, A.H.: Pharmacological implications of microsomal enzyme induction. Pharmacol. Rev. 19, 317-366 (1967).

Fahimi, H.D.: Perfusion and immersion fixation of rat liver with glutaraldehyde. Lab. Invest. 16, 736-750 (1967).

Ghidoni, J.J.: Light and electron microscopic study of primate liver 36 to 48 hours after high doses of 32-million-electron-volt protons. Lab. Invest. 16, 268-286 (1967).

Goldblatt, L.A.: Aflatoxin: Scientific Background, Control, and Implications. New York-London: Academic Press 1969.

Halver, J.E.: Aflatoxicosis and trout hepatoma. In: Aflatoxin: Scientific Background, Control, and Implications (L.A. Goldblatt, ed.). New York-London: Academic Press 1969, pp. 265-306.

Hamilton, R.L., Regen, D.M., Gray, M.E., LeQuire, V.S.: Lipid transport in liver. I. Electron microscopic identification of very low density lipoproteins in perfused rat liver. Lab. Invest. 16, 305-319 (1967).
Harley, E.H., Rees, K.R., Cohen, A.: A comparative study of the effect of aflatoxin B_1 and actinomycin D on HeLa cells. Biochem. J. 114, 289-298 (1969).
Hayes, L.C., Plapp, F.P., Tilzer, L.T., Chiga, M.: Characterization of monosomes produced by Aflatoxin B_1. Chem.-Biol. Interactions 10, 343-347 (1975).
Hendee, W.R., Alders, M.A.: Ultrastructural development of radiation injury in hepatic parenchymal cells of γ-irradiated mice. Lab. Invest. 18, 151-158 (1968).
Kalengayi, M.M.R., Desmet, V.J.: Sequential histological and histochemical study of the rat liver during aflatoxin B_1-induced carcinogenesis. Cancer Res. 35, 2845-2852 (1975).
Lancaster, M.C., Jenkins, F.P., Philp, J.M.: Toxicity associated with certain samples of groundnuts. Nature (Lond.) 192, 1095-1097 (1961).
Miller, E.C., Miller, J.A.: Biochemical mechanisms of chemical carcinogenesis. In: The Molecular Biology of Cancer (H. Busch, ed.). New York-London: Academic Press 1974, pp. 377-402.
Newberne, P.M.: Experimental hepatocellular carcinogenesis. Cancer Res. 36, 2573-2578 (1976).
Newberne, P.M., Butler, W.H.: Acute and chronic effects of aflatoxin on the liver of domestic and laboratory animals: a review. Cancer Res. 29, 236-250 (1969).
Newberne, P.M., Wogan, G.N.: Sequential morphologic changes in aflatoxin B_1 carcinogenesis in the rat. Cancer Res. 28, 770-781 (1968).
Novi, A.M.: Molecular basis of a control mechanism of DNA synthesis in mammalian cells. Klin. Wschr. 54, 961-968 (1976).
Orrenius, S., Ericsson, J.L.E., Ernster, L.: Phenobarbital-induced synthesis of the microsomal drug-metabolizing enzyme system and its relationship to the proliferation of endoplasmic membranes. A morphological and biochemical study. J. Cell Biol. 25, 627-639 (1965).
Palade, G.E., Siekevitz, P.: Liver microsomes. An integrated morphological and biochemical study. J. Biophys. Biochem. Cytol. 2, 171-200 (1956).
Peers, F.G., Gilman, G.A., Linsell, C.A.: Dietary aflatoxins and human liver cancer. A study in Swaziland. Internat. J. Cancer 17, 167-176 (1976).
Phillips, D.L., Yourtee, D.M., Searles, S.: Presence of aflatoxin B_1 in human liver in the United States. Toxicol. appl. Pharmacol. 36, 403-406 (1976).
Porter, K.R.: The endoplasmic reticulum: some current interpretations of its forms and functions. In: Biological Structure and Function (T.W. Goodwin, O. Lindberg, eds.). New York: Academic Press 1961, Vol. 1, pp. 127-155.
Purchase, I.F.H., Steyn, M., Gilfillan, T.C.: Metabolism and acute toxicity of aflatoxin B_1 in rats. Chem.-Biol. Interactions 7, 283-287 (1973).
Rappaport, A.M.: The microcirculatory acinar concept of normal and pathological hepatic structure. Beitr. Path. 157, 215-243 (1976).
Reddy, J.K., Svoboda, D.J., Rao, M.S.: Induction of liver tumors by aflatoxin B_1 in the tree shrew (Tupaia glis), a nonhuman primate. Cancer Res. 36, 151-160 (1976).
Richardson, C.L., Baker, S.R., Morré, D.J., Keenan, T.W.: Glycosphingolipid synthesis and tumorigenesis. A role for the Golgi apparatus in the origin of specific receptor molecules of the mammalian cell surface. Biochim. biophys. Acta 417, 175-186 (1975).
Robinson, D.S., Seakins, A.: The development in the rat of fatty livers associated with reduced plasma-lipoprotein synthesis. Biochim. biophys. Acta 62, 163-165 (1962).
Rosen, S.I., Kelly, G.W., Peters, V.P.: Glucose-6-phosphatase in tubular endoplasmic reticulum of hepatocytes. Science 152, 352-354 (1966).
Sarasin, A., Moulé, Y.: In-vivo effect of aflatoxin B_1 on protein synthesis in rat liver. FEBS Letters 29, 329-332 (1973).
Sarasin, A., Moulé, Y.: Translational step inhibited in vivo by aflatoxin B_1 in rat-liver polysomes. Europ. J. Biochem. 54, 329-340 (1975).
Sato, S., Matsushima, T., Tanaka, N., Sugimura, T., Takashima, F.: Hepatic tumors in the guppy (Lebister reticulatus) induced by aflatoxin B_1, dimethylnitrosamine, and 2-acetylaminofluorene. J. natl. Cancer Inst. 50, 765-778 (1973).
Schabort, J.C., Steyn, M.: Aflatoxin B_1 and phenobarbital inducible Aflatoxin-Δ^2-hydration by rat liver microsomes. Biochem. Pharmacol. 21, 2931-2933 (1972).

Shank, R.C., Bhamarapravati, N., Gordon, J.E., Wogan, G.N.: Dietary aflatoxins and human liver cancer. IV. Incidence of primary liver cancer in two municipal populations of Thailand. Food Cosmet. Toxicol. 10, 171-179 (1972).
Smuckler, E.A., Arcasoy, M.: Structural and functional changes of the endoplasmic reticulum of hepatic parenchymal cells. Internat. Rev. exp. Path. 7, 305-419 (1969).
Stenger, R.J.: Organelle pathology of the liver. The endoplasmic reticulum. Gastroenterology 58, 554-574 (1970).
Svoboda, D., Grady, H.J., Higginson, J.: Aflatoxin B_1 injury in rat and monkey liver. Amer. J. Path. 49, 1023-1051 (1966).
Svoboda, D., Higginson, J.: A comparison of ultrastructural changes in rat liver due to chemical carcinogens. Cancer Res. 28, 1703-1733 (1968).
Van Rensburg, S.J., Kirsipuu, A., Coutinho, L.P., van der Watt, J.J.: Circumstances associated with the contamination of food by aflatoxin in a high primary liver cancer area. S. Afr. med. J. 49, 877-883 (1975).
Wachstein, M.: Cyto- and histochemistry of the liver. In: The Liver: Morphology, Biochemistry, Physiology (C. Rouiller, ed.). New York-London: Academic Press 1963, Vol. 1, pp. 137-194.
Williams, D.J., Rabin, B.R.: Disruption by carcinogens of the hormone dependent association of membranes with polysomes. Nature 232, 102-105 (1971).
Wogan, G.N.: Chemical nature and biological effects of the aflatoxins. Bacteriol. Rev. 30, 460-470 (1966).
Wogan, G.N.: Aflatoxin carcinogenesis. In: Methods in Cancer Research. (H. Busch, ed.). New York-London: Academic Press 1973, Vol. VII, pp. 309-344.
Wogan, G.N., Newberne, P.M.: Dose-response characteristics of aflatoxin B_1 carcinogenesis in the rat. Cancer Res. 27, 2370-2376 (1967).

Blastomycosis

A Review of 152 Cases

J. SCHWARZ and K. SALFELDER[1]

[1] From the Clinical Laboratories, Jewish Hospital, Cincinnati, Ohio and the Department of Pathology, Universidad de los Andes, Merida, Venezuela. The material of this study was made available by the Department of Infectious and Parasitic Disease Pathology, AFIP.

I. Introduction

(North American) Blastomycosis is caused by the dimorphic fungus *Blastomyces dermatitidis*, first described by *Gilchrist* and *Stokes* in 1896. The perfect stage was grown by *McDonough* and *Lewis* in 1967 and is known as *Ajellomyces dermatitidis.*

In the body and on appropriate media at 37°C, the organism presents itself as a round, thick-walled budding yeast cell, characteristically with a broad porus between mother and daughter cells. The yeast cell is multinucleated.

For many years, North America was assumed to be the only place where blastomycosis was found, but recent demonstration of indigenous African cases changed this impression (*Emmons* et al., 1964). Within the United States, more cases are seen in Kentucky, Ohio, the Carolinas, Illinois, Michigan, Wisconsin, Iowa, Tennessee, Arkansas, and the Virginias than in the remainder of the country (*Chick*, 1971). In Mexico, occasionally, and in the provinces of Canada adjacent to the endemic areas of the United States, endemic blastomycosis has been recognized.

Soil has been long suspected as the habitat for the fungus, but recovery from soil has seldom been successful (*Denton* and *Di Salvo*, 1964). The primary infection is, as a rule, pulmonary with frequent secondary foci in skin, bone, male genital system, and, eventually, spares no organ in widely disseminated cases.

The rare cases of primary cutaneous blastomycosis are consequences of accidental percutaneous laboratory infection. These can be clinically easily differentiated from the average case of secondary hematogenous spread to the skin (*Landay* and *Schwarz*, 1971).

Blastomycosis, an important but uncommon mycosis, is hard to analyze since larger numbers of patients are rarely seen by individual observers, even within a time period of 10 years or more. To review significant numbers of patients, it is necessary to organize either cooperative studies (*Busey* et al., 1964), use very long time periods (*Cherniss* and *Waisbren*, 1956; *Kepron* et al., 1972; *Witorsch* and *Utz*, 1968), or accept material for study that was accumulated in a registry-type depository of material, as at the AFIP. The possible accumulation of presumably difficult or atypical cases in such a consultation-type collection, is undeniable, even if there is no yardstick for measurement of the deviation from "average material."

II. Material

We reviewed 152 cases of blastomycosis, accumulated at the AFIP from 1951 to 1972. Previous material (36 cases) was reported in 1951 (*Schwarz* and *Baum*, 1951). After computer recovery, all available cases were reviewed without selectivity. Of the 152 cases, 93 were submitted from the Veterans Administration, 11 from the U.S. Army, 3 each from the U.S. Navy and the U.S. Air Force, 1 from the U.S. Public Health Service, 39 from civilian sources, and 2 came from outside of the United States. The clinical information frequently was limited to localization of the biopsy material, age, sex, and race of the patient. In several of the older cases, few special stains were available. Nevertheless, the material provided fascinating information otherwise unavailable from individual sources. It was our hope to learn about the morphology of the organism and the tissue response from the available material.

III. Case Material (Table 1)

1. Pulmonary Blastomycosis

Lung tissue was available for study in 37 patients, the youngest a girl of seven years, the oldest a man of 81 years. Seven had cavitations, others had hard "tubercles" (mimicking and mistaken for sarcoid), or various forms of granulomatous response. At autopsy, the weight of lungs varied considerably, reaching a maximum in one case of 2970 g for both lungs. An outstanding finding was the frequency of ulceractive bronchitis, which, in part,

Table 1. Age, sex, and race in 152 patients[a] with blastomycosis 1951-1972 AFIP

	White		Black		No Race Given	Total
Age	Female	Male	Female	Male	Male	Total
1-19			1	1		2
20-29		10		5		15
30-39	1	13		13	3	30
40-49		21	1	4	6	32
50-59		18	2	5	3	28
60-69	2	18		4	3	27
70-79	3	2		2	1	8
80-89		1		1		2
No age given		1		1	2	4
Total	6	84	4	36	18	148

[a]Four patients were not tabulated—two lacked information on sex, race, and age, one on race, and one was a 28-year-old male American Indian.

explains the common finding of organisms in sputum. We were impressed by this finding as early as 1951 (*Schwarz* and *Baum*, 1951). Untreated bronchitis no doubt leads to intracanalicular dissemination, so well known in tuberculosis and histoplasmosis (*Vaněk* et al., 1970). Ulcerative bronchitis (granulomatous and/or necrotizing) was seen 13 times. Considering that some lungs had little sampling, it is obvious that this lesion is found in more than a third of patients with pulmonary blastomycosis. Often, the bronchitis was associated with bronchiectasis. Association of pulmonary lesions with diabetes mellitus existed three times, with lymphoma (including leukemias) three times, with amyloidosis twice, and with active histoplasmosis twice.

Great variations were seen in the number of *B. dermatitidis* changing from scarce organisms to lakes of yeast cells—the latter comparable, in a few instances, to the appearance in cryptococcosis (Fig. 1). The similarity was accentuated by minimal tissue reaction. Probably underlying diseases like lymphomas, diabetes, and steroid therapy can be associated with massive multiplication of *B. dermatitidis* in tissues. Other variations referred to the size and staining properties of yeast cells, some of which were confusing and provoked contradictory diagnoses from consultants (Fig. 2). A complicated finding was in a case where (adjacent) caseous foci were found, some with the small ovoid yeast in groups, characteristic of *Histoplasma capsulatum*, and others with typical round organisms having broad-based buds (*B. dermatitidis*). A third (necrotizing) lesion existed containing broad nonseptate hyphae, most likely a Phycomyces species.

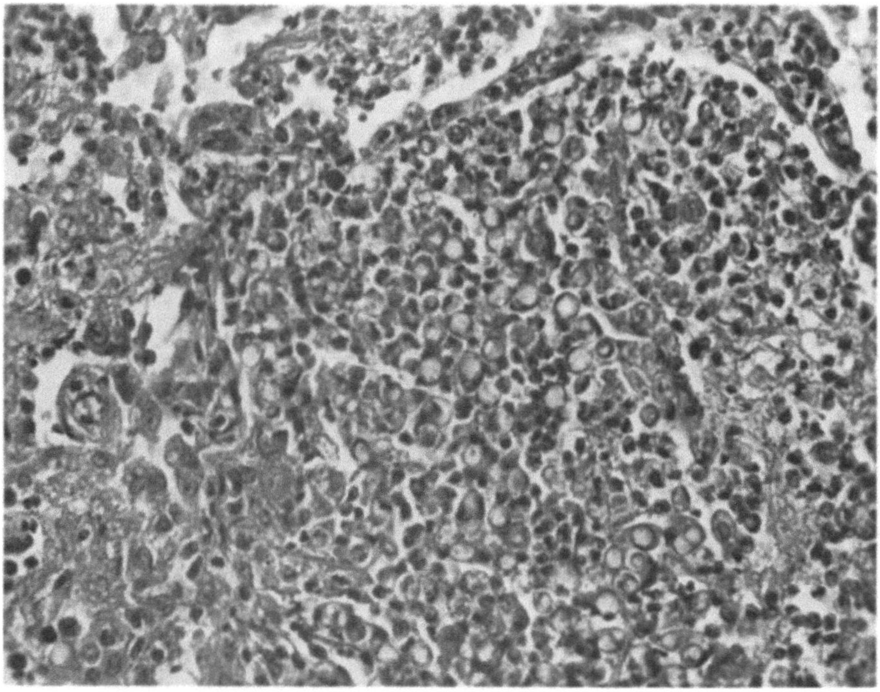

Fig. 1 (Legend see p. 169)

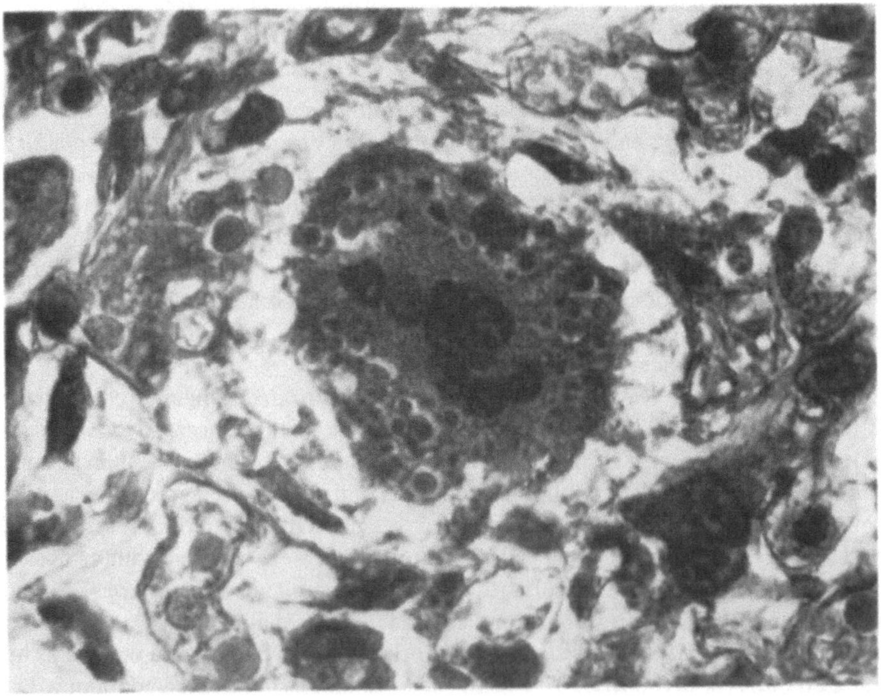

Fig. 2 (Legend see p. 169)

In a 7-year-old girl, uniform fibrocaseous foci of about 5 mm were found (healing "epidemic" histoplasmosis) with similar foci in lymph nodes noted. In addition, interstitial, granulomatous foci with giant cells containing fair numbers of *B. dermatitidis* were seen. Conceivably, the same spore-containing dust producing the pulmonary infections, could have contained both *H. capsulatum* and *B. dermatitidis.*

Cavitation was present in six men and one woman. The size of the cavities varied from small foci of breakdown up to several centimeters, generally with pus and organisms in the cavity. The granuloma of blastomycosis frequently is characterized by a rim of epithelioid cells with central necrosis and/or suppuration. The confluence of such individual granulomata can easily lead to major foci of necrosis with liquefaction, creating the basis for cavity formation. This sequence of event is much easier acceptable than necrosis in a granuloma formed by "hard tubercles." The bilateral nature and the multiplicity of such cavitary blastomycosis also fits this concept.

The healing tendency in many cases of pulmonary blastomycosis was notable. Healing could be traced from carnification of alveolar contents to segmental fibrosis. Hard (sarcoid-like) tubercles with no central necrosis or suppuration were seen only once. In two more cases, a mixture of hard tubercles existed with centrally suppurated nodules. Sometimes, alveolar pleomorphic exudate with organisms was found and only the presence of organisms, sometimes together with occasional tubercles in the interstitium or in isolated alveoli, pointed toward the correct diagnosis. Giant cells varied greatly in number from case to case and were more frequently of the foreign body cell type. Almost routinely, from one to several yeast cells were found within the cytoplasm of the giant cells.

There were two cases demonstrating unbelievably large numbers of yeast cells. The first patient had documented immunosuppression from prednisone therapy, while the second case, although therapeutic information was lacking, was diagnosed as lymphosarcoma.

The difficulties of morphologic identification of the organisms are highlighted by the case of a diabetic (Fig. 3), who had quite atypical yeast cells with three possible interpretations:

1. Atypical *B. dermatitidis*
2. *B. dermatitidis* mixed with *C. neoformans*
3. Atypical *C. neoformans*

The culture grew *B. dermatitidis.* Since *C. neoformans*, as a rule, grows much faster, the recovery of *B. dermatitidis* by culture very likely proves the case to be "simple" blastomycosis. The case points, on the one hand, to the importance of cultures. On the other hand, the need for interpretation of culture results remains—in absence of clearcut fluorescent antibody staining by tissue response, morphology of the organisms, and bias of the observer.

Anatomically, a primary focus in the lung can be recognized conclusively as such only if it is found together with satellite regional lymph nodes. The lymph nodes must show tissue reaction in an identical or similar stage as that of the pulmonary focus. This "ideal" setting will be almost exclusively found at autopsy, but may, even at this time, be obscured by widespread pulmonary involvement, which makes it difficult, if not impossible, to iden-

---

Fig. 1. Overwhelming numbers of organisms in distended alveoli of lobar blastomycosis. The degree of involvement can be properly called: "colonization," H & E x 355. AFIP neg. 74-5916

Fig. 2. Multiple minute budding yeast cells in multinucleated giant cells. Some yeast cells are only 1-2 μ in size; lung. H & E x 970. AFIP neg. 74-5908

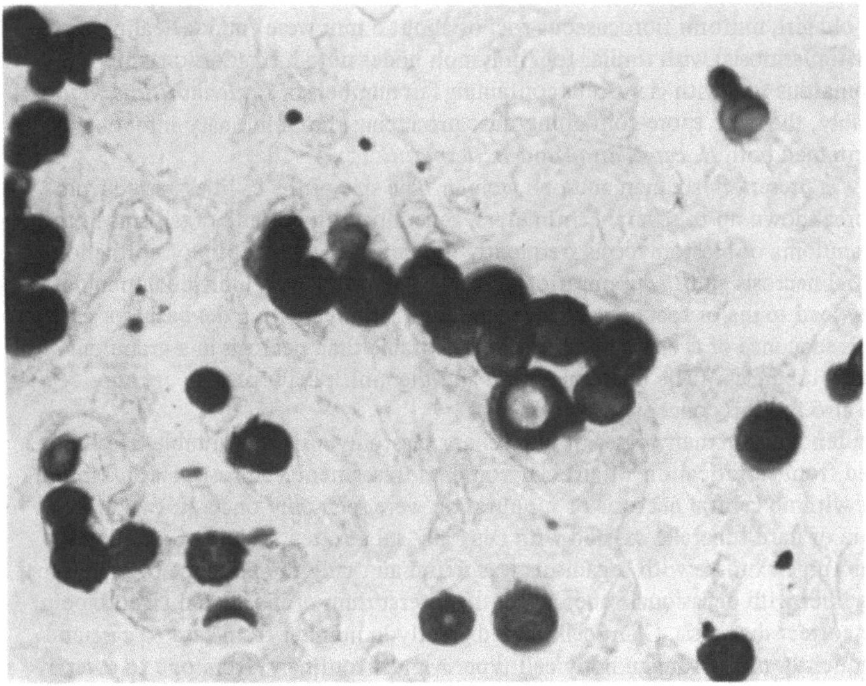

Fig. 3. Chains of yeast cells are commonly seen and considered diagnostic for Lobo's disease (*Loboa loboi*); but they are present in this case of blastomycosis, illustrating one more differential diagnosis. Whenever possible, cultures should be attempted. Grocott x 970. AFIP neg. 74-5915

tify a specific lung lesion as primary. None of the cases reviewed at this time had the material permitting the recognition of a primary complex. Furthermore, the lymph node component in blastomycosis is much less prominent and constant than in tuberculosis or histoplasmosis, two diseases in which a complex is formed with regularity.

One must conclude that incompleteness of the primary complex in pulmonary blastomycosis, and in some of the rare primary cutaneous inoculation cases (*Landay* and *Schwarz*, 1971) has more complicated explanations than are apparent. In addition, the nature of the material precludes pathogenic studies about the true incidence or completeness of the primary complex.

Almost 20% of the cases with available lung tissue had cavities; ulceration of the bronchus was found in 35% of the cases. This important complication should be looked for by endoscopists, not only as source of excellent material for culture and biopsy, but also for evaluation of the prognosis and management of the patient. Healing of such foci will be desirable; progression, on the contrary, will be a highly unfavorable development, heralding the possibility of intracanalicular spread.

The gamut of morphologic response, from hard tubercles to caseation, suppuration, or total lack of response, renders the morphological appearance, at best, helpful and, at worst, misleading. In the lung, a truly "specific granuloma" that could be considered pathognomonic for blastomycosis does not exist. The demonstration of the organism by simple or sophisticated methods is absolutely necessary for diagnosis.

2. Skin

Skin involvement in blastomycosis is so common that it has led to the (mistaken) assumption that the skin is the regular portal of entry of the organism.

In the common cutaneous (secondary) involvement, lymphangitis and lymphadenitis are lacking and the cutaneous lesions are often multiple ulcero-vegetative localizations of a disseminated (hematogenous) spread. Excised, the lesions show marked epithelial thickening, a feature which can be so prominent that it leads to the mistaken diagnosis of squamous cell carcinoma. In reality, the proliferation consists of mature squamous cells, often with acanthosis and frequently pierced by intraepithelial microabscesses. In the latter, and also in the corium, organisms can be found in variable numbers. The number of yeast cells varies from case to case, as does the number of microabscesses, and the amount of production of giant cells (Fig. 4), most of which are of the foreign body type, and which surround one to numerous yeast cells. The type of infection can be generally easily and safely determined from typical thick-walled budding organisms, since the single broad-based bud is unique for *B. dermatitidis*. Special stains will invariably and promptly reveal more organisms than prolonged search on H & E stained sections renders. It has been widely accepted that the common clinical case of cutaneous blastomycosis is secondary to a pulmonary primary infection, even when the frequency of cutaneous involvement and apparent lack of clinical pulmonary disease precipitate relapse to the consideration of "a primary skin infection."

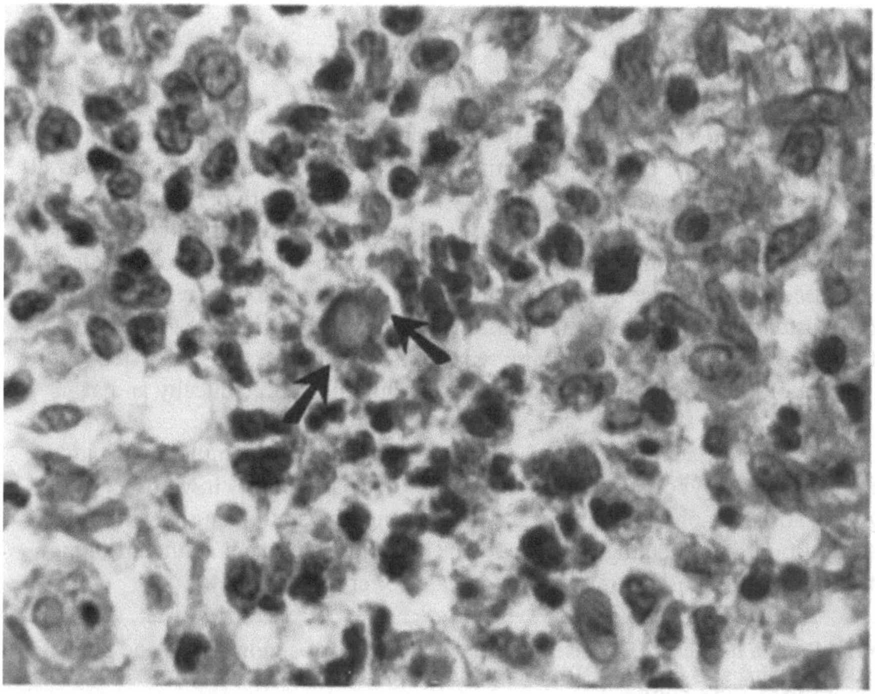

Fig. 4. Skin lesion with solitary organism with short club-like projections. ("Asteroid body," Hoeppli-Splendore phenomenon.) Probably a form of antigen-antibody reaction. H & E x 970. AFIP neg. 74-5913

When rigorous work-up by culture from sputum, bronchial washings, X-rays—using more than a single A-P exposure—and prostatic massage are used, and when any palpable lymph node and mediastinoscopy tissue are taken for culture and biopsy (using adequate stains), a large number of apparently "primary cutaneous" foci can be even clinically proven to be pulmonary in origin. In the rare case where pulmonary foci cannot be verified by clinical methods at the time of the first hospitalization, subsequent appearance of new skin lesions, or involvement of new organ systems (bone, urogenital organs) will justify the renewed search for a primary respiratory infection. In view of the clinical importance and because of their easy clinical recognition, cutaneous blastomycosis will often be represented in biopsy material, leading, hopefully, to the recognition of the entire case. When deep-seated dermal or subcutaneous infiltrates are biopsied—lacking any connection with the skin surface—the hematogenous origin of the lesions becomes adequately demonstrated. Serial sections can be used to convince the most skeptical observer.

Of the 73 cases with skin involvement, 53 had single lesions, ten multiple lesions, and ten multiple lesions as part of disseminated disease. Twenty-two lesions were located on skin, normally covered by clothing, and 20 were on exposed surfaces. Four sinus tracts of the chest wall were fistulas from pleuropulmonary disease. The lower extremities were involved nine times by single lesions, the arms seven times, and the face (including nose, lips, lids, and earlobes) 12 times. Multiple lesions occurred in a great variety of combinations, as face and leg, wrist and buttocks, etc., illustrating the hematogenous character of the cutaneous lesions. Thirty-five cases were in white men, 21 in black men, and the remaining 14 men had no racial identification.

3. Urogenital Lesions

Table 2 shows some of the shortcomings of the material. Epididymitis was found nine times, but in the 11 additional cases of urogenital blastomycosis, epididymis was not available. Similarly, testicular slides were available only in seven cases, with orchitis in one. Seminal vesicle and bladder were not tabulated, since each organ was involved only once and material was seldom available for microscopy. Clinically, prostatic involvement can be demonstrated by microscopy of exudate obtained by prostatic massage and we have made the diagnosis of the existence of blastomycosis occasionally this way. It would seem obvious that demonstration of *B. dermatitidis* in prostatic secretions would suggest, as next step, thorough examination of kidneys, seminal vesicles, and epididymis, both clinically and at autopsy.

Ascending pyelonephritis in the presence of prostatitis cannot be completely excluded, but localization of blastomycotic lesions in the glomeruli clearly points towards a hematogenous origin. Cystitis was observed in a case with huge numbers of organisms without granulomatous response; in the lung of this patient, blastomycetes were abundant in number and with little reaction, as commonly seen in cases of cryptococcosis.

Fig. 5. "Colony" of *B. dermatitidis* occupying the major part of a glomerulus and compressing tufts appearing as a crescent. Round cell infiltrates surround the glomerulus. H & E x 275. AFIP neg. 74-5925

Fig. 6. Large yeast cell (10 μ) in kidney with seven dark dots simulating endospores. Notice difference in size in photograph from same case (Fig. 2). H & E x 970. AFIP neg. 74-5907

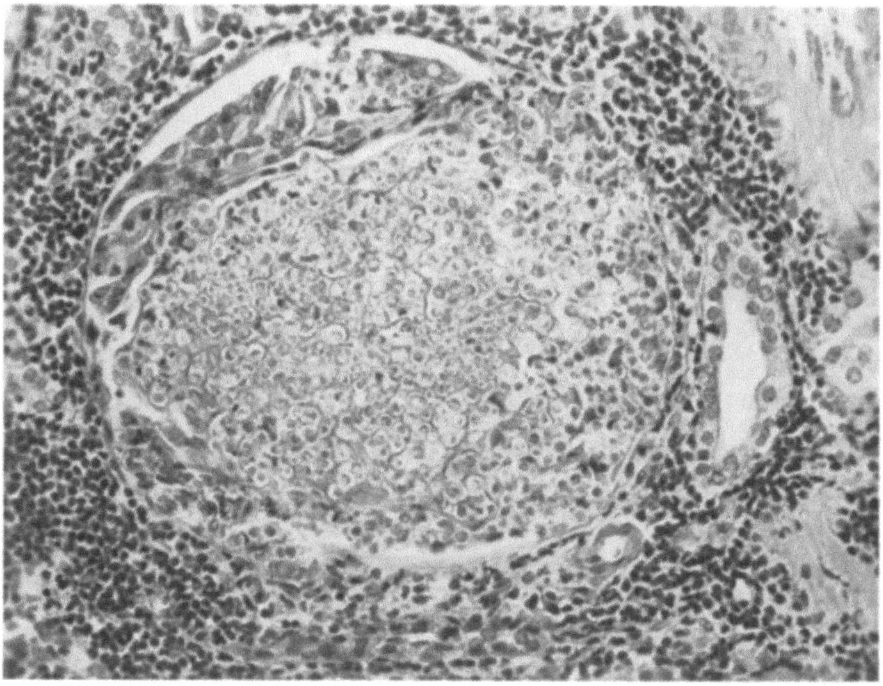

Fig. 5 (Legend see p. 172)

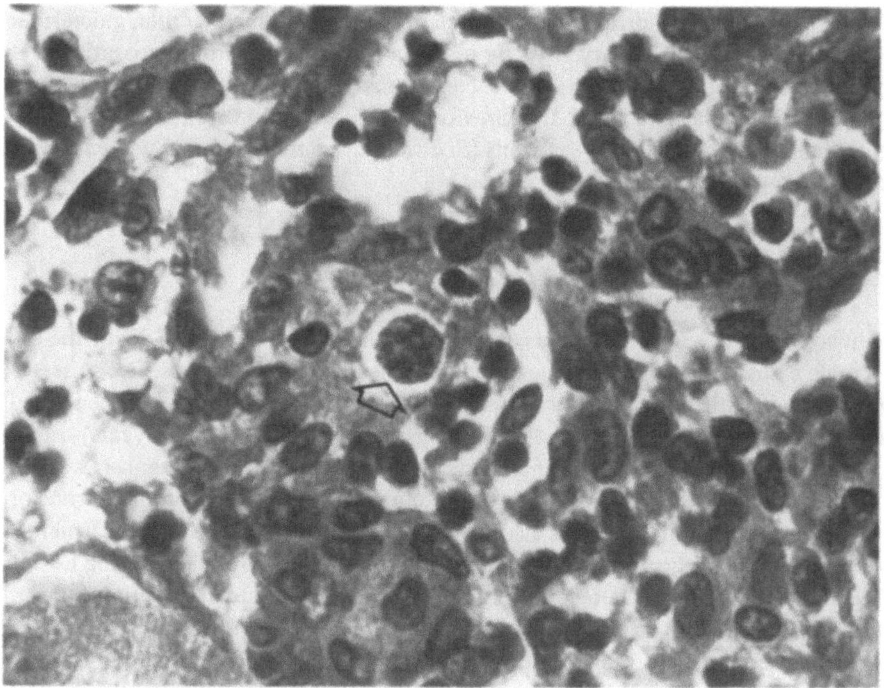

Fig. 6 (Legend see p. 172)

Table 2. Distribution of urogenital blastomycosis

Age	Prostate	Epididymis	Testis	Kidney
38	+	0	0	+
56	+	+	–	–
?	+	+	–	0
61	+	+	–	–
?	+	+	+	+
56	+	0	0	0
32	+	+	0	+
45	+	0	0	+
32	+	0	0	0
40	+	0	0	+
58	+	+	0	+
53	+	+	0	–
48	+	0	0	0
43	+	0	0	0
55	–	+	–	0
67	0	+	0	+
55	–	+	–	0
31	–	0	–	+
68	–	0	0	+
59	–	0	0	+
Total	14	9	1	10

+ = blastomycotic involvement; – = no blastomycotic involvement; 0 = no slides available

One case (Fig. 5) had, in addition to interstitial granulomas in the medulla, glomerular lesions with compression of capillary tufts by masses of yeast cells with comparatively minor lymphocytic periglomerular infiltrates. Numerous yeast cells were seen in the compressed glomerular tufts also (Fig. 6). In a previous series, we had seen multiple casts in renal tubuli completely formed by yeast cells (*Schwarz* and *Baum*, 1951). Such casts were not found in the present material.

4. Prostate

Prostatic involvement was noted 14 times (11.5% of male patients) and in 38% of the disseminated male cases. Prostatitis was associated six times with epididymitis, five times with nephritis, once with testicular and seminal vesicle blastomycosis. Three patients had central nervous system involvement. The average age was 46 (from 32 to 61 years). Eight patients were white, two black, and four lacked racial information. The diagnosis was made once by needle biopsy of the prostate when granulomas with giant cells and numerous organisms were found. A second case was also diagnosed by biopsy from a small fragment of prostate in presence of dysuria, and with multiple skin lesions appearing during hospitalization. The morphology of tissue response varied from clinical nodular granulomas over mixed suppurative lesions to frank abscess formation. One case had sheet-like histiocytic infiltrates without a tendency to nodular granulomas. Giant cells were common, mostly of the multinucleated foreign body type and frequently engulfing yeast cells. Necrosis and caseation were seen five times, often in combination with suppuration. In 10 cases, the prostatitis was part of (known) wide dissemination; in the four other patients, this information was lacking. The number of yeast cells was generally abundant, with great variation in size of the yeast cells in several instances, noted. This variation in size of yeast cells in the prostate was seen sometimes in spite of uniform size in other organs. Some relationship seems to exist between large numbers of organisms (rapid reproduction) and variation in size from barely 2 μ to 10 μ and more.

5. Epididymis

Epididymitis was seen in nine of 121 men (7.4%); a much higher incidence can be calculated if only disseminated cases are considered (9/36 = 24%). In one case, the epididymitis was bilateral and twice it was associated with a scrotal fistula. Associated prostatitis was found six times, orchitis only once, but renal involvement in three cases. The autopsy cases with epididymitis involved six white males, twice it was found in black men, and one patient was not identified as to race. The average age was 52.6 years (from 32 to 67 years). The seven autopsy cases with epididymitis all had widely disseminated blastomycosis, the number of organisms varied from few to innumerable. The greatest number of organisms was seen in a case of lymphosarcoma. This particular case, a 67-year-old white man, had colonization of most organs by large numbers of yeast cells, but only colchicin (for gout) had been recorded as therapy.

The morphology of epididymal involvement ranged from single huge abscesses to caseation, from granulomas of various ages to granulomas with necrotic rather than suppurated centers. In one case, breakthrough from the interstitium into tubuli was clearly visible. Two cases showed great variation in the size of the yeast cells, all others had fairly uniform organisms. The comparative paucity of bilateral involvement brings up the question whether it reflects the true incidence or is falsified by incomplete examination or records.

The seminal vesicles were found only once involved with blastomycosis, but this organ is unfortunately neglected by the average prosector and is difficult to pinpoint clinically. The low figure of seminal vesicle disease smells of neglect.

6. Testis

The fact that the prostate was found involved 14 times and the epididymis 9 times contrasted with the single case of testicular blastomycosis. This patient had additional urogenital foci in prostate, epididymis, and kidney, and this clearly suggested the orchitis as part of a hematogenous dissemination. The paucity of testicular involvement is paralleled by the situation in tuberculosis, where epididymitis is the common localization with occasional to rare extension into the testis.

7. Larynx

Laryngeal blastomycosis was found 9 times. Eight of these cases were white men, while the ninth case had no racial identification. The average age was 51.2 with variation from

38 to 65 years of age. The description of the lesions varied from papillomatous to fungating, to ulcerative and "leukoplakia-like" in appearance. Microscopically, the typical cases showed pseudoepitheliomatous thickening of the mucosa with or without intraepithelial microabscesses. One case had an outspoken "sarcoid" appearance with dry discrete epithelioid cell tubercles. In other cases, the epithelioid cells refused to form nodules and were not recognized as granulomatous. The number of organisms was generally small and their presence had to be verified by special stains. Giant cells tended to be of the foreign body type.

Only four cases had sufficient data to document pulmonary involvement. Only one patient came to autopsy (several years after positive biopsy), but, at this time, had no demonstrable blastomycotic laryngitis. Two more cases were reported "healed." The fact that most specimens were biopsies is in contrast with the majority of other material, except involvement of the skin, which also generally is of surgical rather than of postmortem origin. Hoarseness and laryngeal obstructive symptoms led generally to the biopsy, which was, at least once, submitted as "benign papilloma." One case had three consecutive biopsies before the true nature of the lesion was established. After the second biopsy, the recurrence was obstructing already after two weeks. In this specific case, the epithelial proliferation included cornification and the differential diagnosis had to include squamous cell carcinoma. It was our impression that the process probably still was reactive rather than neoplastic.

8. Central Nervous System

Six cases of meningitis and four of encephalitis were on record. Both groups were exclusively in men. The meningitic cases were 42 and 65 years of age (average 46.5 years). Four meningitides and three encephalitides occurred in white men, two meningitides in black, one encephalitis in a 28-year-old Indian. Eight cases were found at autopsy; two encephalitic lesions were diagnosed from surgical biopsies.

The encephalitic foci were completely necrotic (coagulation) without any tendency toward breakdown. The center resembled the periphery, complete necrosis with loss of practically all cellular detail and absence of inflammatory cells. In the periphery, there was either a scattering of lymphocytes or a narrow rim of histiocytes. If there were giant cells, they were exceptional. The lesions were expansive, compressing the surrounding brain tissue. Several cases had marked perivascular cuffing, almost exclusively lymphocytic, and utilizing special stains, isolated *B. dermatitidis* were seen in the cell accumulations about the vessels. Such cuffing is seen also in candidiasis and is, therefore, not restricted to viral encephalitis (Figs. 7-8).

When combined with meningitis, sometimes vessels in the leptomeninges were completely necrotic. Perineural (cranial or spinal) involvement showed giant cells containing several *B. dermatitidis.*

Fig. 7. Encephalitic cuffing. Yeast cells of *B. dermatitidis* were seen (in small numbers) in Virchow-Robin spaces. H & E x 80. AFIP neg. 74-5928

Fig. 8. Numerous organisms and coagulation necrosis; meninges. H & E x 150. AFIP neg. 74-5911

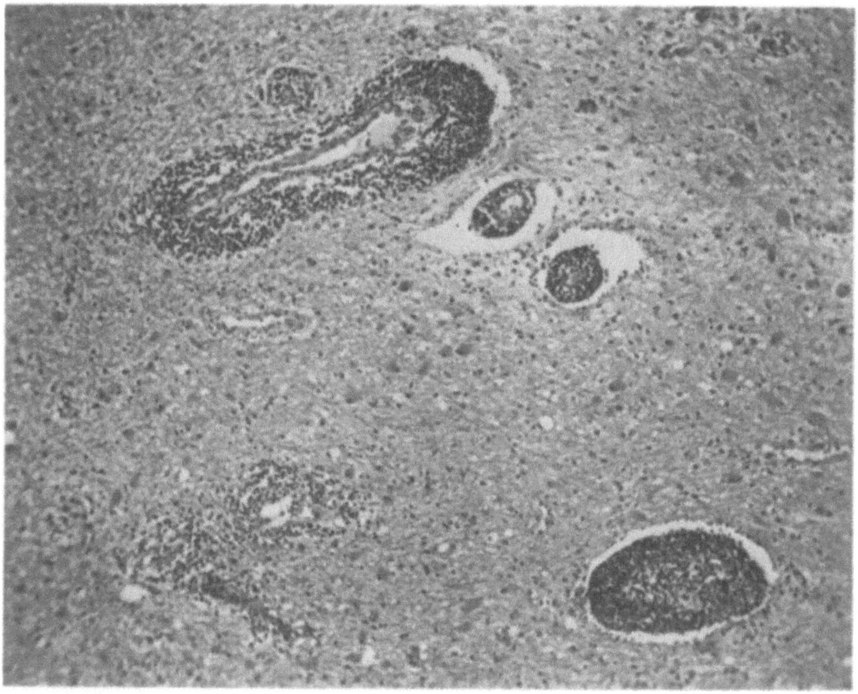

Fig. 7 (Legend see p. 176)

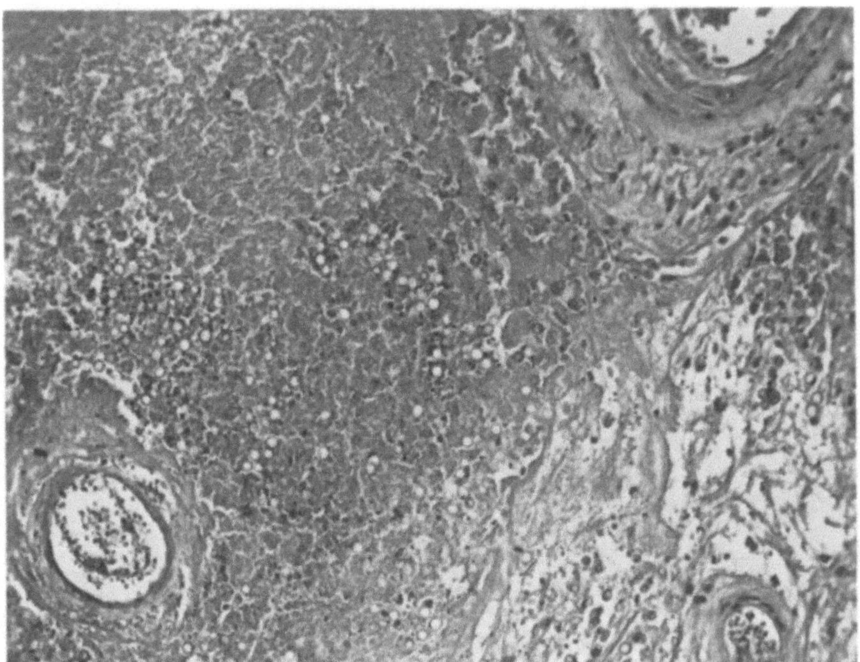

Fig. 8 (Legend see p. 176)

9. Adrenal

Of 18 adrenal glands available, 4 showed blastomycosis, all 4 in males. One had caseous foci, while 3 showed discrete granulomas. All positive cases occurred before 1954.

10. Thyroid

Of 12 available thyroids, 6 had blastomycosis, all in patients with disseminated disease. Numerous organisms and granulomas were the rule and all 6 occurred in males.

11. Heart

One case (Fig. 9) had myocardial foci close to the epicardial and endocardial surfaces (771063). *Witorsch* and *Utz* (1968) did not observe cardiac involvement.

12. Bone

Bone involvement was found 12 times, once in association with arthritis. Independent arthritis was found twice. The bone lesions were located mostly in short bones and the

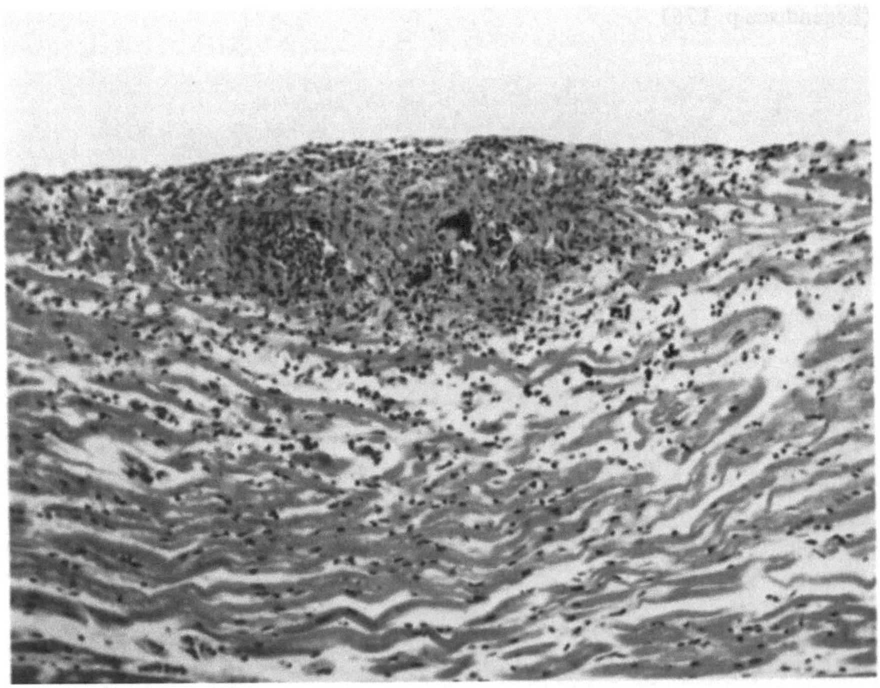

Fig. 9. Subendocardial granuloma in widespread blastomycosis. Cardiac involvement is rare; in this instance, the subendocardial focus may have been feeding organisms into the circulation. H & E x 140. AFIP neg. 74-5918

histology varied from granulomatous to necrotizing, caseous, and suppurative. Bone destruction with sequestration of bone was found in some cases. All were indeed disseminated cases, with the ostitis or osteomyelitis part of the picture.

13. Amyloidosis

Two cases of amyloidosis were present in the material.

A 32-year-old black man (Fig. 10) had diffuse amyloidosis of liver and adrenals, follicular amyloidosis in the spleen, and some amyloid of the kidney, mostly tubular and less glomerular. The organs involved by the amyloid, with exception of the kidney, did not show granuloma of blastomycosis. The prostate, epididymis, and kidneys had abscesses and granulomas, apparently of embolic origin. This was particularly convincing in the epididymis where interstitial granulomas were seen in rupture into the tubular lumina. Pulmonary blastomycotic lesions were widespread with discrete amyloid deposits in the interstitium. The patient also had myocardial involvement with granulomas close to epi- and endocardium. There was a history of five years duration of pulmonary disease, and sinus tracts had formed through the chest wall. Blastomycotic bone involvement was noted in the protocol.

A 32-year-old black man had extensive follicular, almost confluent amyloidosis of the spleen and lymph nodes and glomerular deposits in the kidneys. Adrenals and liver were

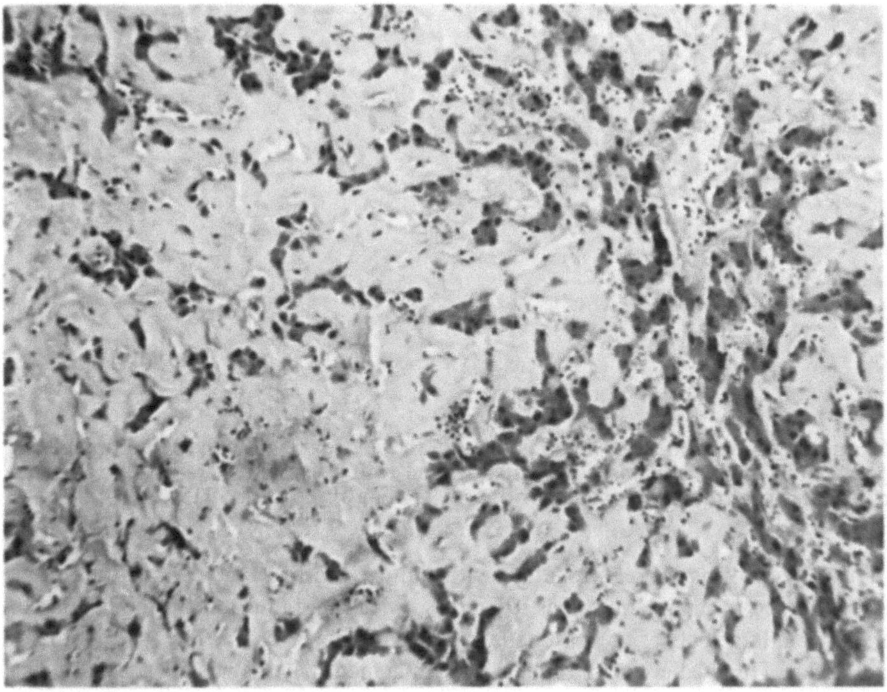

Fig. 10. "Secondary" amyloidosis; liver–a rare but not unexpected complication of longstanding blastomycosis. H & E x 140. AFIP neg. 74-5919

free of amyloid. The blastomycotic lesions were seen in lung and prostate and a granulomatous infiltrate was seen in the peritoneum, invading the external layers of the large bowel. There was no evidence of mucosal involvement of the intestinal tract by blastomycosis.

IV. Morphology of Organisms

B. dermatitidis in tissues is a round yeast cell with thick walls, often budding. The single bud connects with the mother cell through a broad porus or exhibits a broad base when cut at other levels. The yeast cells vary from 5-15 μ, with extremes from 2 μ (microforms) to 30 μ (Fig. 11). The cytoplasm can be basophilic and several nuclei can be visible.

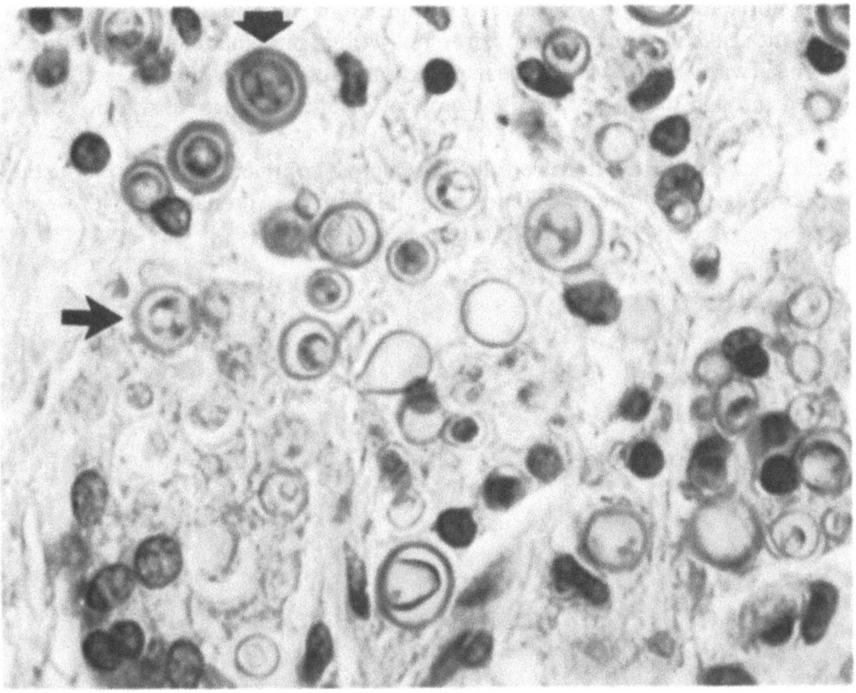

Fig. 11. Morphologic variation can be considerable in one field; small and large organisms, pear-shaped "empty cells" contrast with thick-walled round yeasts with a variety of endoplasmic configurations (arrow); patella. Gridley x 970. AFIP neg. 74-5912

Sometimes, microforms are seen together with standard forms (Fig. 12) but their number varies from organ to organ and seems to increase with rapid multiplication–if this can be concluded from large masses of yeast cells in a given focus or organ. The microforms are as small as 2 μ. Thin walled yeasts, identical with standard forms in size, shape, nuclear content, and mode of budding, can occur side by side with "double" (thick) walled forms (Fig. 13).

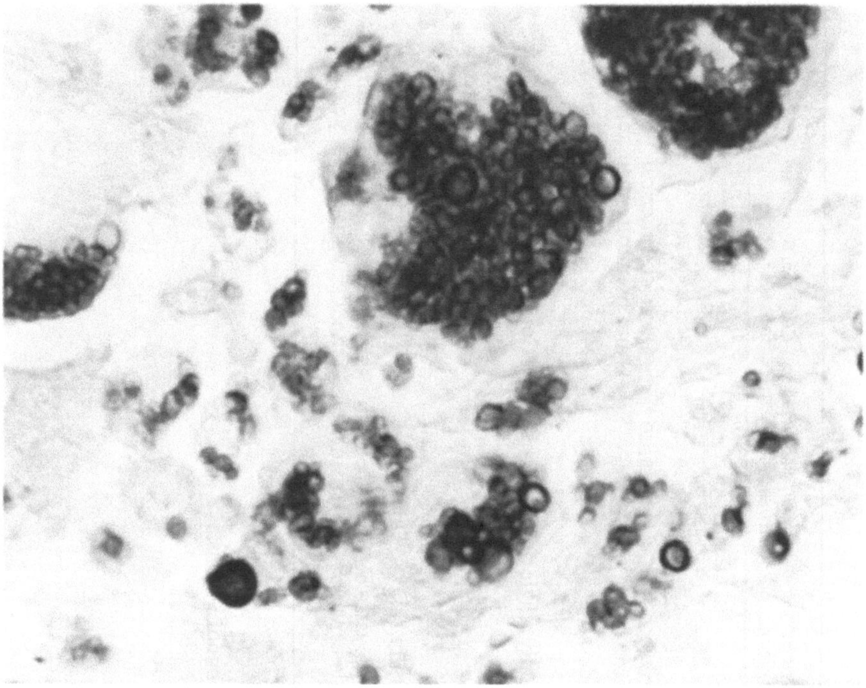

Fig. 12. Clusters of microforms of *B. dermatitidis* in prostate. Precipitous budding may be a partial explanation for the small size of most yeast cells in this instance. Gridley x 970. AFIP neg. 74-5921

Some yeast cells are recognized as strange spherule-like large (30 μ) organisms (Fig. 14), sometimes with structures in the cytoplasm resembling endospores. Odd forms of yeasts—bottle-shaped, ovoid, ovoid with constriction, sickle-shaped—may also be found. Undoubtedly, some of the irregularly shaped larger structures represent wall defective organisms (spheroplasts) (Figs. 15, 16).

When few organisms are encountered, either in skin or in internal organs, they are generally rather uniform in size and, if buds are present, the classical appearance of an "8" is found. The more organisms present in a case, in an organ, or in one focus, the more variable the size and shape. It is our distinct impression that the production and separation of small buds from the mother cell is the result of precipitous development and some, quite often many, of the small cells become reproductive in spite of the reduced size and the thin walls. They often create rather hollow structures, either with typical "8" forms or of more irregular shape. On the other hand, the existence of cases with microforms is undeniable and it is, in our opinion, not established whether these are special (small) mutants or whether the small size of the yeasts is the result of precipitous separation of buds. Six cases had microforms of about 2 μ.

Often, there are great differences in size and staining properties from field to field, organ to organ, and case to case. The thickness of the wall can vary greatly, as does staining of the wall and cytoplasm.

Table 3. Morphologic differentiation of yeast cells in tissues

	Blastomyces dermatitidis	*Paracoccidioides brasiliensis*	*Cryptococcus neoformans*	*Histoplasma duboisii*	*Candida albicans*	*Loboa loboi*
Extreme sizes in μ	2-30	2-60	2.5-20	10-15[a]	2-14	7-14
Average size in μ	5-10	10-30	3 -8	10-15	2- 5	9-10
Shape	Spherical to elliptical	Spherical to elliptical	Spherical to elliptical	Spherical to elliptical	Ovoid to spherical and pseudohyphae	Spherical to elliptical
Variation in size in tissue	Moderate to considerable	Moderate to considerable	Considerable	Low grade	Moderate	Low grade
Number of buds	Generally single	Multiple[b]	Generally single	Generally single	Generally single[b]	Multiple[b]
Porus between mother and buds	Broad	Generally narrow	Narrow	Narrow	Narrow	Generally narrow
Nucleus	Multiple	Multiple	Single	Single	Single	Multiple
Thickness of wall	Mostly thick	Mostly thick	Generally thin	Thick	Thin	Thick
Single most characteristic feature	Single broad-based bud	Multiple buds "pilot wheel"	Mucopolysaccharide capsule[c]	Yeast cells in huge giant cells	Presence of pseudohyphae	Chains of yeast cells

[a]Simultaneous presence of "capsulatum" forms of 2-4 μ possible.

[b]Daughter cells sometimes do not separate, resulting in chains of budding cells.

[c]Positive mucicarmine stain.

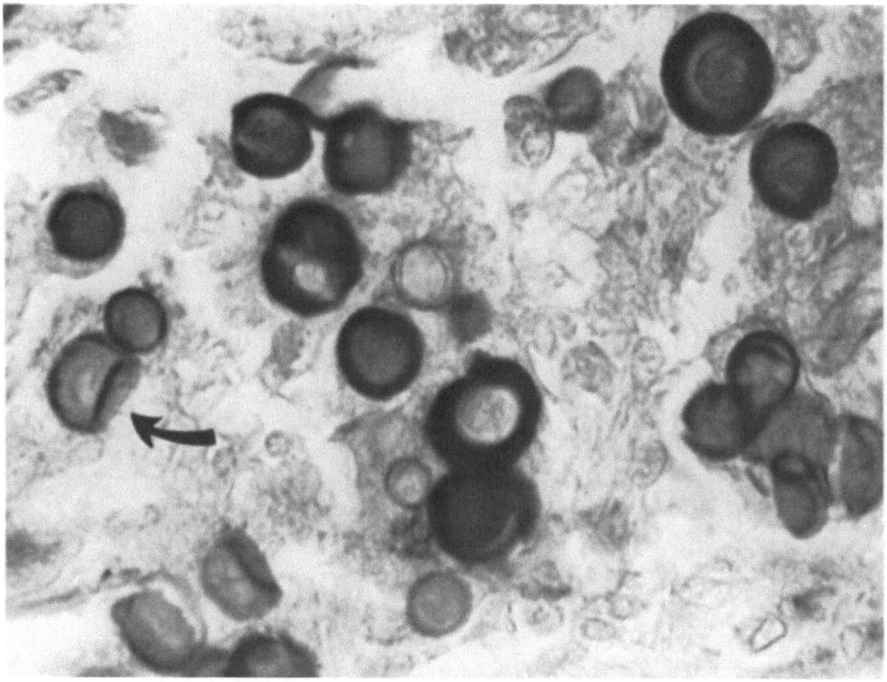

Fig. 13. Thick-walled yeast cells, some budding. Collapsed yeast cells have thinner poorly staining walls (arrow); lung. Gridley x 970. AFIP neg. 74-5906

The African case (*Jelliffe* et al., 1964) shows many classical *B. dermatitidis* and a few strange ones, resembling curved buns with reproductive forms, which are similar to septation rather than to budding. Some of these forms bring to mind pictures of *Schizosaccharomyces* with flat endings at the point of separation of the bud from the mother cells. However, it seems that the morphologic variations are within the range of *Blastomyces*. Wall defective organisms (spheroplasts) become either very irregular and large, or collapse, resulting in the appearance of "punched in" (sickle-shaped) balloon forms. In vitro, extremely bizarre forms can be induced on egg media or blood agar. Old cultures or cultures on old media especially abound with markedly atypical "yeasts." Similar degenerative forms were found on tissue explants (*Goldman* and *Schwarz*, 1966).

A word must be said about the interpretation of the mucicarmine reaction. Some yeast cells of *B. dermatitidis* take a very faint pink hue on overstaining with Meyer's mucicarmine: Intense red color is characteristically and quite uniquely seen with *Cryptococcus neoformans*. We do not accept the faint reaction of some *Blastomyces* as a positive reaction. The yeast cells of *C. neoformans* stain uniformly red but not every cell reacts, but, in every group of *C. neoformans*, a few, and sometimes many, or even all yeast cells, will be found with a bright red color with the mucicarmine stain. Sometimes in *C. neoformans*, the broad mucopolysaccharide capsule stains or red strands radiate from the cell wall to the capsular border.

If cultural confirmation is lacking in isolated cases with atypical yeasts, no decision is possible and should be avoided on morphologic grounds alone.

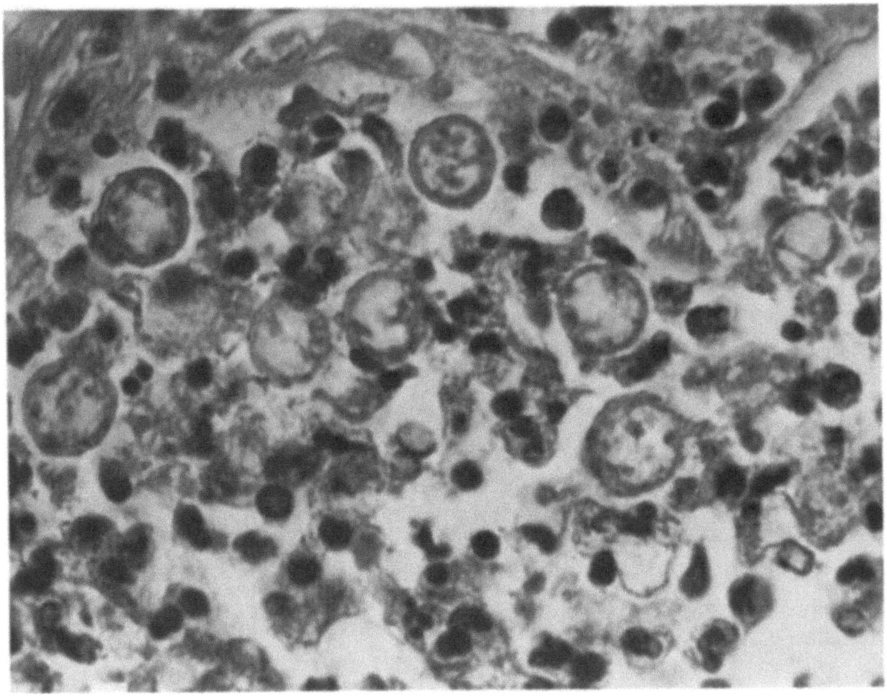

Fig. 14 (Legend see p. 185)

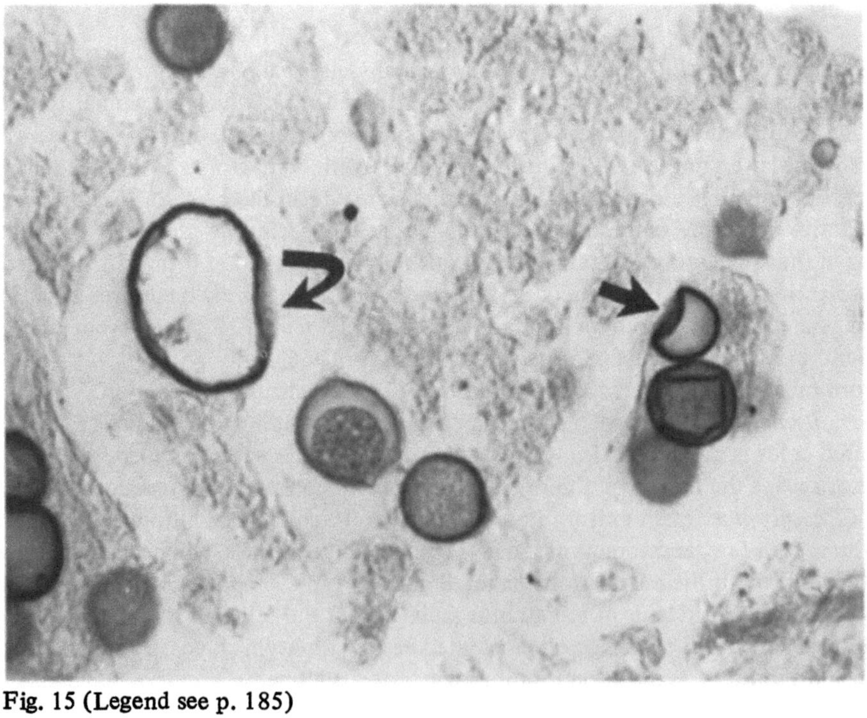

Fig. 15 (Legend see p. 185)

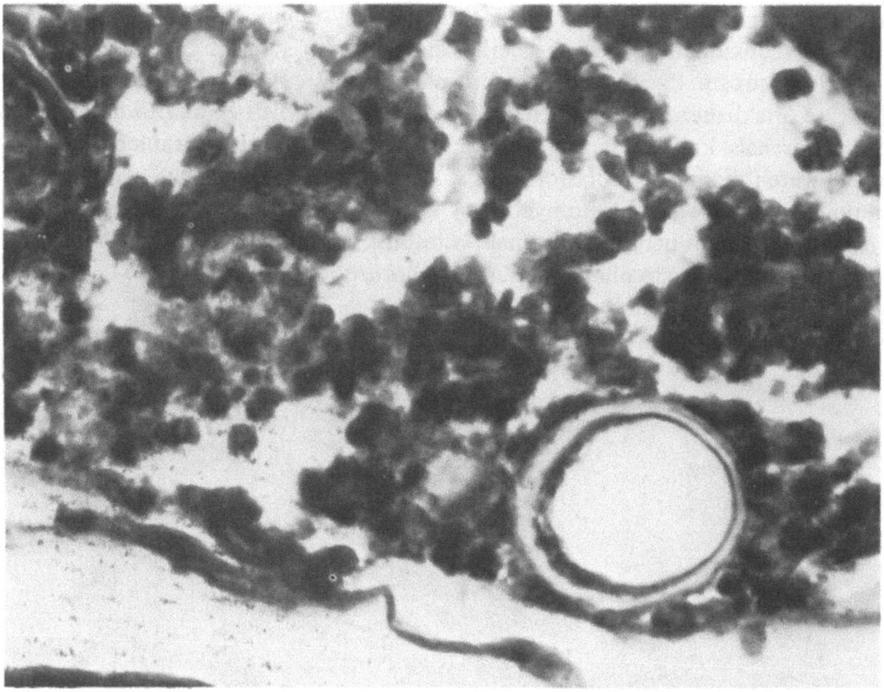

Fig. 16. Giant and thick-walled yeast cell (30 x 27 μ); skin. Neighboring yeast cells were of "typical" size and shape. H & E x 970. AFIP neg. 74-5923

V. Mechanisms of Dissemination

The lung is the ordinary portal of entrance for blastomycosis. Dissemination from the lung occurs generally by way of lympho-hematogenous spread. The presence of fungemia can be readily demonstrated morphologically in view of the large size of the agents,which are much easier visible than bacteria. In five cases, we found *B. dermatitidis* in vessel lumina, free or within blood clots, this finding not necessarily synonymous with widespread dissemination. This unveils the problem why fungemia does not always produce metastatic foci. Such seemingly vague notions like "organ resistance" and organ tropism must be advocated in trying to explain this behavior. Positive and negative tropisms probably have very distinct physicochemical causes, since differences in enzymatic systems, immune-body concentration, carbohydrate content between organs, and even between individual cells, are documented (*Soskin* and *Levine*, 1962).

Fig. 14. Uniform size of large yeast cells, somewhat resembling small spherules of *C. immitis.* Variations in size and staining properties are considerable in blastomycosis; lung. H & E x 970. AFIP neg. 74-5924

Fig. 15. Huge wall-defective yeast cell (25:16 μ) (curved arrow) in lung; other yeast cells are "punched in" (arrow). Gridley x 970. AFIP neg. 74-5927

No large number of patients with blastomycosis undergo systemic attempts at culture. Hence, there are no factual data to answer whether circulation or actual multiplication occurs within the blood stream. Positive blood cultures have been reported. A discrepancy was obvious in the case of a diabetic with huge numbers of yeast cells of *B. dermatitidis* in a large pulmonary vein. Adrenals, kidneys, heart, liver, and spleen were available for microscopic examination and were found free of blastomycosis. Another case (Fig. 17) had organisms in a large pulmonary vein and had blastomycosis in some organs (spleen, prostate, kidney, brain, bone marrow), whereas pancreas, adrenals, pituitary, and liver were spared. Three more cases had only lung tissue available with *B. dermatitidis*, once in veins, once in arteries, and once in both (large) arteries and veins.

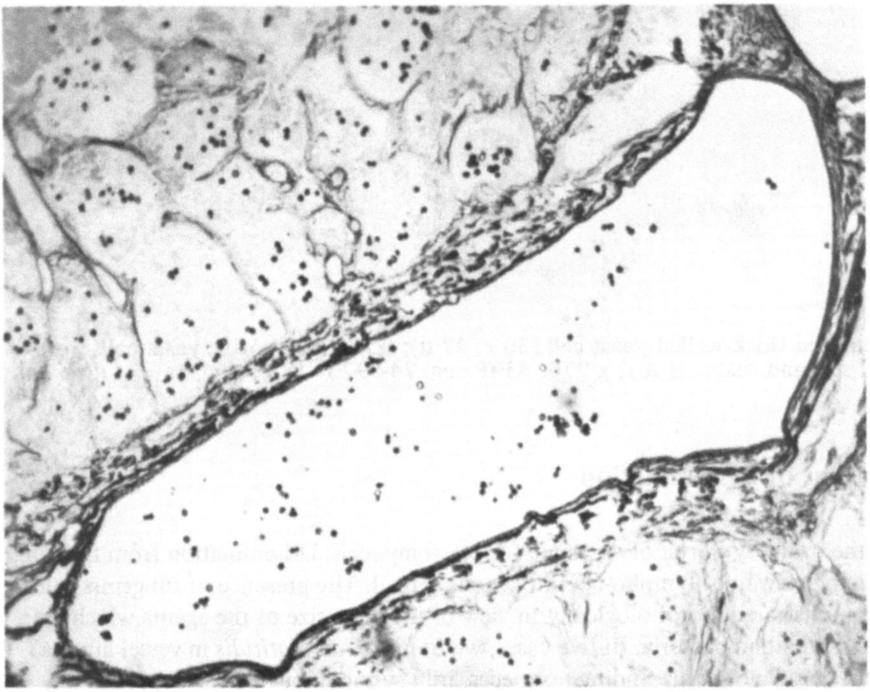

Fig. 17. Numerous blastomycetes in pulmonary alveoli and in large vein. The demonstration of yeast cells in vascular lamina eloquently illustrates fungemia. Gridley x 77. AFIP neg. 74-5920

That immune mechanisms are at work in regulating progression of disease is suggested from a study of the rare cutaneous inoculation cases, which stop at the portal of entry or at the axillary lymph nodes. Of the eight known cases, none has disseminated. Parenthetically, the one culturally proven case of pulmonary laboratory infection (*Baum* and *Lerner*, 1970) became likewise arrested without progression.[2] Illustrating the opposite behavior is

[2] A probable case of laboratory infection by inhalation (*Denton* et al., 1967), developed osteolytic lesions in one fibula, and was treated with surgery and amphotericin B. The possibility of spontaneous infection is not discountable and proof of laboratory acquired blastomycosis is circumstantial.

a patient who was followed over ten years. This man constantly developed new cutaneous foci, a few months after apparent successful, repeated arrest by amphotericin B and/or stilbamidine. Pulmonary and laryngeal blastomycosis coexisted and he was unable to handle the infection.

VI. Tissue Response

In describing the most commonly seen and, therefore, "typical" tissue reaction, it would probably be correct to state that most cases of blastomycosis show epithelioid cell tubercles with giant cells and leukocytic invasion of the central necrotic area. This statement applies especially to the lung and, to a lesser degree, to other internal organs. It seldom is true for skin, which has a unique reaction. Individual cases, however, can present very differently, i.e., hard epithelioid cell tubercles without necrosis, sometimes incorrectly diagnosed as sarcoid. Three such cases were observed, two in lung biopsies and one in a lymph node. Clinically, this confusion leads to grave errors (*Baum* et al., 1973). In general, it must be accepted that a wide variation of morphology exists in the granulomatous diseases and that a specific diagnosis depends on demonstration of the causative agent and not on tissue response alone. The specific character of inflammation, when present, can be extremely helpful in suspecting a given organism, and it will often be possible to identify *B. dermatitidis* in epithelioid cell tubercles with central suppuration in any given organ, if investigated with special stains. Totally unlike sarcoid-like lesions are the necrotizing, strictly exudative cases where polymorphonuclear leukocytes may be found, but few, if any, histiocytes are present. In other instances, for example, in the lung, the alveoli may be filled with and distended by rapidly multiplying blastomycetes with little tissue reaction noted and resembling the "non-reactive" picture often seen in cryptococcosis. Otherwise, the intra-alveolar yeast colonies may be associated with isolated tubercles of epithelioid cells in the interstitium or a sprinkling of multinucleated giant cells of either the Langhans or (predominantly) the foreign body type. In the prostate, lakes of yeast cells can be found apparently in cystic dilatation of glands. Closer inspection may reveal, however, that some of the space occupied by the yeast cells is actually the result of tissue breakdown. The organisms proper also show variation in staining reaction, some representing necrotic organisms. In the kidneys, a great variation of reaction can be seen. These reactions range from caseating granulomas and abscesses to cast formations with little reaction. The finding of innumerable yeast cells in renal tubuli is uncommon, but impressive (*Schwarz* and *Baum*, 1951). Perivascular encephalitic infiltrates and granulomatous and nonspecific neuritis, emanating from the spinal cord for some distance in the endo- and perineurium of peripheral nerves, can be seen. In the skin and in squamous mucosae, the pseudoepitheliomatous proliferation with intraepithelial microabscesses is so characteristic that it can be considered strongly suggestive for blastomycosis until proven otherwise; however, in all examples given, the demonstration of organisms is indispensable for confirmation of the diagnosis.

In general, it must be stated that review of numerous cases proves that the morphology of the organism, especially its size, shows more variation than suggested in standard textbooks. Microforms can be found in the same giant cell which harbors normal-sized organisms. Entire fields, in the given case, may be dominated by the small forms without transition, only to find transitions in another field or another organ. The round size of the microforms, with single broadbased buds, strongly suggests that they represent a variation of *B. dermatitidis*, rather than a dual infection. This suggestion is strengthened by the presence of small and large forms in one cell. Fluorescent antibody staining would be most helpful in a prospective study to confirm the interpretation of microforms and giant yeasts as *B. dermatitidis*.

Giant cells in blastomycosis are more often of the foreign body cell type, a reaction this organism shares with other "large" fungus cells, such as *Coccidioides immitis, Paracoccidioides brasiliensis*, and *C. neoformans*. It is tempting to assume that size, to considerable degree, determines the type of giant cell response. Single to numerous yeast cells of *B. dermatitidis* can be easily detected within the cytoplasm or the giant cells. Accordingly, the size of the giant cells markedly varies up to gigantic types.

VII. Special Pathology of Organs

1. Lung

In a clinical study, 25% of patients with lung lesions had cavities (*Busey* et al., 1964). Two of our cavitary cases had diabetes, a remarkable incidence considering that, of the total of 152 cases, only 4 had diabetes. The tissues of the diabetic have long been known susceptible to necrotizing infection. *Busey* et al. (1964) found diabetes nine times in 198 blastomycotic patients. Other authors (*Chick* et al., 1960; *Zimmerman*, 1955) feel that diabetes is not more frequent in blastomycotic patients than in the general population.

Aspergillomas were described in blastomycotic cavities (*Sarosi* et al., 1971). No such case was found in the present material, but "aspergillomas" frequently are discarded because they are (mistaken for) blood clots. The absence of pertinent cases cannot be necessarily accepted as factual.

The material available in this survey did not include complete lungs with lymph nodes, which would have permitted to establish the presence of a complete pulmonary primary complex. It has been already mentioned that such complexes are found with much greater constancy in histoplasmosis than in blastomycosis or coccidioidomycosis.

Exceptions to this rule occur, however, for instance, in spontaneous histoplasmosis of dogs, where only 40% of the animals have a complete complex, meaning the lymph node component can be absent in up to 60% of cases (*Fattal* et al., 1961). While complete complexes have been observed in man and animals in blastomycosis, undoubtedly, the incidence is much lower than in either histoplasmosis or tuberculosis. Similar findings (of incomplete complexes) were made in coccidioidomycosis, where we concluded that the presence of lymphadenitis already represents a step towards dissemination (*Straub* and *Schwarz*, 1962) and should be viewed as complication rather than a normal development of a primary complex. In dogs with spontaneous histoplasmosis, 60% show no satellite lymph node involvement in circumstances where *H. capsulatum* was cultured from many lymph nodes lacking gross or microscopic lesions (*Fattal* et al., 1961). When we tried to duplicate these findings in men, culturing from cervical and bronchial lymph nodes, *H. capsulatum* was found only once in a disseminated case of histoplasmosis (*Lai* and *Schwarz*, 1972). To our knowledge, no series exists on cultural versus morphologic findings in lymph nodes of blastomycotic dogs. The presence of satellite lymph nodes can be decisive in judging primary inoculation blastomycosis versus secondary skin involvement.

We have pointed out repeatedly (*Landay* and *Schwarz*, 1971; *Schwarz* and *Baum*, 1951) that primary cutaneous blastomycosis is rare and restricted to the rather exceptional cases of traumatic inoculation occurring in autopsy rooms and mycology laboratories. After such accidental inoculation, a "chancriform syndrome (*Wilson*, 1953) occurs, consisting of the (single) chancre, generally with regional lymphadenitis, often linked by lymphangitis (*Landay* and *Schwarz*, 1971).

2. Kidney

All 10 patients with renal involvement were male autopsy cases with widespread blastomycosis. The embolic character of renal blastomycosis is illustrated clearly in three cases without additional genitourinary involvement, which permits exclusion of ascending infection. Three cases had simultaneous prostatitis, one had epididymitis. Two patients had, in addition to renal involvement, blastomycotic prostatitis and epididymitis and one had prostatitis, epididymitis, and orchitis.

Witorsch and *Utz* (1968) did not have a single case of renal involvement (seven cases examined) but had seven times combined prostatic, epididymal, and testicular blastomycosis and three times prostatitis and three times epididymitis alone. *Kepron* et al. (1972) found renal blastomycosis in two of 36 patients with blastomycosis.

Obviously, tissue conditions in the epididymis and prostate must be propitious for the development of blastomycosis, since we know, with certainty, that *Blastomycetes* circulate throughout the body quite frequently in disseminated cases, while "takes" occur only in epididymis and prostate with any degree of frequency. Circulation of *Blastomycetes* is easily documented by the presence of organisms in blood vessels and blood clots.

In contrast, blastomycotic salpingitis is most uncommon, one of the obvious (albeit incomplete) explanations being the rarity of blastomycosis in women (*Hamblen* et al., 1935).

VIII. Pathogenesis of Urogenital Blastomycosis

The pathogenesis of urogenital blastomycosis could be:

1. *ascending* (in the exceptional case of "venereal" infection with *B. dermatitidis*) (*Chick* et al., 1960);
2. *hematogenous (secondary) to the kidney* with tertiary prostatic involvement following in orthograde way the urinary flow to the prostate;
3. *hematogenous to the prostate* with (a) retrograde ascending infection of the kidney possible (but unlikely) in cases of prostatic obstruction, or (b) retrograde infection of seminal vesicles, epididymis, and testis. This must be exceptional, since testis and seminal vesicles are so rarely involved and can be used as index against acceptance of this modality as "rule"
4. *hematogenous (secondary) to the epididymis* and (tertiary) involvement of the prostate (rarely of testis and seminal vesicles). This follows orthograde flow of semen and is an acceptable way of propagation.

To assume that, from the epididymitis, retrograde renal infection occurs (with intermediary prostatitis) appears unlikely, exceptional, and tortuous. Combination of 2, 3, and/or 4 certainly occur. "Primary" prostatitis with lung lesions secondary to prostatic massage has been also claimed (*Burr* and *Huffines*, 1951) but can be dismissed as contrary to well established pathogenetic facts.

Since tuberculosis of the urogenital tract was and is so much more common, it would seem logical to find answers in texts on urogenital tuberculosis, which could be applied—mutatis mutandis—to the pathogenesis of blastomycosis. However, perusal of the corresponding literature reveals what appears obvious bias by some authors for seminal vesicles as beginning focus of hematogenous tuberculosis, whereas others choose in equally opinionated form foci of secondary involvement in the individual organs (*Lattimer* et al., 1970).

It is concluded that the blastomycotic epididymitis is hematogenous in origin because of:

1. Frequent combination with prostatitis
2. Presence of granulomas in the interstitium with rupture into tubuli
3. Being part of widely disseminated blastomycosis
4. Analogy with tuberculosis
5. Occasional bilateral (symmetrical) involvement

Retrograde infection of the epididymis from the prostate can be postulated but must be exceptional. In our material, epididymitis was less frequent than prostatitis but this can be explained by the fact that symptomatic prostatitis will be clinically more prominent (obstruction) than epididymitis. The bilateral involvement of the epididymis (noted once) and the finding of interstitial granulomas breaking into the epididymal tubules lead us to accept the hematogenous route of infection as the more common and more logical, appearing more likely than retrograde infection from the prostate.

1. Larynx

The differential diagnosis of papilloma and carcinoma can overshadow the tissue reaction to *B. dermatitidis* and the use of special stains will be mandatory in the larynx, whenever inflammatory, granulomatous, or pseudoepitheliomatous proliferation with or without intraepithelial microabscesses is found (*Hoffarth* et al., 1973; *Lyons*, 1966).

It would appear that blastomycotic laryngitis is often part of progressive pulmonary disease but hematogenous involvement cannot be excluded. No facts point to the larynx as common or even possible portal of entry. The complete absence of laryngitis in black males should be mentioned since 30% of the men in this series were black.

2. Adrenals

Four cases, found in this material, all occurred before 1954. A possible coincidence with new therapeutic measures could be postulated.

Stilbamidine and its derivatives were introduced in 1951 (*Schoenbach* et al., 1951) and Amphotericin B about 1956 (*Gold* et al., 1955-56), but it is hard to believe that the introduction of these therapeutic agents prevented adrenal involvement, in view of the presence of disseminated cases up to the present. In 58 cases previously reported (*Schwarz* and *Baum*, 1951), we found four cases of adrenal blastomycosis. In contrast, other series had no adrenal involvement at all (*Witorsch* and *Utz*, 1968).

Addison's disease caused by blastomycotic adrenal destruction is on record (*Abernathy* and *Melby*, 1962).

3. Central Nervous System

The literature gives an involvement of the central nervous system in 6% (*Chick*, 1956; *Chick* et al., 1956) and 33% (*Wade* and *Bel*, 1916) in autopsy series. *Fetter* et al. (1967) present, from a review of the literature, the fact that the lesions may be granulomatous or suppurative or a combination of both.

Central nervous system involvement was rare in several series–once *Witorsch* and *Utz* (1968), three times *Cherniss* and *Waisbren* (1956) and twice *Kepron* et al. (1972).

4. Bone

Similarly, wide variations exist in the incidence of bone involvement. *Cherniss* and *Waisbren* (1956) had, in 40 cases of blastomycosis, 18 times bone and joint involvement; *Kepron* et al. (1972) six times in 36 cases; *Witorsch* and *Utz* (1968) 11 times in 40 patients.

5. Comment

The variation in size, shape, thickness of wall, staining reaction, and sheer number of organisms is very impressive when larger numbers of cases are reviewed. In addition to microforms of barely 2 μ, the spectrum of size goes up to 30 μ but some of the large forms are probably wall defective bulging degenerated yeasts (spheroplasts). Round yeasts, ovoid forms, and, rarely, bun-like shapes were noticed. The cytoplasm can stain uniformly purple with H & E or rather sharp-outlined vacuoles appear. The wall may be thin or thick, and a (retraction from fixation) capsule may be visible in tissue sections. The notion that the size of *B. dermatitidis* is more or less constant is not in accord with the review of these 152 cases.

IX. Differential Diagnostic Problems with Identification of *B. dermatitidis* in Tissue Sections

The finding of rare yeast cell(s) without buds does generally preclude a species diagnosis of the offending yeast. The presence of multiple nuclei (demonstrated on well-fixed material by light microscopy or clearly in EM) may tip the balance toward *B. dermatitidis*, since yeasts of comparable sizes, as *C. neoformans* (Fig. 18) and *Histoplasma duboisii*, are mononuclear. The broad-based bud is probably the single most valuable identifying finding and clue for identification. If several such budding thick-walled yeast cells are found within the average range of diameter of the yeast cell, the diagnosis of blastomycosis is morphologically justified. However, isolated broad-based buds can be seen in cryptococcosis and even in candidiasis. In the former, the great variation in the size of yeast cells, the presence of a capsule-leaving organisms floating in a "hole" on H & E, the positive staining with mucicarmine, will generally make a differentiation reasonably easy. In candidiasis (Fig. 19) the majority

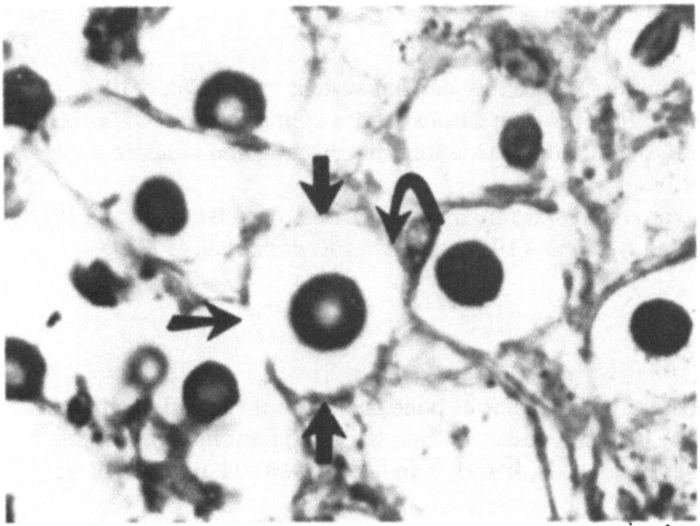

Fig. 18[a]. *Cryptococcus neoformans* is easily recognized if it has such an outstanding capsule as shown (arrows); the intense staining with the mucicarmine procedure is unique for the organism. Lung, mucicarmine x 970

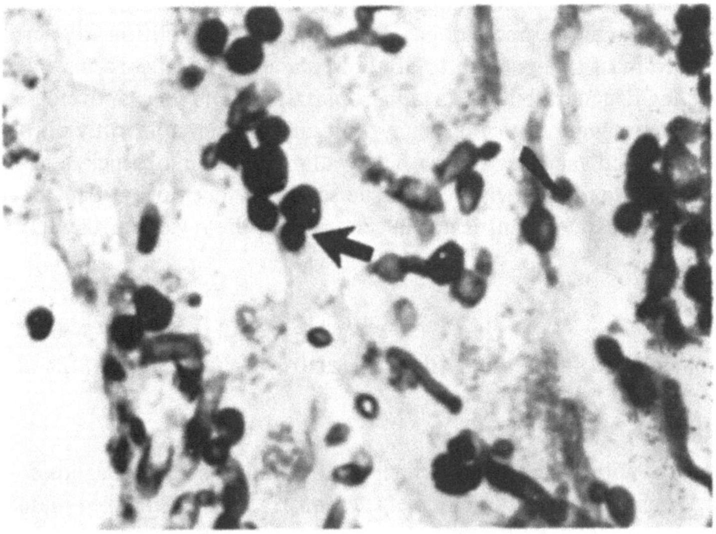

Fig. 19. *Candida albicans* on heart valve; single budding organisms (arrow) can be confused with *B. dermatitidis*; however, the presence of many small ovoid yeasts in combination with pseudohyphae clearly suggests candidiasis. Grocott x 970

of yeast cells will be small and quite often, pseudohyphae will abound. *Candida* stains well with the Gram stain. *Blastomyces* stains poorly or not at all with Gram stain. It is also important to remember that "apparent" thick walls may be simulated by the Grocott

[a] Photographs 18-25 are from the author's files

silver methenamine stain, which makes the outline of cells appear much heavier than other stains do. Comparison with H & E or Gridley-stained material will easily dispel the notion of thick walls and "broad buds" in cryptococcosis and candidiasis. *Paracoccidioides* (Fig. 20), classically, is characterized by multiple buds, but problems arise when only rare cells are present, some of which may show only single buds. Often, the large size of *P. brasiliensis* in itself will be helpful in ruling out *B. dermatitidis*, together with distribution of organ lesions and with the geographic history. Isolated organisms of *H. duboisii* (Figs. 21, 22) could

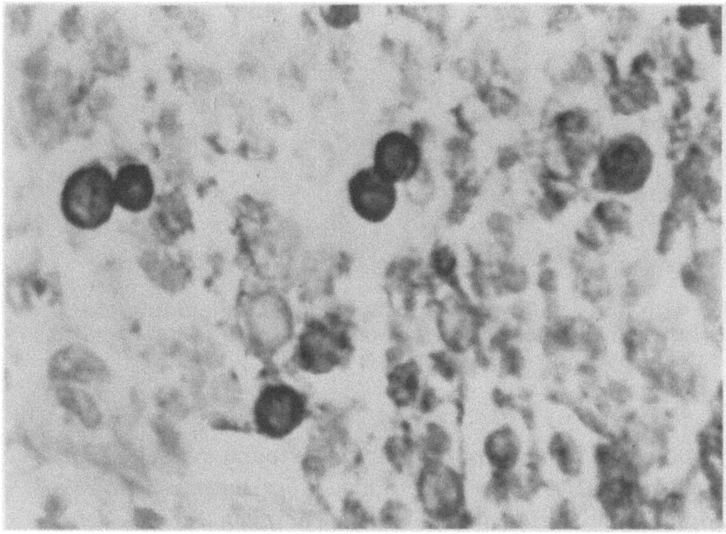

Fig. 20. Yeast cells some with single buds in paracoccidioidomycosis; lung. Gridley x 970

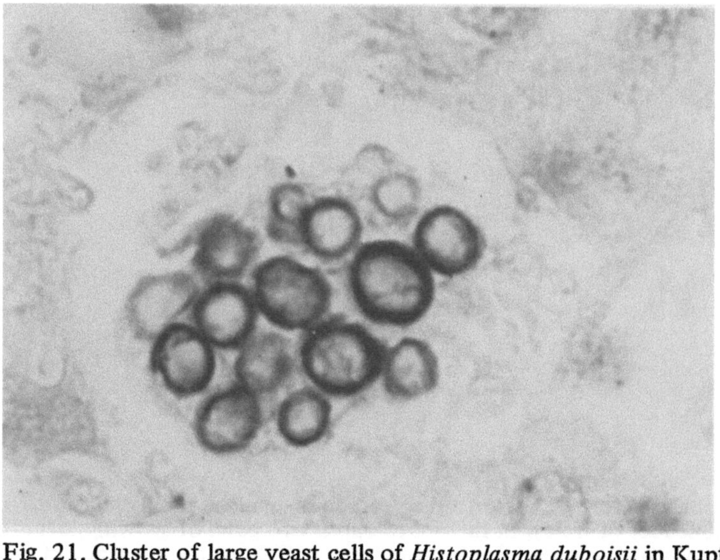

Fig. 21. Cluster of large yeast cells of *Histoplasma duboisii* in Kupffer cell-mouse liver. The special stain in this instance is rather contra-productive (compare with Fig. 22); the H & E-stained slide shows the characteristic large giant cells filled with fairly uniform yeast cells. Gridley x 970

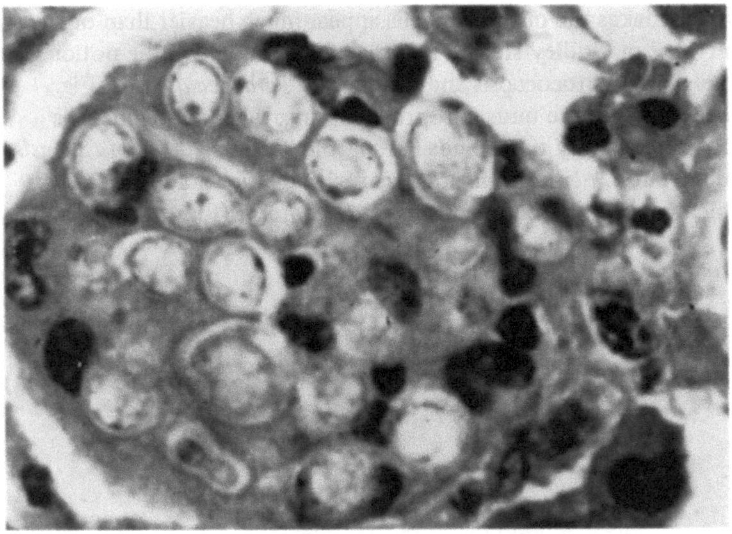

Fig. 22. Huge giant cells filled with fairly uniform yeast cells (some) with budding; the intracellular location in a histiocyte in absence of foreign body giant cells would be most unusual for blastomycosis, but is typical for *H. duboisii*. H & E x 970

be quite confusing, but, generally, large numbers of *H. duboisii* are found in tissues and, most frequently, within large giant cells, which are rather unique for the disease. On EM, the single nucleus of *H. duboisii* is easily differentiated from the multinucleated *B. dermatitidis.*

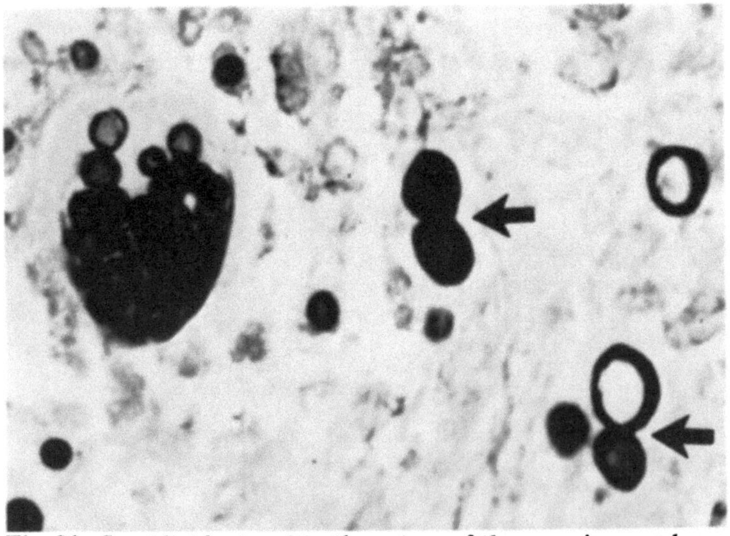

Fig. 23. *Coccidioides immitis*: the nature of the organism can be recognized from the rupturec (endospore-filled) spherule (left half of field); in the photograph, two pairs of growing, overlapping endospores are seen, resulting in pseudobudding (arrows). Without the presence of the spherule, the diagnosis would be (erroneously) suggestive of *B. dermatitidis*. Lung, Grocott x 970

Chains of yeast cells, classically seen in *Loboa loboi* and also in *P. brasiliensis* occasionally are present in blastomycosis (Fig. 13).

Atypical forms of *B. dermatitidis* can be, however, beyond recognition of individual yeast cells. They may have thin walls, may be without buds and cannot be identified morphologically. Culture will be decisive. FAS is not as easily applied for diagnosis in blastomycosis, as, for instance, in histoplasmosis.

Endospores of *Coccidioides immitis* (Figs. 23, 24) can occasionally create problems of identification and, if they are of about 10 μ in size and are lying closely together, overlaps may simulate budding and lead to confusion with *B. dermatitidis*. Search for intact spherules will be the best weapon in establishing the correct diagnosis.

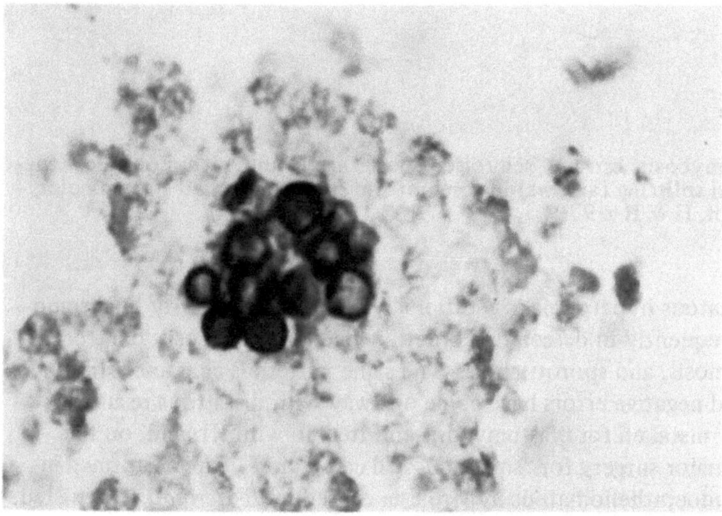

Fig. 24. Cluster of endospores of *C. immitis*; the ruptured wall of the spherule frequently is not found or stains poorly; this cluster cannot be identified per se. Lung, Gridley x 970

Since the cutaneous pathology of chromoblastomycosis (Fig. 25) is similar or identical to blastomycosis, it must be mentioned that the "sclerotic" spores of the organisms creating chromoblastomycosis are of brown color and frequently have an equatorial split, but no budding. It is the brown color which is the single most valuable difference between the spores of dematiaceous fungi and *B. dermatitidis*.

1. Tissue Reaction

The tissue reaction shows some specificity only in the skin and mucous membranes with squamous epithelium where the typical response is a pseudoepitheliomatous proliferation with microabscesses in the epithelium and corium. Organisms are demonstrable in small numbers. Tubercular or "nonspecific" infiltrates are uncommon in cutaneous blastomycosis.

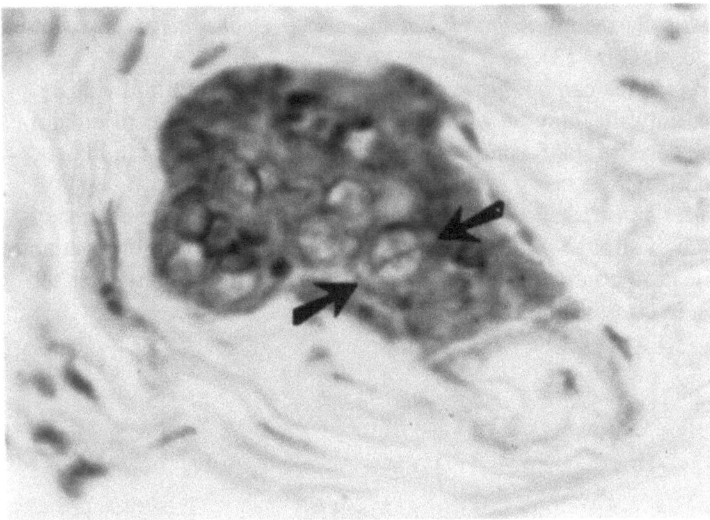

Fig. 25. In chromoblastomycosis, brown "sclerotic" spores are found within or below the epithelium; the horizontal splitting (arrows) in some of the spores and their brown color permit identification. Skin, H & E x 970

The pseudoepitheliomatous hyperplasia is additionally seen with regularity in chromoblastomycosis, and less frequently in descending order in coccidioidomycosis, paracoccidioidomycosis, histoplasmosis, and sporotrichosis. The same pattern is characteristic for bromoderma. Positive and negative errors have come our way with disastrous results in squamous cell carcinoma mistaken for blastomycosis and treated with KI, and, on the other hand, cases where major surgery for "squamous cell carcinoma" were performed in circumstances where pseudoepitheliomatous hyperplasia caused by *B. dermatitidis* existed. Blastomycosis was overlooked because no special stains were made. The epithelium in pseudoepitheliomatous hyperplasia is indeed mature and does not show the mitotic activity and cellular atypism associated with squamous cell carcinoma. However, inadequate biopsies and failure to stain for organisms can create considerable problems. Sometimes, material from oral mucosa or from the larynx shows pseudoepitheliomatous reaction resembling closely the pathology of skin. Crusts on top of eroded cutaneous lesions often contain yeast cells of *B. dermatitidis*—a fact to remember for microscopic and cultural identification. The secondary nature of skin lesions (metastatic from the lung) has been repeatedly discussed and differs from the exceptional cases of laboratory accidents with traumatic inoculation into the skin (*Landay* and *Schwarz*, 1971).

The pseudoepitheliomatous skin lesions are either grossly and microscopically obvious papillomatous (more frequent finding) or create flat, elevated cutaneous plaques, often with greater epithelial thickening than in the papillary cases.

Large masses of organisms were sometimes associated with sparse tissue reaction and the "lakes of organisms" remind the observer of similar findings in cryptococcosis and are often associated with particularly great variation in the size of the yeast cells—possibly, because of precipitous separation of small buds. What immune process governs the rapid multiplication of organisms and the poor tissue response in such instances cannot be answered from a morphologic study. Five patients with large numbers of organisms had the following background: one had diabetes mellitus, one had lymphosarcoma, one was on Prednisone therapy, two had no particular concurrent disorder.

2. Blastomycosis and Underlying Diseases

It is well known that *Candida albicans, C. neoformans*, and *Aspergillus species* proliferate in tissues of immuno-deprived patients and, at least, *C. albicans* is quite common in diabetic patients. The truly pathogenic fungi *C. immitis, H. capsulatum, P. brasiliensis*, and *B. dermatitidis* were never considered in the same light. Experience in transplant patients in the endemic area of histoplasmosis (personal unpublished experience), the occasional development of coccidioidomycosis in transplant patients (*Chandler* et al., 1972), and, finally, our present material showing the comparatively frequent association of lymphomas and diabetes with blastomycosis, require second thoughts about this point. Five of the patients in this review had "lymphomas," three were diagnosed as lymphocytic lymphomas, one had chronic lymphatic leukemia, and one chronic myelogenous leukemia. In addition, two patients had corticosteroid therapy for reasons unrelated to blastomycosis. One of the lymphoma patients had, in addition, prostatic carcinoma. Four other patients had diabetes and, while it appears unrealistic to draw too far-reaching conclusions from these findings, for practical purpose, it apparently is necessary to consider blastomycosis as a possible complicating disease in lymphomas, in patients on steroid therapy, in diabetics, and in terminal carcinoma. Three cases had carcinoma (lung twice and pancreas). The prostatic carcinoma complicating a lymphosarcoma has been mentioned before. Whether the blastomycotic symptomatology anteceded the presently incurable diseases, complicated them, or, in turn, was elicited by the constitutional "weakening," we are unable to decide from the available information.

In summary, then, it must be said that blastomycosis (as do other fungus diseases) appears to have a higher incidence in association with lymphomas, leukemias, cancer, and diabetes, and appears to be influenced by steroid therapy.

Association with other diseases of infectious origin were observed in a 58-year-old black man, where caseous foci existed in abundance in the lungs. Some of the lesions contained the classical morphologic picture of *H. capsulatum* in the form of groups of small ovoid yeast cells of uniform size. Others, with similar tissue reaction, had the round, large budding cells with broad-based buds characteristic of *B. dermatitidis*. The second case was in a seven-year-old black girl, who had numerous fibrocaseous healing foci of uniform size (each about 5 mm), morphologically representing foci of "epidemic histoplasmosis." *H. capsulatum* was found in the individual foci, and foci and organisms were present in satellite lymph nodes. In the interstitium, there were granulomatous foci with foreign body giant cells containing round large yeast in fair numbers. In view of the tissue reaction, the possibility of dual simultaneous infection was considered. The association with tuberculosis occurred but we would prefer not to give numbers for the simple reason that we have no documentation and tuberculosis was frequently mentioned as "history" but no proof existed to exclude the suspicion that the pulmonary symptoms attributed to tuberculosis in reality were already unrecognized blastomycosis. Since acid-fast stains were not available, we only mention the occurrence of this type of dual infection without "providing" figures, which we feel are unsubstantiated. Despite the chronic character of some deep mycoses and specifically of blastomycosis, amyloidosis is not a common complications (*Bassoe*, 1906; *Montgomery*, 1948; *Schwarz* and *Baum*, 1951). The two blastomycotic patients did not receive cortisone, a fact worth mentioning since cortisone accelerates experimental and clinical amyloidosis (*Teilum*, 1964). *Symmers* (1973) found actinomycosis not infrequently associated with amyloidosis (14 cases of amyloidosis in 112 patients with visceral actinomycosis, none in 174 cases of cervicofacial involvement only).

X. Summary

Blastomycosis is an important disease, the source of which is spore containing dust inhaled, resulting in primary pulmonary pathology. Secondary cutaneous foci are the most common extrapulmonary localization. The rare laboratory infections with percutaneous inoculation take a markedly different development (*Landay* and *Schwarz*, 1971).

The variation in size of the organism, *B. dermatitidis*, is considerable and oscillates from 2 μ to as high as 30 μ. Some of the large organisms may actually be spheroplasts.

Association with debilitating or immunosuppressing diseases is reported. Five lymphomas, four diabetics, three carcinomas, and, in addition, two patients on steroid therapy were observed.

Two patients had systemic (secondary) amyloidosis—both chronic cases with widespread blastomycosis. Two cases of active histoplasmosis and blastomycosis, side by side, in the lungs, were noted.

Cavitary blastomycosis is not as uncommon (20%) as we found years ago. Only muco-cutaneous blastomycosis is sufficiently specific in its tissue response to suspect prima facie the disease. But, even in muco-cutaneous localization, and more so in other organs, the demonstration of the organism is mandatory if a rational diagnosis is attempted. Special stains are absolutely indispensable in view of the common paucity of organisms. The Grocott methenamine silver stain, the Gridley procedure, or the PAS are adequate stains in our experience in the sequence given.

Culture or microscopic demonstration of *B. dermatitidis* in material from lesions should be attempted every time. The cultural identification will hinge on the faculty of inducing the yeast phase or in more sophisticated laboratories, by induction of the sexual phase with exposure to testor strains. Amphotericin B therapy is, at present, the most hopeful method and good results can be expected in most instances.

Previously believed to be restricted to the North American continent, bona fide cases have been observed in Africa with the possibility that the disease was brought unwillingly by the victims of human bondage to America. Ajello favors a change of nomenclature from "North American blastomycosis" to plain "blastomycosis." The practicality and desirability of this change is questionable, since, particularly, in the European literature, "blastomycosis" is used for almost any yeast-related disease.

References

Abernathy, R.S., Melby, J.C.: Addison's disease in North American Blastomycosis. New Engl. J. Med. **266**, 552-554 (1962).
Bassoe, P.: Disseminated blastomycosis. J. infect. Dis. 3, 91-101 (1906).
Baum, G.L., Lerner, P.I.: Primary pulmonary blastomycosis. A laboratory acquired infection. Ann. intern. Med. 73, 263-265 (1970).
Baum, G.L., Schwarz, J., Barlow, P.B.: Sarcoidosis and specific etiologic agents; a continuing enigma. Chest. **63**, 488-494 (1973).
Burr, A.H., Huffines, T.R.: Blastomycosis of the prostate with miliary dissemination treated with stilbamidine. J. Urol. (Baltimore) **71**, 464-468 (1951).
Busey, J.F., Baker, R., Birch, L., Buechner, H., Chick, E.W., Justice, F.K., Matthews, J.H., McDearman, S., Pickar, D.N., Sutliff, W.D., Walkup, H.E., Zimmerman, S.: Blastomycosis; a review of 198 collected cases in Veterans Administration Hospital. Amer. Rev. resp. Dis. **89**, 659-672 (1964).
Chandler, J.W., Kaline, R.E., Milam, D.F.: Coccidioidal choroiditis following renal transplantation. Amer. J. Ophthal. **74**, 1080-1085 (1972).
Cherniss, E.I., Waisbren, B.A.: North American Blastomycosis: A clinical study of 40 cases. Ann. intern. Med. **44**, 105-123 (1956).
Chick, E.W.: North American Blastomycosis. In: Baker, R.D.: Human Infection with Fungi, Actinomycetes and Algae. New York-Heidelberg-Berlin: Springer 1971, pp. 465-506.
Chick, E.W., Peters, H.J., Denton, J.F., Boring, W.D.: Die nordamerikanische Blastomykose. Ergebn. allg. Path. path. Anat. **40**, 34-98 (1960).
Chick, E.W., Sutliff, W.D., Rakich, J.H., Furcolow, M.L.: Epidemiological aspects of cases of blastomycosis admitted to Memphis, Tennessee hospitals during the period 1922-1954; a review of 86 cases. Amer. J. med. Sci. **231**, 253-262 (1956).
Craig, M.W., Davey, W.N., Green, R.A.: Conjugal blastomycosis. Amer. Rev. resp. Dis. **120**, 86-90 (1970).
Denton, J.F., Di Salvo, A.F.: Isolation of *Blastomyces dermatitidis* from natural sites at Augusta, Georgia. Amer. J. trop. Med. Hyg. **13**, 716-722 (1964).
Denton, J.F., Di Salvo, A.F., Hirsch, M.D.: Laboratory-acquired North American Blastomycosis. J. Amer. med. Ass.**199**, 935-936 (1967).
Emmons, C.W., Murray, I.G., Lurie, H.L., King, M.H., Tulloch, J.A., Connor, D.H.: North American Blastomycosis: two autochthonous cases from Africa. Sabouraudia 3, 306-311 (1964).
Fattal, A.R., Schwarz, J., Straub, M.: Isolation of *Histoplasma capsulatum* from lymph nodes of spontaneously infected dogs. Amer. J. clin. Path. **36**, 119-124 (1961).
Fetter, B.F., Klintworth, G.K., Hendry, W.S.: Mycoses of the central nervous system. Baltimore: Williams and Wilkins 1967.
Gilchrist, T.C., Stockes, W.R.: The presence of an Oidium in the tissues of a case of pseudo-lupus vulgaris. Johns Hopk. Hosp. Bull. 7, 129-133 (1896).
Gold, W., Stout, H.A.,Pagano, J.S., Donovick, R.: Amphotericins A and B. Antibiot. Ann. 3, 579-586 (1955-56).
Goldman, J.N., Schwarz, J.: Cytology of four yeast-like organisms in tissue explants. Mycopath. Mycol. appl. 29, 161-167 (1966).
Hamblen, C.E., Baker, R.D., Smith, D.S.: Blastomycosis of the female reproductive tract. Amer. J. Obstet. Gynec. 30, 345-356 (1935).
Hoffarth, G.A., Joseph, D.L., Shumrick, D.A.: Deep mycoses. Arch. Otolaryng (Chicago) **97**, 476-479 (1973).
Jelliffe, D.B., Hutt, M.S.R., Connor, D.H., King, M.G., Lunn, H.F.: Report of a clinicopathological conference from Ulago, 30th July, 1963. E. Afr. med. J. **41**, 79-87 (1964).
Kepron, M.D., Schoemperlen, B., Hershfield, E.S., Zylak, C.J., Cherniak, R.M.: North American Blastomycosis in Central Canada. Canad. med. ass. J. **106**, 243-264 (1972).
Lai, D.S., Schwarz, J., Cultural and morphologic findings in cervical and mediastinal lymph nodes at necropsy with reference to fungi. Amer. J. clin. Path. **57**, 212-214 (1972).
Landay, M.E., Schwarz, J.: Primary cutaneous blastomycosis. Arch. Derm. **104**, 408-411 (1971).
Lattimer, J.K., Uson, A.C., Melicow, M.M.: Tuberculous infections and inflammations of the urinary tract. In: Campbell, M.F., Harrison, J.H.: Urology. Philadelphia: W.B. Saunders 1970, Vol. I, pp. 443-479.

Lyons, G.D.: Mycotic disease of the larynx. Ann. Otol. **75**, 162-175 (1966).
McDonough, E.S., Lewis, A.L.: *Blastomyces dermatitidis*. Production of the sexual stage. Science **156**, 528-529 (1967).
Montgomery, H.: Systemic blastomycosis. Med. Clin. N. Amer. **14**, 622-651 (1948).
Sarosi, G.A., Silberfarb, P.M., Saliba, N.A., Huggin, P.M., Tosh, F.E.: Aspergillomas occurring in blastomycotic cavities. Amer. Rev. resp. Dis. **104**, 581 (1971).
Schoenbach, E.B., Miller, J.M., Ginsberg, M., Long, P.H.: Systemic blastomycosis treated with stilbamidine: A preliminary report. J. Amer. med. Ass. **146**, 1317-1318 (1951).
Schwarz, J., Baum, G.: Blastomycosis. Amer. J. clin. Path. **21**, 999-1029 (1951).
Soskin, S., Levine, R.: Carbohydrate metabolism, 2nd ed. Chicago: Univ. Chicago Press 1952.
Straub, M., Schwarz, J.: Histoplasmosis, coccidioidomycosis and tuberculosis; a comparative pathological study. Path. Microbiol. **25**, 421-477 (1962).
Symmers, W.St.C.: Amyloidosis complicating actinomycosis. Brit. med. J. **1973 IV**, 423-424.
Teilum, G.: Pathogenesis of amyloidosis. Acta path. microbiol. scand. **61**, 21-45 (1964).
Vaněk, J., Schwarz, J., Hakim, S.: N.A. blastomycosis. Amer. J. clin. Path. **54**, 384-400 (1970).
Wade, H.W., Bel, G.S.: A critical consideration of systemic blastomycosis with notes of certain special features and report of five cases. Arch. intern. Med. **18**, 103-130 (1916).
Wilson, J.W.: Primary cutaneous coccidioidomycosis–the criteria for diagnosis and a report of a case. Calif. Med. **79**, 233-239 (1953).
Witorsch, P., Utz, J.P.: N.A. blastomycosis: A study of 40 patients. Medicine **17**, 169-200 (1968).
Zimmerman, L.E.: Fatal fungus infections complicating other diseases. Amer. J. clin. Path. **25**, 46-65 (1955).

Subject Index

The numbers set in *italics* refer to those pages on which the respective catch-word is discussed in detail

Index to Volumes 58-64 Current Topics in Pathology

Volume 62

Volume 63

Volume 64

MIX
Papier aus verantwortungsvollen Quellen
Paper from responsible sources
FSC® C105338

If you have any concerns about our products,
you can contact us on
ProductSafety@springernature.com

In case Publisher is established outside the EU,
the EU authorized representative is:
Springer Nature Customer Service Center GmbH
Europaplatz 3, 69115 Heidelberg, Germany

Printed by Libri Plureos GmbH
in Hamburg, Germany